Color Atlas of
Gynaecological Surgery

Volume 6: Surgery of Conditions Complicating Pregnancy

David H. Lees

FRCS(ED), FRCOG
Honorary Consultant Obstetrician and Gynaecologist,
Jessop Hospital for Women, Sheffield

Albert Singer

Ph.D, D.Phil (OXON), FRCOG
Former Reader in Obstetrics and Gynaecology,
University of Sheffield

Consultant Gynaecologist to the Whittington
and Royal Northern Hospitals, London

Year Book Medical Publishers, Inc.
35 East Wacker Drive, Chicago

To our wives
Anne & Talya

Contents

Acknowledgements

This six-volume Colour Atlas of Gynaecological Surgery was produced at the Jessop Hospital for Women, Sheffield as part of a postgraduate project to teach operative surgery by edited colour slides. We are indebted to all who took part in the exercise, but there are some whom we would particularly like to mention.

Mr Alan Tunstill, Head of Department of Medical Illustration, The Royal Hallamshire Hospital, Sheffield Area Health Authority (Teaching), organised the whole of the photography. Mr Stephen Hirst, of the same Department, took nearly all of the photographs; the colour diagrams are all the work of Mr Patrick Elliott, Medical Artist of the Department.

As always, our immediate clinical colleagues in Sheffield gave us every assistance. Mr A N Johnson provided several of the surgical illustrations of hysterectomy for ruptured uterus in Chapter 10 and also allowed us to use a laparoscopic view of tubal pregnancy (Figure 6, Chapter 5). Mr D R Millar supplied up-to-date figures of the results currently being obtained at the Sheffield Trophoblastic Treatment Centre. Dr R K Levick provided the I.V. urogram of uterine dilatation in pregnancy (Figure 6, Chapter 1) and Dr R G Grainger sent us the radiogram of fluid levels in intestinal obstruction (Figure 22, Chapter 6).

Mr P C Steptoe kindly made available Figures 4 and 5 on the laparoscopic diagnosis of ectopic pregnancy in Chapter 5 and Mr W F Walker and the publishers allowed us to reproduce illustrations of intestinal obstruction from 'A Colour Atlas of Surgical Diagnosis (Wolfe). Photography of a specimen of invasive carcinoma of the cervix was provided by Mr I D Duncan of Dundee. Dr Malcolm Anderson of The Samaritan Hospital, London went to great trouble to let us have the histological photographs relating to the subjects of abortion, ectopic pregnancy and trophoblastic disease and we are most grateful.

The illustrations of gestational trophoblastic disease appropriately come from Singapore. Clinical Professor Y M Salmon with her staff at The Kandang Kerbau Hospital, Drs S H Kee, K K Tan and A L Lim, supplied Figures 1 and 5 with helpful accompanying clinical comment which is embodied in Chapter 13. Mr Ian McDonald of Melbourne has allowed us to quote from his writings on cerclage and to use his operation diagrams; we are much indebted to him for help with a difficult subject.

In the realm of sophisticated techniques Dr E Heydermann of St Thomas' Hospital, London has provided colour photographs and relative legends on the immuno-peroxidase staining procedure for early diagnosis of chorionic carcinoma. Professor Goldman of the Department of Radiology at Thomas Jefferson Hospital, Philadelphia supplied details of the ultra-sonic probe used in amniocentesis and Messrs Rocket of London provided illustrations and descriptions of their apparatus for use in out-patient therapeutic abortion.

Dr R G Law of Whittington Hospital, London, deserves special acknowledgement and thanks for producing all of the quite superb ultra-sonograms used in Chapters 2, 5, 7, 13 and 14. The accuracy and value of this diagnostic method is constantly increasing and we consider ourselves very fortunate to have had the co-operation of a colleague so skilled in its use.

The anaesthetists at all levels were very co-operative. Dr A G D Nicholas, Dr D R Powell and Professor J A Thornton were the consultants involved. Of the numerous senior registrars we remember particularly Doctors Bailey, Birks, Burt, Clark, Dye, Mullins, Saunders and Stacey.

Dr Pierre Cotteel, of Lille, generously provided his logical and practical management protocol for Disseminated Intravascular Coagulation (DIC) on page 198. We believe such a regime to be invaluable when laboratory facilities are limited or even non-existent.

Miss J Hughes-Nurse, Mr I V Scott, Miss P Buck, Miss V Brown and Dr H David were the senior registrars and lecturers in obstetrics and gynaecology during the time and greatly assisted by keeping us informed of suitable cases and in the organising of operations. Doctors Katherine Jones, E Lachman, Janet Patrick, K Edmonds, A Bar-Am and C Rankin were involved in the management of the cases and assisted at operations.

Miss M Crowley, nursing officer in charge of the Jessop Hospital operating theatres ensured that we had every facility, and Sisters J Taylor, M Henderson, E Duffield, M Waller and A Broadly each acted as theatre sister or 'scrub' nurse at the individual operations. Mr Leslie Gilbert and Mr Gordon Dale the operating room assistants, were valuable members of the team. We particularly wish to thank the whole theatre staff for their courtesy and efficiency.

Mrs Valerie Prior and Mrs Talya Singer were responsible for typing the manuscript.

In view of the increasing complexity and diversity of the whole project we have continued to enlist the further assistance of our wives. Colour matching, proof-reading, spot typing and slide organisation have all demanded much extra time both at home and when travelling overseas.

The photographs in this book were taken on Kodachrome 25 colour reversal film. The camera was a 35 mm Nikkormat FTN fitted with a 105 mm f2.5 Nikkor auto lens. A PK-3 extension ring was used for close-ups and a 55 mm f3.5 Micro-Nikkor auto lens for general views. Illumination was provided by a Sunpak auto zoom 4000 electronic flash unit, set on full power. An exposure setting of 1/60th of a second at f16 was used.

Introduction

There is probably no substitute for the type of personal tuition provided by teacher and pupil working together in the operating theatre as surgeon and assistant, with knowledge and experience being passed on directly. There is, however, the disadvantage that such a relationship is not available to everyone and is, at best, transient. In addition the learner is frequently not at a stage in his career when he can take full advantage of what is available. The majority, therefore, have to look elsewhere for such instruction.

Textbooks of operative surgery provide the principal source of information, but these are only as good as their illustrations. The occasional colour plate does not instruct and there is something unreal about the well-executed drawings prepared by a medical artist to the specification of the author. The one worthwhile teaching aid is the simple line diagram or sketch, which demands considerable skill and ingenuity and allows the student to see and follow what is required. But to carry that information in one's mind and apply it in practice is another matter. In surgery, with all its accompanying distractions, the real life structures are frighteningly different from those which the simple diagrams have led one to expect, and these same structures obstinately refuse to adopt the position and behaviour expected of them.

Cine films are excellent but the cost of their production in time and money is high, besides which they are clumsy to use. This series of atlases offers what we consider to be the next best thing: a series of step-by-step colour photographs accompanied by an appropriate written commentary. This form of presentation follows almost exactly the colour slide plus commentary method most often used to teach surgery. Using slides, of course, it is necessary to have projection apparatus and access to a library or bank of suitable material. The method adopted in this series – of using high quality colour reproduction processes – retains the advantages of the slide and commentary method while avoiding its drawbacks.

The present series of atlases sets out to provide detailed instruction in the techniques of standard gynaecological operations. Its methodology is straightforward. The technique of each operation is clearly shown, step-by-step, using life-size photographs in natural colour, and with liberal use of indicators and accompanying diagrams. Where a step is repetitive or there is a natural sequence of steps, grouping has sometimes been used, but the natural size of the structures is maintained.

The accompanying commentary is concise and is printed on the same page as the photograph or photographs to which it refers. Every effort has been made to include only necessary material, but in situations where experience and special training have provided additional information and knowledge, that has been included.

The illustrations are selected and the accompanying commentaries so arranged as to carry the reader forward in a logical progression of thought and action in which he becomes involved. Occupied with one step he is at the same time anticipating the next, and in due course confirms his foresight as logical and correct. The photographs are those of a real patient having a real operation and the picture seen is exactly what the reader will see in the operation theatre when he does it himself. Interest is concentrated on the one step of the operation being taken at that time.

In any form of medical teaching there is the inevitable problem of pitching instruction at the level required by the audience and the presumption that the reader has insight into the specialist knowledge of the author is just as irritating as being patronised. We do not think there is a problem in this context because an atlas is by definition a guide and therefore for general use. It is just as likely to be consulted by a junior house surgeon about to assist at his first hysterectomy as by a senior colleague seeking an alternative method of dealing with a particular problem. That, at least, is the spirit in which it has been written.

Certain assumptions have had to be made to avoid verbosity, tediousness and sheer bulk of paper. It is hoped that the reader will be kind enough to attribute any omissions and shortcomings to the acceptance of such a policy. No one should be embarking on any of the procedures described without training in surgical principles, nor should he attempt them without knowledge of abdominal and pelvic anatomy and physiology.

Several areas have purposely been avoided in preparing the Atlas. There is no attempt to advise on the indications for operative treatment and only in the most general terms are the uses of a particular operation discussed. Individual surgeons develop their own ideas on pre- and post-operative care and have their personal predilections regarding forms of anaesthesia, fluid replacement and the use of antibiotics.

Even on the purely technical aspects the temptation to advise on the choice of instruments and surgical materials is largely resisted and it is assumed that the reader is capable of placing secure knots and ligatures. Each volume of the Atlas contains a photograph of the instruments used by the authors and some of these are shown individually. Most readers will have their own favourites but the information may be useful to younger colleagues. We do not consider the choice of suture material to be of over-riding importance. The senior author has used PGA suture material since its inception and although generally preferring it to catgut does not consider it perfect. It has disadvantages and can be very sore on the surgeon's hands but it does have advantages in that it is particularly suitable for vaginal work and for closing the abdomen.

There are, of course, several methods of performing the various operations but those described here have consistently given the authors the best results. It need hardly be reiterated that the observance of basic surgical principles is probably more important than anything else.

The Atlas is produced in six volumes, each of which relates approximately to a regional subspecialty. This is done primarily to keep the size of the volumes convenient for use but also to allow publication to proceed progressively.

From what has been written it might appear that the authors think of gynaecologists as necessarily male. The suggestion is rejected: the old-fashioned usage of the inclusive masculine gender is merely retained for simplicity and neatness. Anyone questioning the sincerity of this explanation would have to be reminded that every gynaecologist must, in the very nature of things, be a feminist.

Introduction to Volume 6

Surgical conditions complicating pregnancy

Some form of ante-natal care is available to almost all pregnant women. The general and obstetric history is documented, observation is continuous and the commoner complications of pregnancy are recognised and the appropriate non-surgical treatment instituted when that is required. Specialist advice will or should have been arranged where there is a background of diabetes, severe cardiac disease, thyrotoxicosis and other general systemic diseases. Such conditions would come under the general heading of *obstetric care* and do not concern us in the compilation of an atlas on the surgical complications of pregnancy. This present volume illustrates and explains the technique of those surgical procedures which become necessary during the course of pregnancy, whether for an abnormality in pregnancy itself or for an associated condition occurring in that special context. An obvious example of the former is a ruptured ectopic pregnancy while the latter might take the form of an acute appendicitis or a twisted ovarian cyst.

The considerations which influence the form in which the volume is presented are these:

The section on anatomy was previously kept short and served only to recall important features which had a bearing on surgical management. Pregnancy, however, is responsible for such major changes in the anatomical position and relationship of all the pelvic and abdominal organs that the surgeon has to reconsider the whole matter of surgical access and plan to avoid new hazards which may arise. The major anatomical alterations in pregnancy are obvious; the physiological changes are less apparent but no less fundamental and in many ways more important. For this reason the usual section on anatomy has been replaced by one which reviews both the anatomical and physiological factors.

With regard to purely clinical matters, termination of pregnancy has become a very important subject and regardless of the stage of gestation it may become immediately necessary. On the basis of much research and the numerous clinical reports available certain methods of termination are now accepted as standard for particular stages of pregnancy and these are illustrated and described in Chapter 2. As part of the management of spontaneous abortion in Chapter 3 the conditions of septic abortion and endotoxic shock are singled out for detailed consideration because these dangerous complications are still very common.

In the chapter on the acute abdomen emphasis is placed on the importance of being especially alert to the insidious and sometimes rapid development of peritonitis and intestinal obstruction. Despite knowledge of these matters and the very best intentions on all sides, tragedies still occur.

Management of ovarian cysts and uterine fibroids in pregnancy present very similar problems and are considered in the same chapter. Retroverted incarcerated gravid uterus has been added to this section.

Prior to considering caesarean section and a group of dangerous conditions which necessitate hysterectomy, it was thought appropriate to include a short chapter on the prevention and control of blood loss when operating on the pregnant patient. The spectre which confronts experienced and inexperienced surgeons alike is that of massive and apparently uncontrollable haemorrhage. A frank estimate of the causes and effects of haemorrhage in pregnancy with a logical explanation of how to prevent matters getting out of control and how to retrieve the situation if they threaten to do so is the best antidote to such fears.

Caesarean section is illustrated and described in some detail because of its outstanding importance in obstetric management and because there are many occasions when the purely gynaecological surgeon will have to do the operation. Chapter 10 concerns uterine rupture in pregnancy or labour and cases of continuing post partum haemorrhage. The indications and contraindications for total and subtotal hysterectomy are discussed before describing the important steps in relation to each of these operations.

A separate short section (Chapter 11) deals with the effects of blunt and of sharp trauma on the pregnant uterus and since much of the former relates to automobile accidents that aspect has been dealt with in some detail. Most gynaecologists will from time to time be asked for their opinion in cases of multiple crash injuries so that it is very important to understand clearly the principles involved.

In Chapter 12 the management of the positive cervical smear in pregnancy was thought to merit a broader approach than the purely surgical one. The operative techniques involved are simple and already familiar to anyone dealing with such cases; a primary decision concerns what to do rather than how to do it. In Chapter 13 also it was felt to be unsatisfactory and incomplete to deal with the surgical treatment of hydatidiform mole and chorio-carcinoma without reviewing current thought and practice on the whole subject of gestational trophoblastic disease. It is only by assessing the important primary chemo-therapeutic modality and its effectiveness that one can arrive at a balanced decision on the place of surgery.

Amniocentesis is a surgical procedure which may look out of place in this company but it is a necessary operation in patients of a certain age group and the method, while not difficult, is rather precise.

Emergency obstetrical surgery (in the United Kingdom at least) has developed in such a way that the consultant or specialist anaesthetist has effectively taken control of matters in addition to his prime responsibility of anaesthesia. These include resuscitation, fluid replacement, central venous pressure monitoring and control of acidosis and blood coagulation problems. The anaesthetist is continually involved in safeguarding the well being of both mother and fetus and this is to the advantage of all concerned. Dr A D G Nicholas, Consultant in Obstetrical Anaesthesia at the Jessop Hospital for Women, Sheffield, has contributed Chapter 15 on these important matters. It will be informative to those who enjoy the benefits of working with specialist colleagues but is particularly aimed at those who have to shoulder total responsibility for what is often a desperate situation in unfavourable circumstances.

While it is hoped and generally assumed that the induction of analgesia and anaesthesia will be in the hands of a trained individual it is also recognised that there are circumstances where that is not so and the surgeon may be expected to have at least a working knowledge of such procedures, their complications and their correction. This is provided in Chapter 15. As has also been pointed out in the introduction to previous volumes, it is assumed that the surgeon is aware of the general and specific aspects of the pre-operative assessment of the patient. It is not intended to go into this further except to mention that there are important possible hazards in pregnancy which must be recognised before surgery is instituted. We have in mind such conditions as anaemia of various kinds, sickle cell disease and high risk groups for the development of thrombo-embolic disease. The condition of the cardiac and respiratory distressed patient, e.g. the chronic smoker, has also to be assessed and safeguarded.

Appendices have again been used as an economical method of presenting certain detailed information on some subjects covered in the general text. References to the literature have also been presented in this form.

1: Surgical anatomy

1. Developmental anatomy: abnormalities encountered in pregnancy

It is generally taught that few of the possible congenital maldevelopments have much bearing on pregnancy. If severe, the patient is likely to remain infertile, and if mild, the effects on the course of the pregnancy and delivery are seldom dangerous. The authors, however, take the view that even if they are not dangerous in the acute sense, these congenital aberrations can give rise to various complications, some of which may be difficult to understand or recognise unless the clinician has a working knowledge of why they occur. Such knowledge gives a feeling of confidence in management and enables one to explain the situation to the patient and to her husband.

An outline of Mullerian duct development is given in Volume 4 of the Atlas (pages 9 to 11) and the various types of non-fusion in the genital tract are illustrated in Volume 5 (pages 38 to 39). The reader may wish to revise his knowledge by reference to either or both of the sections.

Any degree of fusion failure, from two completely separate uterine cavities to a subseptate uterus, may occur; the two extremes are shown diagramatically in **Figures 1** and **2**. The wide variety of intermediate types, however, provides most of the serious complications of pregnancy, and these include persistent transverse lie with the ovum occupying both cavities; delay in labour is likely to supervene and the lower segment may not develop. The placenta sometimes occupies one cavity and the fetus the other, so that a retained placenta can be extremely difficult to remove even when the obstetrician has come to realise the true state of affairs. An accessory horn predisposes to uterine torsion and may prevent engagement of the fetal head in labour, besides giving problems in lochial drainage. A rudimentary horn may on occasion be occupied by the pregnancy and a situation of impending or actual rupture of what is an ectopic pregnancy results.

It is not proposed to go into detail about the numerous and perhaps unlikely sequelae of congenital uterine abnormalities; enough has been said to indicate the importance of knowing what is possible and what can be the subsequent effects.

Congenital vaginal abnormalities which may affect pregnancy are the persistent vaginal septa. An incomplete longitudinal septum may be recognised for the first time at delivery when it can impede descent of the fetal head. It is a simple matter to incise it with scissors but haemostasis must be attended to as it can be very vascular. Transverse congenital stricture due to imperfect canalisation at the junction of the upper and middle thirds of the vagina may cause obstruction in labour and necessitate delivery by caesarean section. On the other hand an apparently obstructive septum in early pregnancy may soften to a remarkable degree and allow an easy vaginal delivery.

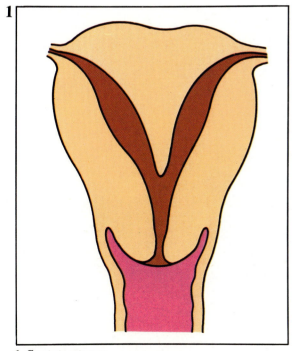

1 Septate uterus

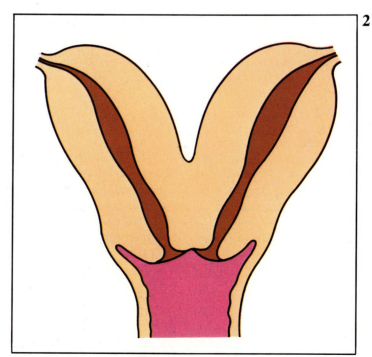

2 Double uterus-bicornis, bicollis

2. Anatomical and physiological changes in pregnancy: their influence on surgical management

Uterine growth and the consequent alteration in intra-abdominal anatomical relationships is only the more obvious manifestation of changes which affect every body system in pregnancy. These changes result from the altered hormonal activity dictated by the needs of the fetus and the preparation of the mother for delivery; they affect function more than morphology.

There is a physiological hypervolaemia with a distinct softening and friability of the tissues which presents the operator with conditions quite different from those in the non-pregnant patient. The manifestations of pregnancy are sometimes similar to, and easily confused with, certain pathological states in the non-pregnant woman, so that the surgeon must be alive to the danger of interpreting a physiological state as a pathological one. In addition to the above, many laboratory values are considerably altered in pregnancy and are no longer reliable indicators of inflammatory or disease processes. In treatment, also, the condition of pregnancy and its requirements have to be taken into account in the matters of fluid replacement and maintenance of hormonal equilibrium.

Cardiovascular changes in pregnancy

(1) Cardiac output
The cardiovascular system undergoes very considerable alteration in pregnancy and this is not surprising since the cardiac output rises by 1.0 to 1.5 litres per minute in the first 10 weeks of pregnancy and is maintained at that level till term[1,2].

The maximum increase in oxygen consumption is approximately 18 per cent above the non-pregnant level[3] and the increase in minute ventilation is similar. Heart rate, arterial and venous pressures and peripheral resistance are all affected while blood volume and composition are both greatly altered.

(2) Heart rate
There is a physiological tachycardia in pregnancy which reaches its maximum in the third trimester when it is 15–20 beats above non-pregnant levels[1]. This has to be taken into account in any clinical investigations of the pregnant patient and especially in relation to infective conditions.

(3) Blood pressure
Blood pressure normally tends to fall by 5 to 15 mm/Hg during the second trimester and rises again nearer term[4]. It is elevated in the presence of toxaemia of pregnancy and this can be a possible source of confusion for the obstetrician assessing antepartum haemorrhage. Accidental antepartum haemorrhage should not be excluded as a diagnosis simply because of a normal blood pressure reading since the relatively

enormous retroplacental blood loss in some cases can lead to a drop in systolic and diastolic pressure. It should be emphasised that blood pressure greater than that in the non-pregnant is always abnormal and is usually due to toxaemia or pregnancy although it may result from stressful anxiety.

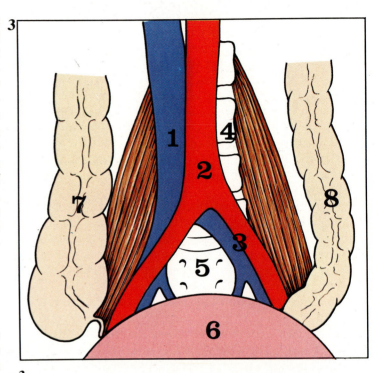

3
Diagram of aorta-caval area subjected to pressure by the heavy pregnant uterus when the woman is supine in late pregnancy. The structures are numbered thus: 1. inferior vena cava, 2. aorta, 3. common iliac vessels, 4. vertebra, 5. sacrum, 6. bladder, 7. ascending colon, 8. descending colon.

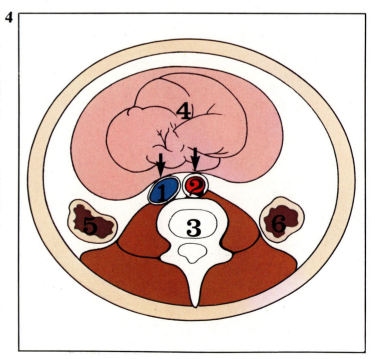

4
Diagram to illustrate the mechanism of inferior vena caval occlusion and aortal pressure. The arrows indicate the area of pressure on the main vessels by the uterus. The structures are numbered thus: 1. inferior vena cava, 2. aorta, 3. vertebra, 4. fetus in utero, 5. ascending colon, 6. descending colon.

(4) Venous pressure

Peripheral venous pressure is unchanged in the upper trunk but in the legs and lower trunk it increases due to pressure of the uterus on the inferior vena cava in late pregnancy. This explains the tendency to develop varicose veins and haemorrhoids and since the effect is temporary it implies that treatment of such conditions should be medical rather than surgical. There is a reported progressive fall in central venous pressure in pregnancy with values of less than half of those for the non-pregnant by the third trimester[5]. This is clearly of importance in central venous pressure monitoring of haemorrhagic cases.

(5) Peripheral blood flow

Peripheral blood flow increases in pregnancy as a result of diminished peripheral vascular resistance. The normal response to shock stimuli is vaso-constriction but this does not necessarily occur in pregnancy. It is suggested either that sympathetic nerve activity is depressed by oestrogen or that there is a lessened response to angiotensin in pregnancy. Whatever the reason, it has to be remembered that a pregnant woman in shock may not exhibit the usual physical signs of that condition.

(6) Effect of maternal position on cardiac output (Supine hypotensive syndrome or inferior vena cava syndrome)

Women in late pregnancy may develop profound hypotension if in the supine position for a length of time; this may lead in turn to impaired uterine blood flow. The major cause of this hypotensive syndrome is compression of the inferior vena cava and major pelvic veins by the heavy gravid uterus (**Figures 3** and **4**) and as much as 30 per cent of the circulating blood volume may be trapped in the venous system[6]. It was shown[7] that changes from supine to left lateral position could account for a 25 per cent increase in cardiac output in late pregnancy. That the uterus may also compress or partially occlude the abdominal aorta and reduce uteroplacental blood flow has been demonstrated[19] (See also Chapter 15, page 187.) This will not be recognised unless the fetal heart rate is being monitored and aortic compression will not be indicated by any change in blood pressure readings on the upper arm. The fact that the condition can be relieved by turning the patient to either side suggests that the aortic involvement is fully as important as that of the inferior vena cava and perhaps the term supine hypotensive syndrome is more correct. Sometimes the condition is spectacularly evident while in other women it is not obvious. In the latter instance the circulation is presumably returned through unusually developed collateral azygos and vertebral veins and is adequately maintained.

Haematological changes in pregnancy

(7) Blood volume

The plasma volume in pregnancy increases by 20–100 per cent, averaging 40 per cent[2,9]. It starts to increase about the tenth week of pregnancy and rapidly rises till the 34th week after which the increase is slower. The increase in erythrocyte volume is relatively less, so that unless the woman is given iron during pregnancy the haematocrit falls and this is seen as the 'physiological anaemia' of pregnancy. This hypervolaemic effect means that a pregnant woman may lose a large amount of blood before symptoms of hypotension develop and also that a massive amount of blood or fluid may be required to reverse the situation. This is one of the reasons why central venous pressure recording is so essential in resuscitation and the management of bleeding from any cause during pregnancy.

(8) Red blood cells and white blood cells

Because of the differential rates of increase in plasma and erythrocyte volume, the haematocrit and haemoglobin levels fall in pregnancy. At 34 weeks if the woman is not being given iron supplements the haematocrit will be around 33 per cent and the haemoglobin 10–11 gm/dl. Such factors have to be remembered in assessing blood reports in all cases of haemorrhage.

The white blood cells are increased in pregnancy during the second and third trimesters and especially during labour. Levels of 18,000/cu.mm in late pregnancy are usual and may rise to 25,000/cu.mm in labour. The increase is largely in neutrophils and by contrast the population of lymphocytes declines by 10–15 per cent during pregnancy. It is obviously important to know of such factors in cases of suspected infection in pregnancy.

(9) ESR

With the increase in serum fibrinogen and alpha and beta globulins the blood sediments vary rapidly in pregnancy. The mean sedimentation rate is 78 mm/hr so that ESR is of little or no value in the diagnosis of disease during pregnancy.

(10) Coagulation factors

Blood fibrinogen levels rise during pregnancy to be twice normal at term and factors VII, VIII, IX and X are all increased; factors II and V are little changed. Bleeding time, clotting time and prothrombin time are all unchanged in pregnancy[10].

Despite increased levels of some clotting factors and the venous stasis of pregnancy caused by the enlarging uterus it is difficult to demonstrate increased incidence of spontaneous venous thrombosis during pregnancy, and this is encouraging in view of the large number of late pregnancy patients who require prolonged bed rest[10]. Antepartum venous thrombosis and thrombophlebitis, however, occasionally occur. The situation changes immediately following delivery with a greatly increased incidence of spontaneous thrombosis.

Table 1 compares the pregnant and non-pregnant values of the more commonly required biochemical tests and serves as a useful reference when assessing the information provided by laboratory investigations in pregnant patients.

TABLE 1

HAEMATOLOGICAL CHANGES IN PREGNANCY. LABORATORY FINDINGS IN NON-PREGNANCY AND LATE PREGNANCY.

	NON-PREGNANT	THIRD TRIMESTER
1. Haemoglobin	12–16 gm%	10–13 gm%
2. W.B.C.s	4,500–10,000/cmm	5,000–14,000/cmm
3. Platelets	175,000–250,000/cmm	200,000–350,000/cmm
4. Plasma volume	2,400 ml	3,700 ml
5. Red blood mass	1,600 ml	1,900 ml
6. Blood volume	4,000 ml	5,250 ml
7. Polymorphs (%)	54–62/cmm	60–85/cmm
8. Lymphocytes (%)	38–45%	15–38%
9. E.S.R.	Less than 20 mm/hr	30–90 mm/hr
10. Fibrinogen (plasma)	300 mg%	450 mg%
11. Glucose	90–110 mg%	90–110 mg%
12. Uric acid	2–6.4 mg%	2–5.5 mg%
13. Creatinine	0.6–1.2 mg%	0.4–0.9 mg%
14. Bilirubin	0.1–1.2 mg/100 ml	0.1–0.9 mg/100 ml
15. Serum iron	75–150 mcg	65–120 mcg
16. Iron combining capacity	250–450 mcg	300–500 mcg
17. Blood urea nitrogen	10–18 mg%	4–12 mg%
18. pH (arterial)	7.3–7.44	7.41–7.46
19. Chlorides (mEq/L)	98–109 mEq/L	90–105 mEq/L
20. HCO_3	24–30 mM/L	19–25 mM/L
21. Sodium	135–145 mEq/L	132–140 mEq/L
22. Potassium	4.0–4.8 mEq/L	3.5–4.5 mEq/L
23. Carbon dioxide	24–30 mM/L	19–25 mM/L

Hypovolaemia and hypoxia in particular relation to the fetus

This huge subject particularly concerns the specialist obstetrician but the gynaecological surgeon should have a general understanding of the effects of hypoxia on the pregnant woman and on the fetus. Only the more obvious surgical considerations are mentioned here. There are numerous publications on the subject including a very concise review by Brinkman and Woods[11] and much of the short summary given here is taken from that source.

Clinical hypovolaemia occurs when cardiac output and perfusion pressure are inadequate to provide normal function to vital organs. Hypoxia is a relative oxygen deficiency in which the tissues fail to receive an adequate supply of oxygen. Hypovolaemia usually results from acute blood loss but may also occur in cases of 'obstetric' shock. The pregnant patient is inevitably affected by hypoxia and the effects on the fetus follow.

The usual causes of haemorrhage are placenta praevia, abruptio placentae, ruptured uterus and external trauma, and the body response is a generalised vaso-constriction and increased vascular resistance. Cerebral and cardiac blood flow are maintained at the expense of the blood supply elsewhere. Clinical evidences of hypovolaemia are restlessness, anxiety, pallor, sweating, tachycardia and a fall in blood pressure. When 50 per cent of the blood volume has been lost, the pulse cannot be felt and blood pressure is not recordable. If the hypovolaemia is not corrected and hypoxia increases neural compensatory mechanisms fail, peripheral vaso-dilatation occurs and toxic metabolites escape from the capillaries to cause further plasma loss. The condition rapidly becomes irreversible.

The effect of maternal hypoxia on the fetus is to initiate a primary hypoxic response to reduced utero-placental perfusion but there is no certainty about what happens because of the difficulty of studying the effects on the fetus in utero. Utero-placental perfusion must be affected but we are dependent on experimental work on animals (sheep) for information on the likely effects[12, 13, 14]. It was shown[13] that reducing maternal arterial oxygen tension to 40 mm/Hg decreased placental flow while increasing maternal heart rate and causing a small drop in blood pressure. It was also found[12] that in the severely hypoxic animal the uterine fraction of the cardiac output fell from the normal 17–20 per cent to 12–14 per cent of output, and at a time when cardiac output was increasing utero-placental perfusion was decreasing. The effect of maternal hypoxia on the fetus in later pregnancy has, of course, been the subject of study in obstetrics. Thus it was demonstrated[15] that the fetal response to acute hypoxia is similar to that of the adult and is characterised by variable changes in blood pressure, a significant rise in pulmonary vascular resistance and a reduction in cardiac output. It should be added that experiments in sheep have shown that there can be as much as a 75 per cent reduction in uterine blood flow without a significant fetal cardiovascular effect[16].

Management is directed towards controlling the bleeding, restoration of circulating blood volume and ensuring that blood pH is regulated by intravenous sodium bicarbonate. Administration of oxygen to the mother does not seem to be very effective; even 100 per cent oxygen given in experimental animals does not change the depressed fetal oxygen pressure or improve cardiac performance. Restoration of maternal blood volume abolishes most of the fetal changes although fetal heart output is elevated for a time. Fetal oxygen consumption returns to normal and acid base balance is restored.

Hypovolaemia and hypoxia may result from shock associated with obstetric conditions such as air embolism, amniotic embolism and the dehydration of prolonged labour. The hypoxic effects on mother and fetus are not dissimilar to those of haemorrhage but management is clearly very different and one of the main dangers can be the giving of too much rather than too little blood.

Effects of pregnancy on the urinary tract

The urinary tract undergoes considerable morphological and functional change during pregnancy, and considering its common embryological origin and close anatomical relationship with the genital tract, this is not surprising.

Renal pelves and ureters
Dilatation of the renal pelvis and ureter appears early in the second trimester of pregnancy and persists in some degree for 3 to 4 weeks after delivery. It is more frequent and obvious on the right side; on both sides it extends distally only as far as the brim of the pelvis. Some believe that mechanical pressure by the uterus, iliac artery or ovarian vein is the primary mechanism; others see the effect as entirely due to hormones and particularly progesterone. The truth is likely to lie in a combination of mechanical and endocrine factors. The ureters are also lengthened and displaced laterally during pregnancy (see **Figure 5**).

From the obstetric and surgical point of view, knowledge of these changes should ensure that a diagnosis of urinary abnormality such as hydronephrosis should not be wrongly arrived at because of radiological findings. It has always been generally accepted that the dilation causes urinary stasis which provides suitable circumstances for urinary infection in pregnancy. Some[17], however, say that urinary stasis does not necessarily occur and others[18] have not been able to show a relationship between severe upper urinary tract change and infection.

The lateral displacement of the ureters should not be thought of as a safety factor by the surgeon who has to do a caesarean hysterectomy. The uterus is greatly widened where the uterine arteries approach it and in fact they lie more closely than usual to the ureters which are of course immobilised in their ureteric tunnels. It behoves the surgeon to keep very close to the lateral aspect of the cervix when doing a total hysterectomy and in desperate circumstances where speed and blood conservation are essential a supravaginal hysterectomy may be a wiser procedure.

Bladder
The bladder is displaced anteriorly and superiorly by the lower uterine segment and cervix to become partially abdominal in position. The urethra is correspondingly elongated. The bladder base is broadened and the space between the ureteric orifices is widened and appears convex on cystoscopic examination. There is muscular hypertrophy and increased vascularity but it is not certain that capacity is increased. These changes are of importance to the surgeon making a cystoscopic examination for urinary symptoms in pregnancy; the general hyperaemia at the trigone and the other changes mentioned must be recognised as normal in the circumstances.

5
Radiograph (intravenous pyelogram) of patient in late pregnancy. Both renal pelves (1) and ureters (2) are dilated, with the dilatation extending only as far as the brim of the pelvis (arrowed). The 4th lumbar vertebra is numbered (3) and the fetal vertebral column (4). Despite appearances this was not a case of hydronephrosis.

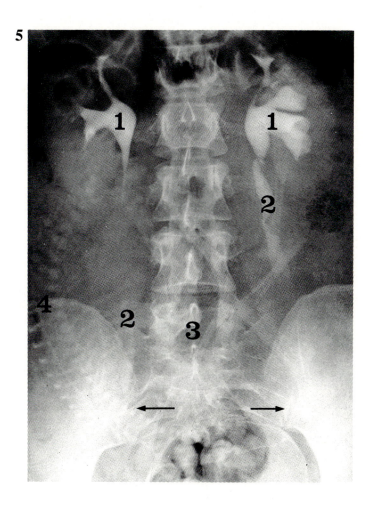

Effects of pregnancy on the alimentary tract

Practically the whole length of the alimentary canal is displaced to some extent during pregnancy and activity of the plain muscle of the gut wall is depressed by the raised progesterone blood levels. The pregnant woman as a result suffers from certain general symptoms related to these factors, and the surgeon must keep them in mind when investigating suspected abdominal conditions during pregnancy. Thus nausea and vomiting occur in about 50 per cent of pregnant women during the first trimester. Heartburn and flatulence are common in later pregnancy as a result of pressure on the stomach from the pregnant uterus or possibly from a hiatus hernia. Constipation is very common.

Displacement of the alimentary tract may be the reason for the development of dangerous associated conditions. The stomach is compressed but retains its position unless there is a diaphragmatic hernia; the duodenum also is relatively fixed. The small intestine which is normally spread throughout the whole peritoneal cavity and which by gravity tends to fall towards the pelvis is displaced upwards by the uterus and lies in the upper abdomen. No harm results unless there are adhesions between the small bowel and pelvic structures such as the broad ligament or pouch of Douglas. In such circumstances a loop of bowel may be held by its apex and put on the stretch, thus leading to acute kinking and possible obstruction. The same applies if the intestine is unreduced in an umbilical, inguinal or femoral hernial sac. The surgeon must always treat known hernia with suspicion during pregnancy and keep in mind the possibility of pelvic adhesions.

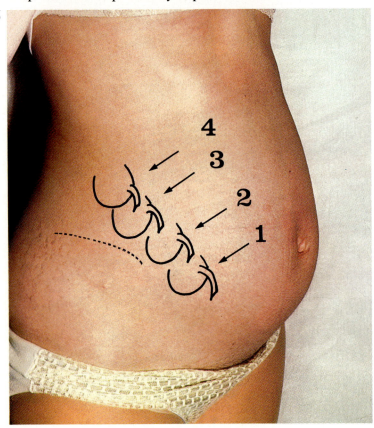

6

The caecum, the ascending colon and the hepatic flexure are all pushed laterally into the iliac fossa and paracolic space by the broad pregnant uterus while the splenic flexure, descending and pelvic colon are pushed to the left at the same levels. As in the case of the small intestine there are dangers of obstruction resulting from fixation or adhesion in hernial sacs and especially at the umbilicus. Such umbilical obstructions may occur when the growing uterus has so stretched the gut that the lumen is flattened and easily occluded. They can also occur immediately following delivery when a loop of large or small intestine which is adherent at umbilical level drops into the pelvis and creates an acute kink at the hernial site.

The most important intestinal change of position in pregnancy is that of the caecum and the appendix. As the caecum is pushed ever more laterally to the right iliac fossa by the growing uterus, it is also pushed in a cephalad direction, with the result that in late pregnancy the base of the appendix is very much higher and more lateral than in the non-pregnant woman. This is shown in diagrammatic form on **Figure 6**. This is a matter of great importance to the surgeon both in the diagnosis and treatment of acute appendicitis in pregnancy.

The site of tenderness on abdominal examination is much higher and more lateral than usual and there is no prospect of gaining information from a rectal examination since the appendix is far beyond the reach of the examining finger. The displacement and disturbance of intraperitoneal relations by the growing uterus means that the omentum is not able to seal off a necrotic or ruptured appendix and early general peritonitis is very liable to develop. It is for this reason that early diagnosis is so important.

As far as operative treatment is concerned the surgeon has to plan the incision so that it falls over the base of the appendix in its displaced position and allows its removal with minimal disturbance to the peritoneal surface. At the same time it is obviously desirable to avoid the mass of the uterus both because of its vulnerability and because it interferes with access. For good measure the pregnant patient has usually accumulated a layer of subcutaneous areolar fat which makes it difficult to locate the incision with accuracy and necessitates a longer cut than one would wish if the muscle and peritoneal openings are not to be made at the bottom of a rather deep hole. The correct incision is an oblique one of McBurney type but higher and more lateral than a normally placed incision of that name. These points are dealt with in greater detail when describing the operation on page 81.

6 Surface marking the appendix in pregnancy
The changing position of the base of the appendix as pregnancy advances is shown on the photograph. The surface markings arrowed and designated (1) (2) (3) and (4) show the position at 12, 18, 24 and 36 weeks respectively.

Metabolic changes during pregnancy

There are profound changes in general body metabolism during pregnancy. There is a progressive weight gain till about the 37th week of pregnancy after which it remains static or drops slightly. This is recognisable as a general deposition of fat, but much of the latter is in fact fluid associated with a marked sodium retention. There is a degree of sugar intolerance and also a lowered renal threshold to it, so that the pregnant woman may have 'alimentary' or lowered renal threshold type of glycosuria.

The growth of the uterus during pregnancy

By the very fact of its increase in size the uterus produces problems which may concern the surgeon. Initially 7 cm long and weighing 70 grams it increases to 36 cm in length and weighs more than 1 kg. The enormous increase in arterial blood supply which accompanies this growth is seen by comparing **Figures 8** and **9** and **Figure 10** is an arteriogram illustrating uterine vascularity at 12 weeks. The overlays on **Figure 7** emphasise the rapid rise in the level of the uterine fundus during pregnancy. The resultant pressure on,

and displacement of, adjoining structures has been seen, but there may also be special uterine problems when the uterus lies in retroversion in early pregnancy or when it contains fibroids. By greatly altering the level of the attached ovaries, it may also affect potential complications from ovarian cysts.

Thus a uterus which is retroverted at the beginning of pregnancy usually corrects its position even if this is partially effected by sacculation to bypass the sacral promontary but in a proportion of cases it is unable to grow towards the abdomen in its true axis and becomes trapped in the pelvis as an incarcerated retroverted gravid uterus. The reasons for this, the subsequent development and the management of the clinical condition are discussed on page 103.

In pregnancy fibroids enlarge in apparent proportion to the size of the uterus itself; in fact the increase is due more to oedema than to fibromyomatous cell growth. The enlargement interferes with the blood supply and may lead to red degeneration in the tumour during the second trimester. The clinical picture is well known to obstetricians and its management and that of fibroids in general is discussed on page 101.

7 Height of uterine fundus at various stages of pregnancy
Surface markings of the uterine fundal level at various stages of pregnancy are shown. The numbers 1, 2, 3, 4, and 5 show the height of the fundus at 12, 18, 24, 36, and 40 weeks respectively.

As the uterus enlarges into the abdomen during pregnancy the broad ligaments are elevated with it and especially at their medial ends. This means that the ovaries lie at a very much higher level in late pregnancy than they normally do and the same applies to the much elongated fallopian tubes. This change is important in relation to sizeable ovarian cysts which in the normal course of events might be expected to interfere with delivery. There is always the possibility of their being drawn up in the train of the broad ligament to escape from the pelvis and lie well above the presenting part at term.

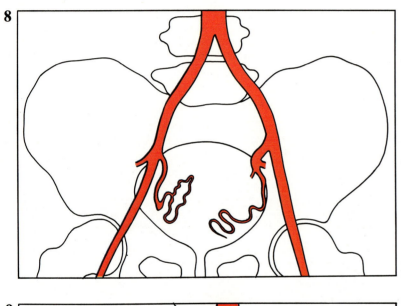

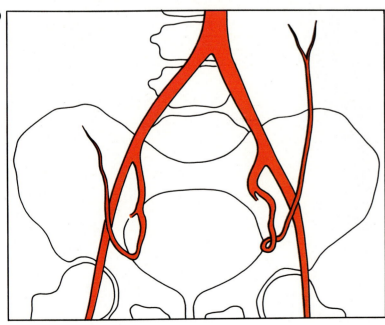

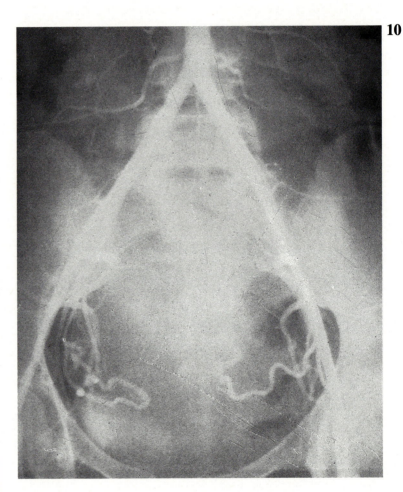

8 to 10
Figures 8 and **9** are drawings based on radiographic tracings to show the increase in uterine artery calibre and length from early (**Figure 8**) to late (**Figure 9**) pregnancy. The radiograph (**Figure 10**) emphasises the enlargement even at 12 weeks.

16

Surgical instruments

The authors' attitude to surgical instruments has been restated in each volume of the Atlas. It is assumed that most readers will have become accustomed to the instruments of their own choice and there is no desire to dissuade them from their use. For those who want guidance a set of simple and straightfoward design in use at the Jessop Hospital for Women, Sheffield is shown below; these have served a succession of exceed-ingly good and careful surgeons over a number of years. With regard to nomenclature the designations attached are those that have been 'handed down' to us; some readers will know their favourites by other names.

Instruments necessary for use in obstetrical surgery are shown as a separate set overleaf.

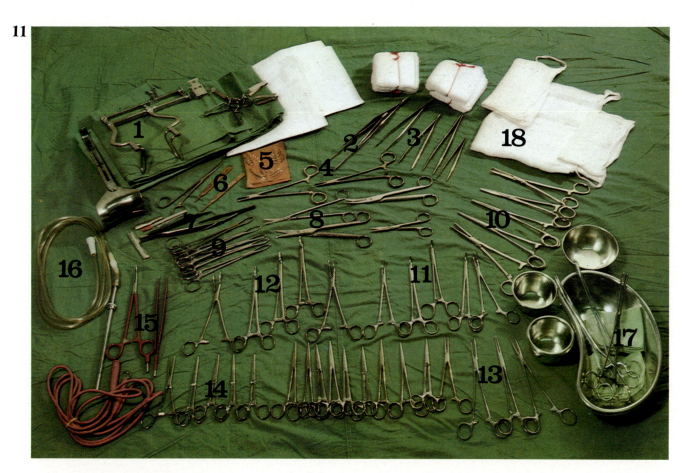

11 Standard abdominal instruments
1 Self-retaining retractor
2 Ureteric dissecting forceps
3 Dissecting forceps
4 Needle holders
5 Assorted needles
6 Scalpels
7 Michel clip forceps
8 Scissors
9 Littlewood's forceps
10 Straight Oschner forceps
11 Curved Oschner forceps
12 Miles-Phillips' forceps
13 Allis' tissue forceps
14 Spencer-Wells forceps
15 Diathermy forceps
16 Sucker
17 Sponge forceps and catheterisation equipment
18 Intra-abdominal packs and swabs

Some additional instruments are essential in obstetric work. These include forceps with which to deliver the fetus abdominally and control the wound edge at caesarean section. Axis traction forceps should perhaps have been shown but it is assumed that they are always available in a gynaecological operating room. Who can deny having suffered the mild embarrassment of delivering the baby on the operating table through a fully dilated cervix when a full-scale caesarean rescue had been mounted?

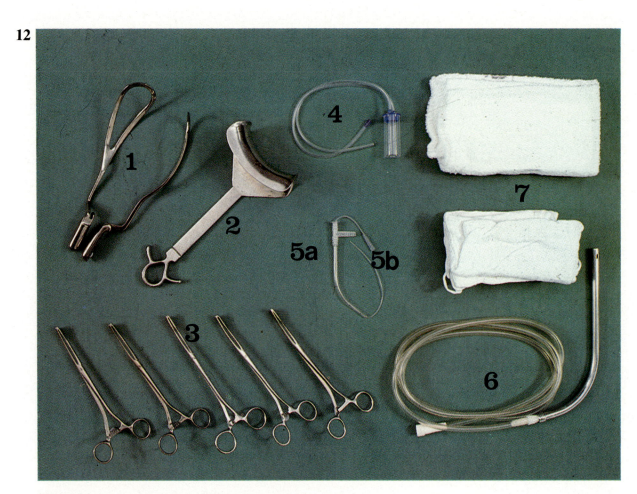

12 Additional instruments for obstetrical surgery
The items are numbered as follows: 1. short obstetric forceps (Wrigleys), 2. Doyen's retractor, 3. Green Armytage forceps, 4. mucus neo-natal aspirator, 5a. neo-natal endo-tracheal tube 5b. with mucus aspirator, 6. metal sucker and tubing, 7. large and small intra-abdominal packs (optional use, see page 199).

2: Therapeutic (induced) abortion

Abortion is the termination of pregnancy prior to the time of fetal viability and since no absolute determination of viability exists abortion has been defined as the termination of a gestation of 24 weeks or less, resulting in the delivery of a fetus weighing less than 500 grams. It can be either spontaneous or induced, the former type is considered in the following chapter, the latter in this. It is estimated that nearly one million pregnancies per annum are induced in the United States and this constitutes a major problem not only for gynaecologists but for society in general.

There are various methods and techniques used for the termination of pregnancy and all have their advantages and disadvantages. In this chapter they will be considered according to the trimester of pregnancy in which they are employed. In the first trimester abortion is predominantly induced by the suction technique; very rarely the sharp curette is employed. In the second trimester several techniques are employed and these range from dilatation and evacuation of the conceptus to extra-amniotic injection of abortifacient agents.

Many of these techniques are more suitable for local than general anaesthesia.

However, the choice of method would depend on the experience of the surgeon, the attitude of the patient and the facilities available. Effective use of any of the methods mentioned presupposes adequate training of the operator. Many doctors, for example, form the erroneous impression that because diagnostic dilatation and curettage is relatively simple and safe, they can use the technique to terminate pregnancy without any complications. In fact termination of pregnancy can develop into an extremely complicated and worrying procedure so that a background of correct training and clinical experience is important. This is especially so when using local anaesthesia. In this situation a degree of rapport with the patient having a termination is essential, and this can sometimes be difficult to establish. The doctor is aware that in most instances induced abortion is a highly emotional and psychologically traumatic event, and due allowance must be made for the patient's general reaction.

I. Techniques for induction of abortion

Suction curettage

In this method the pregnancy is removed via a pliable or a rigid cannula connected to a suction device developing a pressure in the region of 740–750 mm/Hg. Almost 95 per cent of first trimester abortions are dealt with in this way and the fact that it is universally preferred to sharp curettage reflects the clinical advantage of suction over curettage. Thus it can be performed under local anaesthetic rather than general; it is a more rapid method with more efficient emptying of the uterine contents, results in reduced bleeding and has fewer of the other complications normally associated with first trimester abortions. It is significantly safer and simpler than sharp curettage, but it is not without complications. These are discussed later.

Dilatation and evacuation

This operation can be technically difficult and should only be performed by skilled clinicians. It is usually done for pregnancies beyond 12–14 weeks. Many are done under a para-cervical block with the prior use of laminaria tents to achieve cervical softening and dilatation. A large suction curette is used to rupture the membranes and extract the amniotic fluid. Ring forceps are then used to remove fetal parts and suction curettage is intermittently applied to remove remaining fetal debris. It can be done quickly and avoids some of the problems of abortifacients but major complications may arise and these will be discussed later.

Injection of abortifacients

(i) Intra-amniotic
This procedure involves the transabdominal infusion into the amniotic space of abortifacients; these take the form of hypertonic saline, prostaglandins, or urea. Augmentation with oxytocin injected intravenously usually shortens the internal from induction to abortion. Controversy still exists as to the safety of each agent, but prostaglandins appear to be associated with fewer cardiovascular effects and clotting factor disturbances than other methods.

(ii) Extra-amniotic
This method seems to be safer than the intra-amniotic one and requires the introduction of a catheter into the extra-ovular space. The abortifacient used can be either prostaglandins or saline.

Non-surgical methods

Recently prostaglandins have been introduced into the vagina in suppository or tablet form. These eliminate the inherent risks of the surgical techniques but they are yet to be universally employed as an accepted substitute.

II. Complications

Gestational age appears to be the major factor in determining the mortality and morbidity associated with induced abortions. It is estimated that the incidence of abortion-related deaths has decreased significantly over the last 10 years; in the United States a rate of 4.2 deaths per 100,000 procedures in 1972 can be compared to 1.1 per 1000,000 in 1976. This decrease has been attributed to the increased numbers of the early abortions that are associated with safer techniques and the increasing experience of the operator. Deaths, however, do occur and risk of dying from an abortion when performed on a gestation under 8 weeks in the United States is estimated at 0.7 per 1000,000. If the abortion is carried out on a pregnancy between 9 and 10 weeks the relative risk is increased by a factor of 2.9; by 5.9 for an 11 to 12 weeks gestation, 10.7 for 13–15 weeks pregnancy and 28 for 16–20 weeks gestation.[1]

The morbidity associated with abortion may be immediate or long term. The former depends on the type of procedure used but is usually related to uterine perforation, infection or retention of pregnancy products. Long term sequelae are more difficult to assess and there is controversy on the magnitude of the harmful effects that may result from abortion.

Immediate complications

(i) Uterine perforation
This is one of the most serious complications of surgical abortion and its incidence is reported as between 0.5 to 1.7 cases per 1,000 procedures. Its frequency depends on the experience of the operator. The majority occur in extremely anteverted or retroverted uteri and are caused by the uterine sound or by a dilator. Prevention of perforation depends essentially on the correct assessment of the uterine position and the correct handling of instruments. The preoperative insertion of laminaria tents or vaginal prostaglandins removes the need for forceful mechanical cervical dilatation and will reduce the perforation risk[3,4]. A perforation may be clinically suspected when the instrument fails to encounter the expected resistance of the uterine wall or by the occurrence of heavy bleeding during or after the procedure. If local analgesia is being used the patient may experience a severe sharp lower abdominal pain.

When a perforation is supposed a sound should be passed to locate the site of penetration or rupture. If the damage has been caused by a large calibre instrument or if part of the omentum or bowel has been withdrawn into the uterus, then an immediate laparotomy is required. If there is doubt about perforation, laparoscopy will determine the site as well as confirming that perforation has taken place and is recommended by many surgeons. In all cases the bladder is catheterised to exclude damage to that organ.

(ii) Haemorrhage
An estimated blood loss of more than 200 ml results from suction curettage in approximately 25 per cent of cases[5]. The loss is dependent on the gestational age of the pregnancy, rising sharply after nine weeks. Blood loss can be dramatically reduced by the simultaneous or prior injection of an ecbolic usually in the form of synthetic oxytocin, ergometrine or a combination of the two.

(iii) Cervical laceration
A cervical tear or laceration is easily diagnosed and occurs in between 1 and 5 per cent of cases. It can result from excessive tension on the tenaculum and this may be avoided by the use of two such instruments. It may also be caused by forced mechanical dilatation. Preoperative cervical priming with laminaria tents or a vaginal suppository containing prostaglandin PGE_2 reduces this risk.

(iv) Infection
The reported rate of post abortal infections which range from localised pelvic infections to life threatening conditions such as peritonitis and septicaemia[5] is between 0.7–3 per cent. The rate will depend to some extent on the conditions under which the procedure is undertaken. The routine use of prophylactic antibiotics, usually doxycycline and metronidazole, is advised by many surgeons since there is evidence of an increase in the incidence of tubal obstructive disease in women who had induced abortions which were associated with infection[6].

(v) Incomplete abortion
This occurs in less than 1 per cent of cases and its incidence depends on the expertise of the operator. Vaginal bleeding is the major symptom of an incomplete induced abortion and the treatment is to complete the evacuation of uterine contents.

(vi) Rhesus sensitisation
There is always a risk of sensitisation in susceptible women so that it is strongly advised that Anti-D immunoglobulin be adminstered prior to the patient's discharge. Before the 12th week of gestation a dose of 0.5 cc is sufficient to cover any fetal cell leakage, but after 12 weeks it is advised that 1 cc of immunoglobulin be given.

Long term adverse effects

Until about a decade ago the effect of induced abortion on future fertility was thought to be extremely serious and tubal damage resulting in infertility was reported as being 10 times the normal risk. There was a reported increase in the incidence of ectopic pregnancy, premature delivery and even stillbirth. Subsequent studies have questioned many of these initial findings, but today it seems to be established that there is a long term risk to all women undergoing induced abortion.[2] This risk (and the short term complications) depend very much on the different circumstances and countries in which the event occurs. Abortion is still illegal in many parts of the world, and in these circumstances the long term complications would obviously be greater.

So many associated factors are involved that it is almost impossible to interpret the risks in statistical form. Thus many women having abortions come from lower socio-economic groups and are heavy smokers; common factors which themselves jeopardise pregnancy. It is also clear that termination of a young woman's first pregnancy may have different effects from those of an abortion undertaken in an older woman. At surgical level the method of termination and the degree of cervical dilatation produced will influence long term morbidity. It is well known that dilatation of the cervix to more than 10mm can be harmful and this is commonly exceeded prior to the introduction of suction curettage.

In a recent large American study[7] in which 3,500 cases and 28,000 controls were analysed it was suggested that nulliparous women had an increased risk of late miscarriage especially if the abortion had been undertaken by dilatation and curettage. If a woman had had two or more terminations, then her chances of late miscarriage increased threefold. In a large multi-centre study in Europe[8], increased risk of late miscarriage and prematurity was found in those whose termination had been undertaken by dilatation and curettage but not in those who had had a vacuum aspiration. In a large Danish study[9] abortion did not cause subsequent late miscarriage and did not affect placental function values nor birth weight in subsequent pregnancies. Threatened abortion and retained placenta, however, were commoner. Cervical dilatation to more than 12mm was associated with low birth weight and retained placenta. There was no increase in secondary infertility although in other studies it was not uncommon especially if infection had occurred.

Section 2: First trimester therapeutic (induced) abortion

Suction evacuation of uterus

Performed under local or general anaesthesia this is the commonest method of terminating a first trimester pregnancy. Accurate assessment of uterine size and position is an essential safety factor and the correct choice of dilators is most important.

Stage I: Clinical examination and instruments

It is important to correlate the findings on bi-manual examination with the estimated duration of pregnancy and this is especially so when assessing pregnancies that according to dates should be about 12 weeks in size. If the gestation is more than 12 weeks then suction curettage is unsuitable; thus it is essential to make an accurate estimate based on uterine size. Menstrual histories are notoriously inaccurate and women occasionally give dates that conveniently keep the pregnancy within the well recognised 'safe' 12 weeks. Clinical miscalculations are usually in the form of underestimates and the operation becomes more difficult than anticipated; approximately 5 per cent of pregnancies thought to be under 12 weeks of gestation are actually more advanced.

Factors which may lead to an over-estimation of pregnancy include fibroids, multiple pregnancies, hydramnios, obesity and abdominal wall tension.

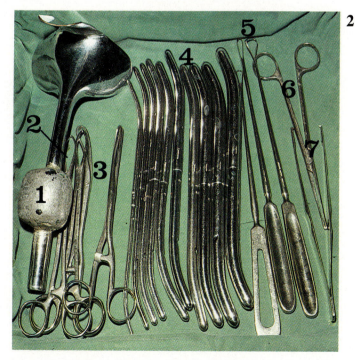

1 Bi-manual examination to assess uterine size and position.

2 Instruments
The tray of instruments comprises the following: 1. Auvard speculum, 2. cervical volsellum – tenaculum forceps,

3. ovum forceps (Bierer, Heywood-Smith or Sopher), 4. Hegar's dilators (other suitable dilators include Pratt, Bierer and Hawkins Ambler's), 5. sharp curettes, 6. and 7. forceps for specimen retrieval.

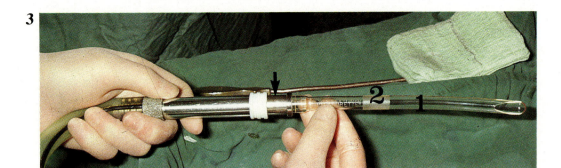

3 Suction curette

The transparent vacuum curette (1) is attached to a suction handle. The operator's thumb is placed over a small aperture (arrowed) which controls the suction produced in the curette. A continuous vacuum of above 60 cm Hg is necessary for effective evacuation. The markings on the curette (2) indicate the uterine depth. Curettes frequently have cm markings on the flexible tubing which also indicate the length of the uterus. A useful formula for interpreting the centimetre readings is applied thus: cavity depth (cm) −2 = number of weeks from last menstrual period (LMP). Thus a uterus that is 12 cm long (by 'sound' measurement) would have a size appropriate for 10 weeks LMP. The tip or leading part of the curette varies in size from 8–12 mm and is either straight or curved. The curved tip seen here is preferable since it conforms to the curvature of the uterine cavity. The selection of tip size usually depends on gestational stage; all extractions performed before 8 weeks from the LMP require the 8 mm tip to avoid over-dilatation of the cervix. A uterine size of 10 weeks would necessitate a 10 mm tip and a 12 week uterine size would indicate the need for a 12 mm tip.

Stage II: Assessment of uterine cavity size

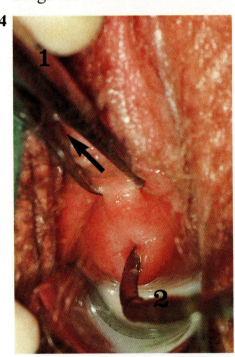

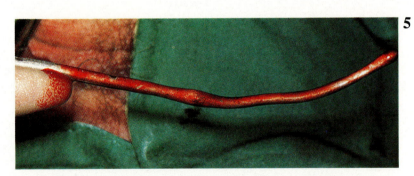

4 Application of volsellum to cervix and sounding of uterus

A single-toothed Braun volsellum (1) has been applied to the cervix in this case. Gentle traction is exerted on the instrument (in the line of the arrow) so as to align the uterus. This is particularly important if the uterus is acutely retroverted or anteverted and will reduce the risk of perforation of the lower uterine segment during dilatation or sounding. Occasionally it is necessary to apply two volsella or tenacula to steady the cervix; one may be placed on the anterior and the other on the posterior lip. A Sim's uterine sound (2) has been passed through the cervix to determine uterine depth.

5 Assessment of uterine depth

The Sim's uterine sound has now been withdrawn and the depth of the uterine cavity measured.

Stage III: Cervical dilatation

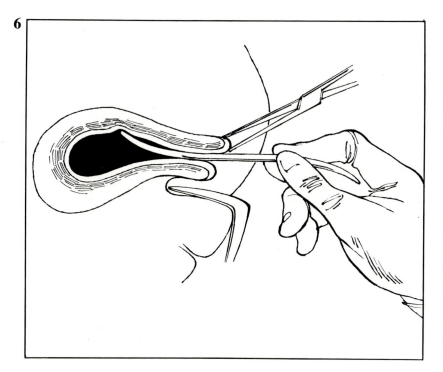

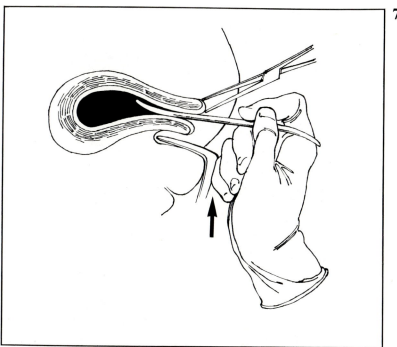

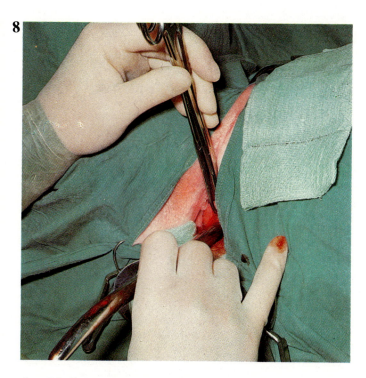

6 and 7 Safe method of cervical dilatation

The cervix is dilated by metal dilators of increasing size. This procedure may be difficult to perform because of a resistant cervix, and uterine perforation can occur. It is important that the uterus be held firmly and for this, 2 tenacula may be needed. If pre-operative vaginal prostaglandins or a

8

A Hegar double-end uterine dilator is being used to dilate the cervix. Note the position of the operator's hand to avoid excessive entry of the dilator into the uterine cavity.

laminaria tent had been inserted the problem is eased. It was previously accepted that the cervix should be dilated to the number of Hegar dilator that equalled the gestational age of the pregnancy, i.e. No. 8 for 8 weeks, No. 9 for 9 weeks. This rather simplistic approach can be recommended as only a rough guide and in fact more accurately represents the maximum dilatation for the particular stage of pregnancy. This particularly applies in the nulliparous patient.

The cervix is dilated to accommodate the appropriate suction curette and the sizes used have been discussed previously. The surgeon must decide which suction curette is to be used and that determines the degree of dilation required. The desire for minimal mechanical dilatation and trauma to the cervix must be set against the need for a suction curette of adequate size to evacuate the uterine contents effectively and completely. If one uses a too large suction curette, then cervical injury may occur; on the other hand a too small curette may result in an incomplete abortion.

Stage III: Cervical dilatation

6 and 7 Safe method for cervical dilatation

In **Figure 6** the surgeon is holding the dilator in a potentially dangerous manner. Once resistance of the internal cervical os has been overcome there is nothing to counteract and stop the forward thrust of the instrument and perforation of the anterior wall of a retroposed uterus is possible. In **Figure 7** the attitude of the hand holding the dilator prevents such an occurrence. This is seen in practice in **Figure 8** where uncontrolled forward movement is obviated (as indicated by the arrow) since the flexed hand forms a buffer to impinge on the perineum. Dilators should be introduced for only a short distance beyond the internal os. In dilatation of the nulliparous cervix, Pratt or Hawkin and Ambler dilators are favoured since they require less force to produce dilatation. Forceful dilatation increases the possibility of cervical laceration and future cervical incompetence.

9

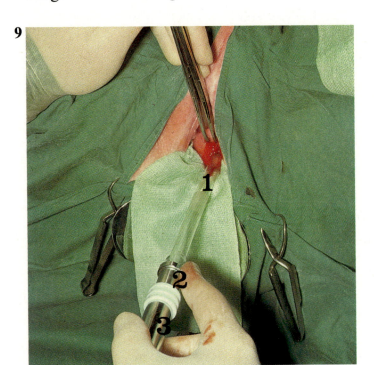

10

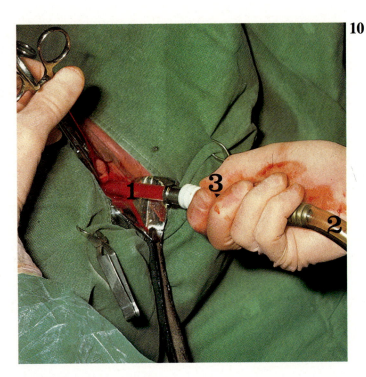

11

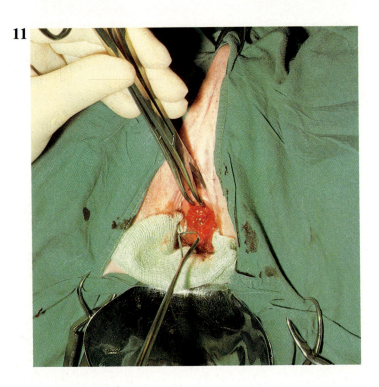

11 Sharp curettage

Sharp curettage is performed after suction aspiration. This is to eliminate any risk of an incomplete abortion. Sheets of decidua or additional gestational tissue are frequently obtained; occasionally the embryo itself or an additional embryo is removed. The operator cannot ensure that the cavity is empty without completing this procedure. The suction curette is reintroduced and rotated slowly for an additional 30 seconds. Additional gestation tissue may still be retrieved at this stage.

9 and 10 Suction curettage

Once the cervix has been dilated, suction curettage can commence. The curette is inserted into the uterine cavity and suction applied. The curette is rotated carefully within the cavity in a downward spiral motion and the tissue examined as it is aspirated from the uterus. This is easy if a transparent vacuum curette is used. Once the uterus has been completely evacuated the surgeon feels the uterus contract around the curette tip and notes the characteristic grating sensation. Air bubbles appear in the transparent tubing at this time. In **Figure 9** the curette (1) is inserted into the uterus and the suction has been turned off so that the tip does not adhere to the uterine wall. Suction can be controlled by shutting off the machine or manipulating a valve on the handle as necessary. This latter manoeuvre is shown with the operator placing his finger over the aperture valve (2) which is situated on the suction handle (3).

The rather fragile suction tip of the curette is preserved by not repeatedly bending it against the fundal wall. Tip inspection should be routine; if it breaks off it can be retrieved with a metal curette. In **Figure 10** suction has been applied and contents are being aspirated via the curette (1) along the heavy tubing (2) which is connected to the suction machine. The operator's finger (3) has been placed over the suction valve aperture. The avoidance of over-zealous suction or curettage will prevent the development of post-abortal uterine synechiae and post-abortal amenorrhoea (Asherman's syndrome). On completion of the procedure, significant uterine contraction may have reduced cavity depth by 2 cm below that of the initial sounding.

Stage V: Inspection of gestational products and estimation of blood loss

The tissue aspirated should be carefully examined, and in those patients with a late (advanced) gestation, the fetal parts should be identified and accounted for. It is helpful to estimate the tissue volume which should correlate with the size of the gestation. It is estimated that approximately 14 cc of tissue volume are present in a 7–8 week gestation and 21 cc in a gestation of 9–10

weeks. There is a fairly wide fluctuation in these volumes and they can only give an approximate estimate of the completeness of the procedure.

In the equipment seen in **Figure 12** the gestational products accumulate in a small gauze bag (1) in the main aspiration bottle. The bag is removed at the end of the procedure and water is run through the tubing of the pump so as to identify the contained gestational tissue. The bag is then detached and rewashed manually with cold water. After the water is squeezed out, it is emptied on to a transparent dish so that the fetal parts can be determined. The operator attempts to separate decidual, fetal and placental tissue and determine whether the amount of tissue indicates that the procedure is complete. If the fetal parts are not complete, if no gestational tissue is seen, or if there is too little placental tissue, the surgeon may choose to repeat the operation. In a pregnancy of more than 10 weeks it should be possible to identify the major structures of the fetus including the cranium, vertebral column, rib cage and limbs. A suspicion of retained products necessitates immediate resuctioning and, if necessary, curettage. The use of the smaller calibre tip may facilitate removal in an already contracted uterus. Occasionally re-dilatation and exploration with ovum forceps is necessary to remove tissue from high in the fundus.

If no tissue is obtained on suction curettage of the cavity, an explanation may be found in one of the following:

1. *A false passage* created by excessive dilatation of a rigid cervix. Avoidance of forceful dilatation reduces the likelihood of this complication. If a false passage is diagnosed and uterine perforation has not occurred, it may be possible to postpone the procedure and use vaginal prostaglandins or a laminaria tent in an attempt to dilate the rigid cervix.

2. *Uterine perforation.* This usually occurs in the severely retroverted uterus when penetration of the anterior aspect of the lower uterine segment follows precipitate entry of a sound or dilator through the cervix and into the cavity. If the operator feels that perforation has occurred and suction is operating, withdrawal of the cannula should be postponed until the pressure in the tubing is equalised. This is done by turning off the machine and disconnecting the tubing from the bottle, which will release the suction. If this is done, then the serious complicating of omentum or abdominal contents being drawn into the perforation site is avoided. Management of the suspected uterine perforation during suction aspiration has been discussed previously.

3. *Ectopic pregnancy.* If only minimal decidual tissue has been obtained by suction, then ectopic pregnancy must be suspected. A radio-receptor assay of the beta sub-unit of human chorionic gonadotrophin (HCG) should be made. If re-examination reveals signs which suggest ectopic pregnancy, then laparoscopy should be undertaken.

4. *A uterus excessively large for dates.* No tissue may be obtained since the suction tip is too small for tissue retrieval. In obese patients the uterus may be enlarged to over 12–14 week size without it being clinically obvious. The techniques used for second trimester evacuation may need to be used.

5. *False positive pregnancy test.* The uterus may be enlarged and soft, thus apparently supporting the false result.

6. *Congenital abnormalities.* A septate uterus should be kept in mind if the above possibilities have been eliminated. Such an anomaly is sought with blunt sounds and a curette, and, in rare cases, a uterine didelphys with a double vagina or cervix may be present. Deflection of a mid-line septum by the vaginal speculum may conceal a second vaginal opening, and this should be checked.

Estimation of blood loss

Blood loss can easily be estimated by reference to the contents held in the suction bottle. Blood loss during the procedure is related to gestational age and increases sharply after 9 weeks. Most surgeons give an ecbolic agent. This may take the form of an injection of oxytocin 20 I.U. in 500 ml of 5 per cent dextrose and water prior to and during evacuation, or 5 I.U. in solution during the procedure, or an intravenous injection of 0.2 mg–0.5 mg of ergometrine prior to the commencement of cervical dilatation. A combination of both (i.e. synthetic oxytocin 5 I.U./ml with ergometrine 0.5 mgm) seems to also be highly effective in reducing blood loss. A loss of over 200 ml may indicate that there are retained gestational products or that the uterus is not contracted. If there is bleeding and the uterus is known to be empty, then possible trauma to the cervix or to the body of the uterus must be considered.

A histological examination of the products of conception should always be made. Absence of villi in a small specimen may point to a diagnosis of ectopic pregnancy or unsuspected trophoblastic disease may be discovered in the specimen. Apart from these purely clinical considerations, it is an essential medico-legal safeguard to have a precise record and evidence of what was done.

Second trimester therapeutic (induced) abortion

Approximately 60 per cent of abortion related deaths in mothers occur as a result of termination of pregnancy in the mid-trimester. Only 15 per cent of all the abortions in the United States, for example, are performed during this time, so that the death rate in the group is very high and makes it a procedure to be undertaken with the utmost care. Determination of a safe and effective mid-trimester abortion technique remains a major gynaecological problem. The most commonly used techniques during this time are:

1 Intra-amniotic instillation of saline, prostaglandins or urea.
2 Extra-amniotic introduction of prostaglandin or saline either continuously or as intermittent dosage.
3 Dilatation and evacuation.

Hysterotomy and hysterectomy may also be performed.

Mid-trimester abortions done by any of the three methods listed should be inpatient procedures in a hospital which has appropriate facilities. All patients must be properly counselled and aware of the proposed procedure and its effects. Local analgesia is normally used in these cases and this means that the patient is fully aware of what is being done. The views and feelings of involved clinical and para-clinical staff must obviously be considered when choosing the method to be used.

The patient's blood is taken for typing and cross matching in case a blood transfusion becomes necessary. It is particularly important that the exact gestation time be calculated, and this is most accurately done by ultrasonography. Such a precaution helps avoid problems that may be encountered in the delivery of a too large or too mature fetus. All rhesus negative patients must receive a full dose of rhesus immune globulin to prevent possible immunisation.

Intra-amniotic instillation of abortifacients

(1) Hypertonic saline
This remains a popular method of inducing abortion in a gestation of more than 15 weeks. The intra-amniotic instillation of hypertonic saline solution possibly stimulates uterine activity through the endogenous release of prostaglandins with resulting fetal expulsion. It requires preliminary amniocentesis and the patient must therefore be at least 16 weeks pregnant. Possible complications of the method are major; the most serious being acute cardiovascular collapse as a result of inadvertent intravenous saline infusion which results in hypernatremia. The induction of a disseminated intravascular coagulation (DIC) mechanism has been reported in a small percentage of cases and the accidental injection of the hypertonic saline solution into the uterine wall can destroy both decidua and myometrium.

(2) Prostaglandins
Many abortions between the 16th and 20th week of gestation are induced by the intra-amniotic instillations of prostaglandin $F_2\propto$. As in the first method, the prostaglandins induce uterine activity which results in expulsion of the conceptus. Fortunately prostaglandins are not associated with the risk of hypernatremia and DIC so that this agent is considered to be safer as well as equally effective. A recent multi-centre study showed that the death rate with intra-amniotic prostaglandins was lower than that for intra-amniotically injected saline[10]. The rate for the former was 13.1 per 100,000 compared with 17.2 per 100,000 for the latter. There is some evidence that prostaglandins are associated with a slightly higher morbidity rate than saline and also with an increased risk of the fetus being born alive. The possibility of a liveborn birth is of concern to many clinicians as the medico-legal consequences are serious. Many surgeons therefore feel that its direct effect on the fetus and fetal tissues makes saline the agent of choice for pregnancies of 20 weeks or more.

(3) Urea
Intra-amniotic instillation of urea is a popular method of inducing mid-trimester abortion. Urea stimulates uterine activity in a manner somewhat similar to that of saline. It results in the immediate death of the fetus and thus avoids the problem of a live birth.

Therapeutic regime

Hypertonic saline
The method involves the withdrawal of approximately 50–100 ml of amniotic fluid and its replacement by an infusion of 200 ml of 20 per cent saline.

Prostaglandins
Prostaglandin $F_2\propto$ is used in a dose of 40 mg. A test dose of 5 mg in a 1 ml solution is given initially and 5 minutes later the remaining 35 mg in a 7 ml solution is injected by slow infusion.

Urea
A solution of 80 gm of urea in 132 ml of 5 per cent dextrose in water is slowly instilled via a drip into the amniotic cavity; 200 ml of amniotic fluid previously having been aspirated. The drip is halted two or three times during the infusion and the urea bottle is lowered to below the level of the patient to ensure that there is a satisfactory flow. Because of the rather prolonged abortion time for urea alone (i.e. 50 hours), the addition of prostaglandins in the form of 5 mg of $PGF_2\propto$ is recommended. This has resulted in a reduction of the abortion time to an average of approximately 16 hours. Urea is a potent diuretic and patients are encouraged to drink fluids to prevent dehydration. Coagulopathy has been reported with urea, and the precautions taken when infusing hypertonic saline should be observed.

Oxytocin
The intra-amniotic use of prostaglandins or saline with a simultaneous infusion of oxytocin has been recommended to reduce the interval from instillation to delivery. It is recommended that the delivery of 10 units of oxytocin per hour, starting within 2 hours of the saline instillation, shortens the abortion time from 35 to 20 hours. Others have reported that an oxytocin infusion at a rate of 1 to 4 units per hour and initiated within 6 hours of instillation also reduces the delivery time.

It has been standard practice in some centres to combine intra-amniotic instillation techniques with the pre-operative use of laminaria tents which induce slow mechanical dilatation of the cervix. A dramatic shortening of the abortion process has been reported[11]. These tents are usually inserted about 18 hour before the intra-amniotic injection.

Intra-amniotic instillation of abortifacients – technique

Stage 1: Injection of local analgesic

The patient is counselled prior to the procedure and is therefore aware of what is going to happen. The bladder is empty and the abdomen prepared with antiseptic solution. A local analgesic agent consisting of 1 per cent lignocaine is injected subcutaneously into the proposed amniocentesis site which has been determined by ultrasound.

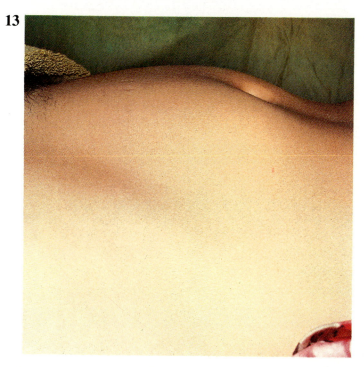

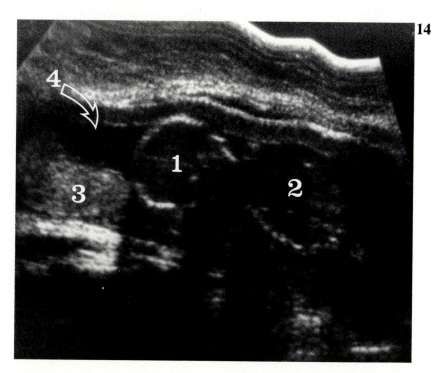

13 Abdomen prior to injection
This 42-year-old patient has a fetus which has been shown to have severe genetic defect (previous amniocentesis). The gestation has progressed to 22 weeks size as determined by ultrasound.

14 Ultrasonography of gestation
Ultrasonography shows the fetal skull (1) and fetal body (2). The placenta situated on the posterior uterine wall extends to the fundal area (3). A clear space occupied by amniotic fluid is easily seen at (4). This is the area where the injecting needle will enter.

15 Introduction of subcutaneous local analgesic
A small weal of 1 per cent local analgesic (lignocaine) has been introduced to a site directly above the clear liquor space seen on ultrasonography.

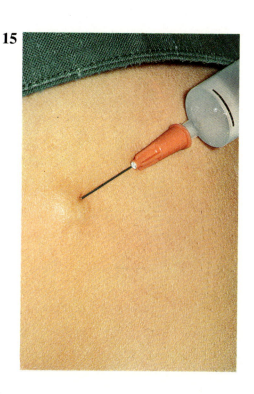

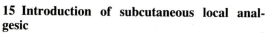

16 Infiltration of local analgesic into anterior abdominal wall
Careful instillation of between 5 and 10ml of local analgesic into the anterior abdominal wall proceeds along the path of the needle insertion. Continual withdrawal before injection is undertaken so as to avoid the risk of intravascular injection of local analgesic agent.

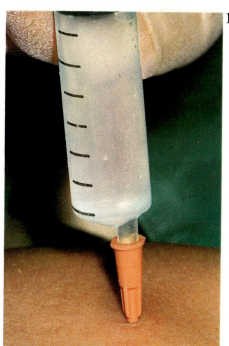

Stage II: Insertion of the amniocentesis needle

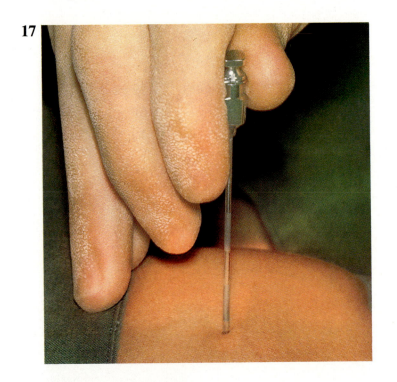

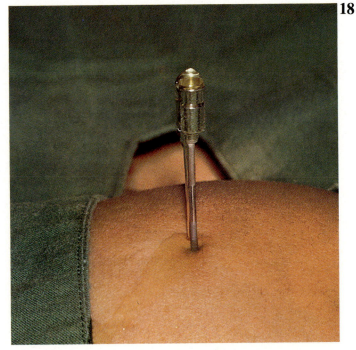

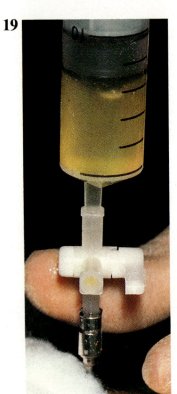

17 and 18

When local analgesia is effective, a 16 or 18 gauge 8.75 cm spinal needle is inserted into the amniotic fluid space (**Figure 17**). In **Figure 18** the trocar has been removed and the free flow of clear amniotic fluid indicates that the needle has been correctly placed. If amniotic fluid cannot be easily obtained, or if fluid is very blood-stained, the procedure should be abandoned and no attempt at re-instillation made for at least 24 hours. This is particularly advisable when saline is to be used. If a second attempt fails and fluid cannot be obtained, the patient should be discharged and re-admitted in a week for a fresh attempt. Such precautions avoid the risk of intravascular injection of the abortifacient.

19 Removal of amniotic fluid

When the needle is in the correct position, a 3-way tap with a 20 ml syringe is attached and the liquor slowly withdrawn. For intra-amniotic instillation of saline approximately 50–100 ml of amniotic fluid is aspirated initially. In the case of prostaglandins most surgeons do not consider it necessary to withdraw any amniotic fluid before instillation.

Stage III: Injection of abortifacient

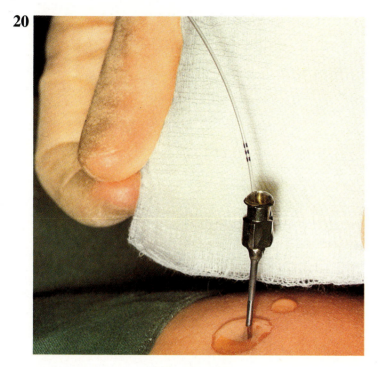

20 and 21 Injection of abortifacient
After aspiration of the liquor a very fine polythene spinal catheter is passed into the amniotic space. An adequate length of catheter should be used. In **Figure 20** the catheter is threaded through the needle and in **Figure 21** the introducing needle is withdrawn over it and the fine catheter left *in situ*.

The abortifacient can now be injected, the dosage has been discussed previously (page 26). When prostaglandin $F_2\propto$ is introduced intra-amniotically a test dose of 1 ml (5 mg) is given initially and 5 minutes elapse before the remaining 7 ml (containing 35 mg of $PGF_2\propto$) is given by slow injection. If acute gastro-intestinal symptoms develop, the amount of drug to be infused can be reduced. If this occurs, only 20 mg need be given when the pregnancy is between 16–18 weeks and 25–30 mg for a pregnancy between 18 and 20 weeks.

If after initial introduction of the saline solution the patient develops abdominal pain, headaches or tingling of the fingers (symptoms suggestive of intravascular injection of sodium chloride), then the procedure should be immediately terminated and the patient carefully observed. A rapid infusion of 1 litre of dextrose in water is suggested if passage of more than small amounts of saline solution is suspected. The patient should be checked for vital signs immediately and she should be kept at bed rest for one hour.

Extra-amniotic injection of abortifacients: technique

The insertion of substances into the extra-ovular or extra-amniotic space is effective in inducing uterine contractions. Prostaglandins, especially the PGE_2, have been used very successfully in this respect. They promote efficient uterine contractions and also develop efficient cervical dilatation by a presumed local effect on the cervical connective tissue. Complications of the technique are less than those with intra-amniotic injection of prostaglandins and no case has been reported of cervical damage caused by prostaglandins injected by this route. Prostaglandins can be given as a continuous infusion or, as recently described, by an intermittent and highly effective regime[13]. Normal saline can also be injected into the extra-ovular space[14] and it appears that its instillation in this site induces a rise in local endogenous prostaglandins with resultant onset of contractions. Preliminary data from a recent study[14] showed that the mean induction delivery time was 15.4 hours. This is only slightly longer than is quoted for prostaglandins when given by continuous infusion, but is much more than the recently reported 10.7 hours for the intermittent dosage regime. It is of particular value in those patients in whom prostaglandins, oxytocin and hypertonic saline are contra-indicated. Its exact mode of action is not clear. Approximately 300–500 ml of saline is given as a once only injection; the amount being related to the uterine size. There is no apparent difference in the length taken to deliver parous or nulliparous women.

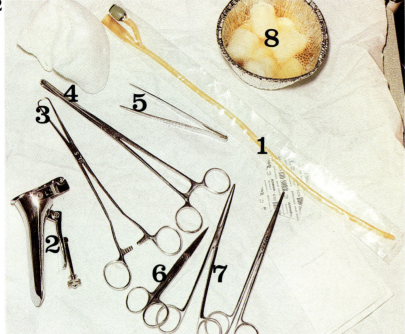

22

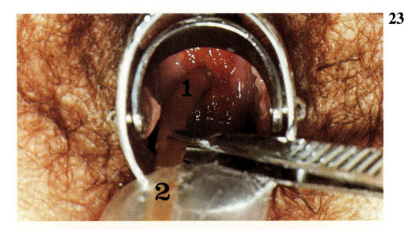

23

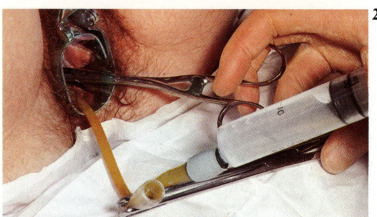

24

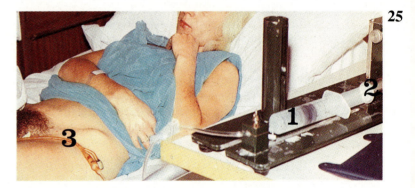

25

22 Instruments
Instruments for the extra-amniotic instillation of either prostaglandins or saline are shown: 1. 14–16 size Foley catheter with a 30 ml balloon and spigot, 2. Cusco vaginal speculum, 3. single toothed tenacula, 4. sponge forceps to assist insertion, 5. non-toothed dissecting forceps, 6. scissors, 7. small sinus forceps, 8. antiseptic solution. Three sets of 20 and 40 ml sterile syringes are provided on a separate tray.

23 Introduction of catheter to extra-amniotic space
The cervix has been cleaned with an antiseptic solution and the end of the Foley catheter (1) is introduced into the cervical canal. Only a small portion of the catheter projects beyond its sterile sheath (2). A pair of non-toothed dissecting forceps then pushes the catheter slowly into the extra-ovular space; the catheter previously being inserted through the os until resistance was felt. It has been filled with 10 ml of normal saline to obliterate the dead space within it. Once the catheter is in the extra-ovular space, the 30 ml balloon is filled with normal saline and the catheter gently retracted. This enables the balloon to position itself at the level of the internal os and so prevent leakage of saline. A double balloon catheter (Porges – France) specially designed for this purpose can be introduced through the cervix to a depth of 8 cm within the extra-ovular space without rupturing the membrane[14]. There is a distal balloon on the catheter which is inflated with 25 ml of saline before the catheter is gently withdrawn, so that the inflated uterine balloon rests against the internal os. The second or proximal balloon is now positioned in the vagina and will press against the external os when inflated with 30 ml of saline solution. When the two balloons are inflated and positioned, the extra-ovular space is sealed and leakage from the area is minimal.

24 Injection of abortifacient
A test dose of 3 ml of prostaglandin PGE_2 corresponding to 100 mcg/ml is about to be injected. Five minutes after this dose, and if no systemic effects from the prostaglandins are evident, then the full amount can be given via a constant infusion pump, usually at a rate of 0.5–1 ml/hr* (100 mcg/ml solution).

*A 100 mcg/ml solution of PGE_2 is obtained by diluting 0.5 ml of the prostaglandin (Prostin, Upjohn Ltd) with 50 ml of saline dilutent.

25 Constant infusion pump for prostaglandin
The patient has already had a test dose without any untoward response and the total dosage is now loaded into a syringe (1) which is connected to a constant infusion pump device (2). The Foley catheter is easily seen (3) and this is conveniently connected by a plastic infusion tube to the syringe.

Intermittent extra-amniotic injections of abortifacients
The intermittent injection method has considerable advantage in that it does not need a constant infusion device and can be easily administered. Recently prostaglandin E_2 has been prepared in a gel form for injection into the extra-ovular space[13] and this makes it much easier to administer. Without anaesthesia a 12 gauge Foley catheter is inserted for a distance of 5 cm through the cervical os and 8.75 ml of gel injected slowly. The catheter is then flushed through with a further 5 ml of sterile tylose gel and removed. If abortion does not occur, a further 3.5 mg of PGE_2 is given every 6 hours until it does. In this recent study[13] the mean time to abortion was 10.7 hours (range 3.3 to 26.3) and 89 per cent of the patients needed only two injections. There were no failures with the technique in 110 patients. One-fifth of the patients did have some mild gastrointestinal upset and three-quarters of them needed one or more doses of analgesia. The method has obvious advantages over the previously described intra-amniotic prostaglandin infusions.

*A 4 per cent of methylhydroxyethyl powder (Tylose MH 300P, Hoechst) was prepared with isotonic saline and autoclaved and PGE_2 3.5 mg in isotonic saline added aseptically.

Special aspects of early and advanced therapeutic abortion

Termination of pregnancy before 8 weeks and after 16 weeks demands particular knowledge and skills because of the peculiar problems posed by such gestations. Early pregnancy with a small sized uterus is suitable for termination in the office or out-patient department and should result in minimal trauma or inconvenience to the patient. These advantages may, however, be offset by complications related to the problem of cervical dilatation and the difficulty of adequately counselling an emotional patient who will be conscious throughout the proceedings.

Similarly the enlarged and vascular uterus of over 16 weeks size presents problems of cervical dilatation and there is the added risk of damage to the uterus, cervix and vagina when removing a large fetus and placenta. The psychological and emotional stresses in this group are well known.

Fortunately there are three basic techniques in current use which help with these separate problems. Thus damage to the cervix in both early and late pregnancy may be avoided by the preoperative use of laminaria tents. Termination of the very early pregnancy has been facilitated and made very safe by the small-bore suction catheters of Karman type while carefully controlled use of dilatation and evacuation has made late abortion as safe as is possible in our present state of knowledge.

In this section three aspects of early and advanced therapeutic abortion will be reviewed. These are:
1 The use of the laminaria tent in early and advanced abortion,
2 Therapeutic abortion of the early pregnancy,
3 Therapeutic abortion of the advanced pregnancy: use of dilatation and evacuation.

Use of the laminaria tent

There are many situations, especially in early and late termination, where the undilated cervix presents a problem to the gynaecologist. Metal dilators used on a tight cervix may cause laceration or rupture and long term cervical incompetence. A gentler alternate is to use a laminaria tent. These are made from seaweed plants that grow in the North Pacific and North Atlantic oceans (Laminaria Japonica, L. Digitata). They have been used for many years but became unpopular in the 1950/60's when the dangers of associated infection were considered unacceptable. However recent advances in sterilisation with high energy gamma radiation has eliminated this danger and they are again popular.

Laminaria is hydroscopic and when wet it dilates to 3 to 5 times its diameter over a period of 6 to 8 hours. In the dry state the tents look like smooth twigs or sticks about 6 cm in length. There are three sizes with diameters of 3–5 mm, 6–8 mm and 8–10 mm. A cord is looped through the proximal end and just beyond it a plastic disc prevents the laminaria from slipping through the cervix into the uterine cavity.

The size of the tent selected for insertion is related to the degree of dilatation required and to the size of the canal. Usually only one insertion lasting 12 to 18 hours is required; it has been shown that the major degree of swelling occurs in the first 5 hours after injection. It seems as though 4 hours is the minimum time required for adequate dilatation. Tents used in early abortion cases are inserted on the day before operation.

Insertion can be facilitated by moistening the tent with sterile lubricating jelly or antiseptic ointment. A transient syncopal effect may sometimes occur during insertion. If the cervix is stenotic and resists the introduction of the tent, the anterior lip of the cervix may be grasped with a single tooth volsellum, and as countertraction is applied the thin laminaria can easily be manoeuvered into the cervical canal. Some gynaecologists routinely give prophylactic antibiotics while the tent is *in situ*.

Many studies attest to the value of tents in reducing the morbidity associated with first trimester abortion.[15,16] Their use in mid-trimester abortion is well documented. They may be inserted before a surgical evacuation of the uterus or concurrently with the intra-amniotic infusion of hypertonic saline or prostaglandin $F_{2\alpha}$[11,17]. The infusion – expulsion time interval for these latter abortions is reduced on average by 20–30 per cent with no corresponding increase in complications. Their employment with the dilatation and evacuation procedure is discussed on Page 36.

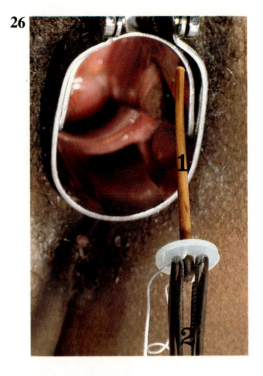

26

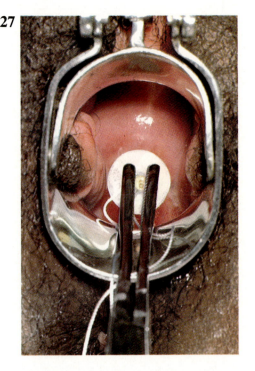

27

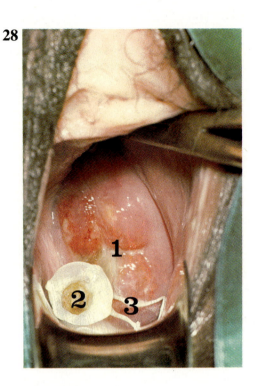

28

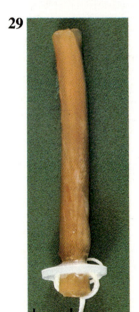

29

26 and 27 The technique of insertion

After bimanual examination and determination of the uterine position, a speculum is inserted into the vagina and the cervix cleaned with an antiseptic solution. If the cervix is already partly dilated as in this case (**Figure 26**) a laminaria (1) of 3–5 mm size can be inserted by holding the proximal end with a sponge holder (2). In **Figure 27** the laminaria has been passed into the cervix of this primigravid patient who was 10 weeks pregnant. Once in position with the plastic disc against the external os several 10 × 10 cm gauze packs are inserted into the vagina to maintain it in position. Otherwise the laminaria may be expelled or slip down the vagina when the patient stands up.

28 and 29 Laminaria tent removal

After 18 hours the tent is about to be removed. In **Figure 28** it is seen to be in its original position. The cervical canal is at (1) and the tent at (2). It is removed by gentle traction on the attached cord (3). In **Figure 29** the tent is seen to have increased in width from 3–5 mm to 7–10 mm after only 18 hours *in situ*.

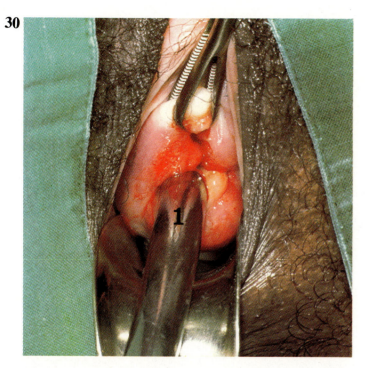

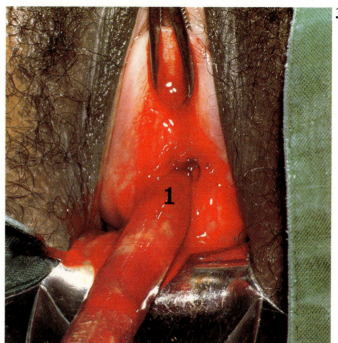

30 and 31 Suction curettage after laminaria tent insertion
With the tent removed in **Figure 30** a Hegar's uterine dilator
of 10 mm size (1) is easily inserted into the cervical canal. In
Figure 31 a 10 mm suction curette (1) is seen evacuating the
gestational products.

Therapeutic abortion of the early first trimester pregnancy

The increasing demand for therapeutic abortion has
created a need for a safer method for those presenting
before the 8 to 9th week of gestation. This has been
partly achieved by the development of suction catheters (i.e. Karman, Vabra), of a design which minimises the risk of uterine and cervical damage and
where the procedure can be done under local analgesia. The Karman catheter is suitable for early
pregnancy termination and sizes of 4, 5, 6, 8, 10 mm are
available. It has a soft flexible design and its blunt
leading surface ensures that the catheter deflects and
collapses rather than perforates the uterus when it is
pushed against the fundus. Requirements for analgesia
are minimal as the small sized catheter can be passed
into many uteri without prior dilatation.

Local analgesia has advantages over general anaesthesia but there are also some disadvantages. Thus the
conscious patient needs counselling and reassurance
not only before but also during the procedure and the
surroundings and atmosphere in which the operation
takes place must necessarily be congenial and friendly,
especially for the apprehensive young nullipara. A
paracervical or an intracervical block may be employed; the authors favour the latter method. In this a
2 per cent solution of either lignocaine or chloro-
procaine hydrochloride with 1 : 200,000 epinephrine is
used. The epinephrine reduces blood loss by contract-

ing uterine vessels. The effect of injection is instan-
taneous and avoids the delay of absorption when using
a paracervical block. A recent study[5] of nearly 54,000
terminations in the United States, 18,000 of which were
performed under local analgesia, showed that abortion
was safer when performed under local as compared
with general anaesthesia. The latter was associated
with a 1.7 times increase in uterine perforation and an
8.2 times increase in intra abdominal haemorrhage.
The rate of endometritis and retained products was
identical in the two groups.

Bleeding during termination of early pregnancy can
be reduced by the use of an ecbolic injection of
ergometrine (0.5 mgm) and synthetic oxytocin, 5 u/ml
given as cervical dilatation begins[18]. The use of this
preparation was associated with a reduction in post
operative nausea and vomiting.

The recent practice of inserting a 10 mgm vaginal
pessary of prostaglandin (PGE_2 – a 4 gm lipid based
pessary, Witepsol, E75) – 4 to 6 hours prior to surgery
not only aids cervical dilatation but also significantly
reduces blood loss. These two methods, the ecbolic
and the vaginal pessary, should be employed to reduce
operative morbidity in early abortion. However the
patient must be warned to expect headache and
abdominal pains for 48–72 hours after the operation.

Suction termination under local anaesthesia

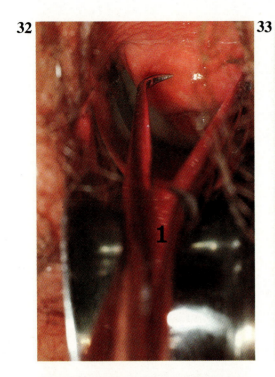

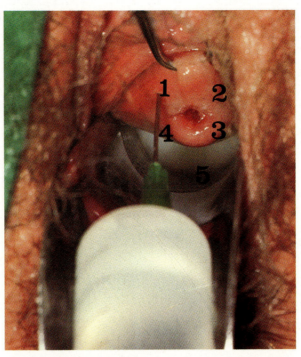

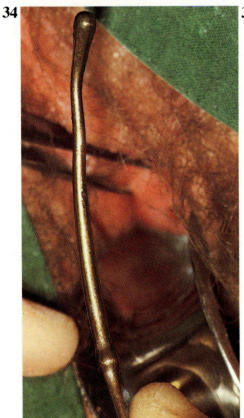

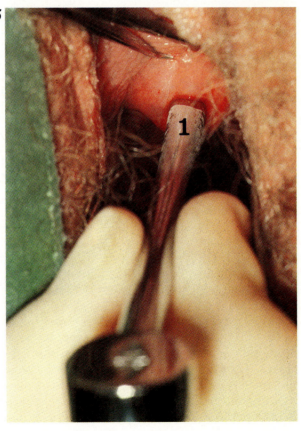

32 Application of volsellum
A tenaculum (1) is about to be applied in the 12 o'clock position of the cervix in a pregnancy of 8 weeks duration; 4 ml of local analgesic have been inserted in this position to numb the area. The tenaculum steadies the cervix.

33 Injection of intracervical local anaesthetic
20 ml of a 2 per cent solution of either lignocaine or nesacaine is injected into the four quadrants of the ectocervix (numbered 1–4). The tenaculum is steadying the cervix and a Sim's vaginal speculum (5) is in place.

34 Estimation of uterine depth
After effective analgesia has been obtained, a uterine sound is passed and the depth of the uterine cavity determined. On this measurement will depend the size of the uterine aspiration (suction) catheter to be employed.

35 Cervical dilatation
If pre-operative prostaglandin suppositories or laminaria tents have not been used to procure cervical dilatation, some form of dilatation may be necessary (using Hawkin Ambler tapered dilators as seen at (1)). When using very small sized (4–6 mm) suction curettes it may be unnecessary to perform dilatation.

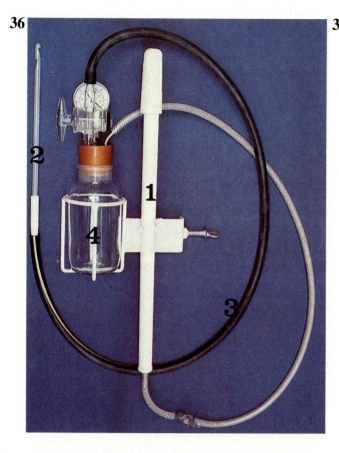

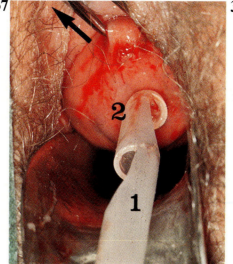

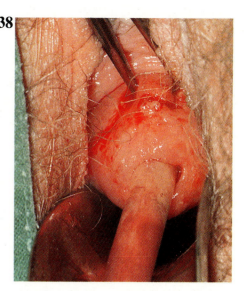

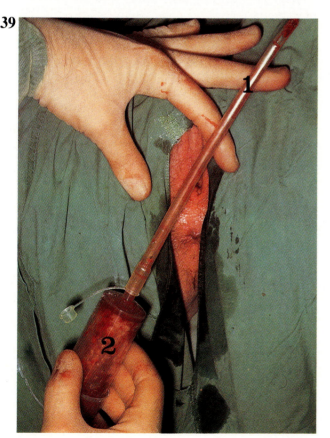

36 *Portable intra-uterine suction apparatus
For office or outpatient termination, it is an advantage to possess a simple and effective aspiration apparatus. One such type is seen here; it is almost noiseless in operation, does not require electricity and creates a high and reliable vacuum via a simple hand pump (1). A 6 mm Karman catheter (2) is connected via 8 mm rubber suction tubing (3) to a central reservoir bottle (4).

*Lewis portable intra-uterine aspiration apparatus, manufactured by Rocket of London, England.

37 Suction curettage using small diameter (Karman) catheter
A 6 mm Karman catheter (1) is about to be inserted into the dilated cervical canal (2). At this stage an ecbolic injection is given. Counter-traction on the volsellum is applied in the direction of the arrow as the catheter is inserted. This manoeuvre lessens the chance of uterine perforation.

38 Suction aspiration of uterine contents
A suction vacuum of between 500–600 mm Hg has been applied and this has resulted in the aspiration of gestational products. A gentle rotational movement is adopted so as to expose all the areas of the uterine cavity to the eye of the catheter. The appearance of air bubbles in the suction tubing and a characteristic 'grating' sound indicates that emptying is nearly complete.

39 Suction curettage using small diameter (Vabra)* catheter
This 6 mm conically shaped catheter (1) is used to terminate early pregnancies under local anaesthesia. The reservoir (2) of the apparatus is designed so that obstruction does not occur when gestational tissue is aspirated. A suction vacuum of 500–600 mmHg is required. The contents once aspirated can be despatched in the reservoir for histological assessment.

*(Vabra abortion instrument manufactured by Ferrosan Ltd, Sborg, Denmark).

Cervical dilatation and suction evacuation (D & E) of the products of conception is the most frequently employed technique of the early mid-trimester abortion, and accounts for nearly one-quarter of all those done after the 16th gestational week. Despite its popularity it is a technique associated with controversy and is not recommended for the 'occasional' operator. In competent hands it is safe with morbidity rates significantly less than those for other procedures employed at this time (e.g. hypertonic saline induction). A recent study [19] compared 6213 D & E induced mid-trimester abortions with 8662 saline inductions and reported a significantly lower failure rate for the former, i.e. 0.11 per cent as against 2.52 per cent for saline induction. Major complications were 0.69 per cent for D & E against 1.78 per cent for saline. Other studies [20,21] report success rates of 99 per cent for the D & E operation with an overall morbidity rate of 2.5–2.8 per cent.

The technique may be used to an upper limit of 20–21 weeks gestation. Ultrasonography should be performed to determine the exact fetal size and all women must be carefully counselled, prior to this operation. Dilatation and evacuation can only be performed in those centres in which the staff are fully aware of the procedure and are willing to accept the rather unpleasant aspects of fetal destruction. The majority of D & E procedures are performed under a paracervic or intracervical block as already described (page 34).

Pre-operative cervical dilatation is usually induced by laminaria tents; some gynaecologists employing a 'cervical block' for their insertion. For an evacuation of a pregnancy larger than 15 weeks, tents (sometimes 3 or 4) of 7–8 cm length and at least 3–5 mm wide are employed. They are left in place for 18 hours, when they are removed and the operation performed.

The safety of the technique depends on the use of correct instruments (**Figure 40**). These include Bierer forceps (1) for grasping the anterior cervical lip,

Sopher forceps (2) for removing the products of conception and an Evans curette (3) which is designed to minimise the risk of uterine perforation.

Before embarking on the operation itself an intravenous injection of Diazepam (10 mg) is given to effect rapid sedation and partial abolition of the memory of the procedure. After removal of the laminaria tents and insertion of local analgesia, the Bierer forceps are applied. Their small teeth (1a) and pelvic curve make them ideal for manipulating the cervix; the membranes are then perforated and the liquor aspirated. At this stage an ecbolic injection is given to reduce subsequent bleeding.

Extraction is begun by using the Sopher forceps; their serrated teeth (2a) allowing an adequate grip on the tissue to be removed. The placenta is removed first, if possible, followed by the fetus. The specimen is examined for completeness, thereafter curettage is performed with the Evans curette. It is long and blunt with a broad rim (3a) and is ideal for this purpose. A final suction curettage with a 12 mm catheter is suggested by some operators. Bleeding is reduced by the injection of the ecbolic agent at the time of membrane rupture.

The major complications of D & E in approximately 5000 cases [20] between 14–18 weeks of gestation were: (1) Uterine perforation (4 per 1000 cases), (2) blood loss requiring transfusion (1 per 1000 cases) and (3) infection (3 per 1000 cases). Long term complications such as cervical incompetence and reproductive difficulties have still to be assessed. The mortality rate [21] from D & E was 9.9/100,000 compared with that from prostaglandin (intra-uterine) infusion of 13.1/100,000 and for saline induction of 17.2/100,000. For the experienced gynaecologists D & E is a safe procedure and the most suitable for the evacuation of an advanced mid-trimester pregnancy.

40   **41**

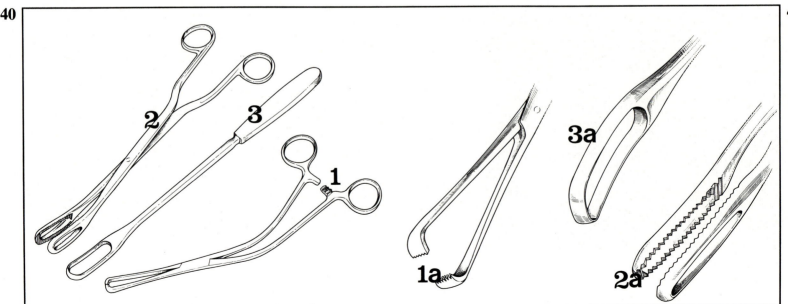

Abdominal hysterotomy

Abdominal hysterotomy has been recommended as the method of choice for termination of pregnancy in cases of severe cardiac disease, severe hypertension, certain haemoglobinopathies, prior caesarean section and uterine scars, large fibroids and ovarian cysts, and after failed amnio-infusion[22]. Another report [23] adds malignancy of the cervix and clotting problems to a similar list. In both instances, however, the authors had employed intra-amniotic instillations of hypertonic saline as the alternative non-surgical procedure. Such measures are now recognised as potentially dangerous and have largely been superseded by the use of prostaglandins. Improvements in such methods would undoubtedly remove several of the conditions from the list of indications for surgery.

Even so, the operation is still in use and some experienced clinicians prefer it to the admitted uncertainties and delays associated with any form of medical induction. It would be impossible to give absolute indications for the operation without reference to individual cases, but a combination of factors sometimes point to it as the method of choice. We have in mind as an example the emotionally charged circumstances of an elderly primipara faced with the abortion of a fetus with Down's syndrome. Many would consider it unkind to add to her burdens a period of drug instillation, the trauma of a miniature labour, possible subsequent evacuation of the uterus and yet with the prospect of having to face a laparoscopic sterilisation 3 days later. It might be considered more humane and medically preferably to achieve definitively the same end result while the patient is under a short general anaesthetic.

For these reasons and because it is likely to remain in use until a really satisfactory prostaglandin regime has been agreed, the technique of abdominal hysterotomy is illustrated and described below. Sterilisation will be required in practically all cases of abdominal hysterotomy and the reader is referred to Volume 2 of the Atlas (Chapter 5, pages 202 to 209) for a detailed description of the available methods.

Operative technique

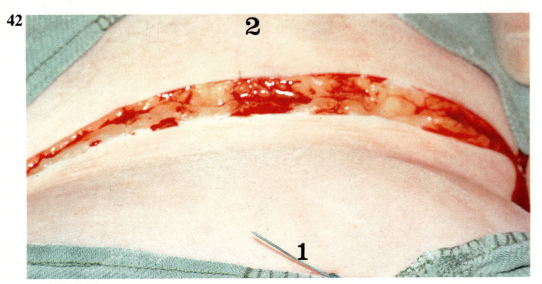

42 Lower abdominal transverse incision
The incision is in the skin crease and slightly curved upwards. It is approximately 10cm long with the ends 5cm below the level of the anterior superior iliac spines. The direction of the umbilicus is indicated by the numeral (1), that of the symphysis pubis by (2).

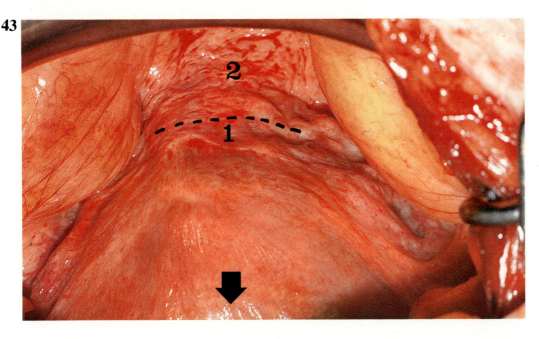

43 Operative approach with the abdomen opened
The uterus is held in the direction of the broad arrow to expose the loose peritoneum covering the lower segment or isthmus (1) and the bladder (2). It is clear that transverse incision into the lower segment must be limited in length but a large opening is not required. The intended peritoneal incision is indicated by a broken line.

44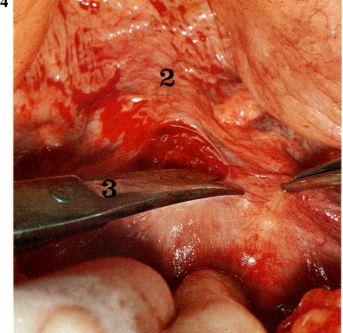

45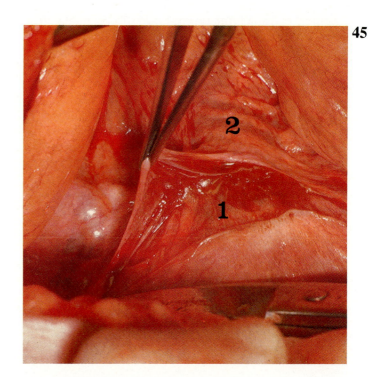

46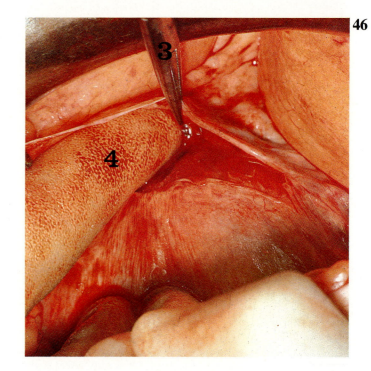

44 to 46 Opening utero-vesical pouch and reflection of bladder from the lower segment

The curved scissors (3) have been inserted under the loose peritoneum for definition of the layer and are shown dividing it on the right side in **Figure 44.** The process has been repeated on the left side and the peritoneal incision is complete in **Figure 45.** The lower segment or isthmal region of the uterus (1) is bare of peritoneum in this photograph; the bladder is again designated (2). In **Figure 46** the lower peritoneal edge is held by dissecting forceps (3) while the surgeon's forefinger (4) separates the bladder from the lower uterus.

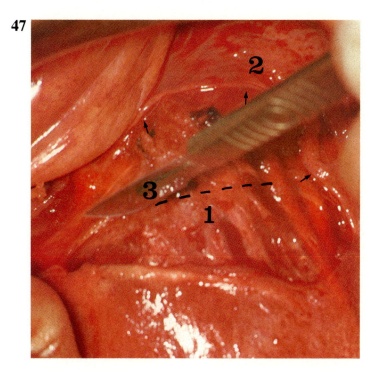

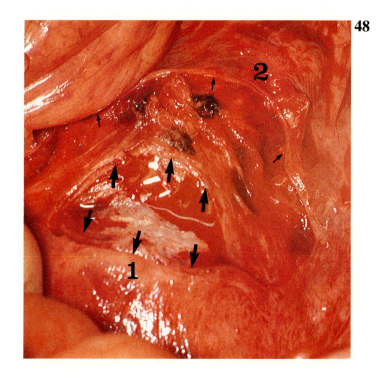

47 to 49 Transverse incision into lower uterine segment
The reflected peritoneal edge is indicated by fine arrows in
all three photographs; the bladder is numbered (2) and the
lower uterus (1). In **Figure 47** the scalpel (3) is about to
incise the lower uterus transversely in the region of the
isthmus along the broken line. This has been done to a depth
of 1.5 cm in **Figure 48** and the wound edges are indicated by
medium sized arrows. The aim of the surgeon is to expose
the membranes without incising them and in **Figure 49** a
gentle stroke with the scalpel in the middle of the incision
exposes the membranes very clearly (long arrow).

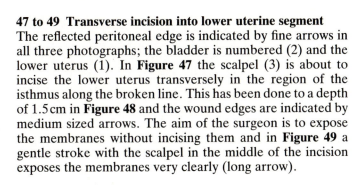

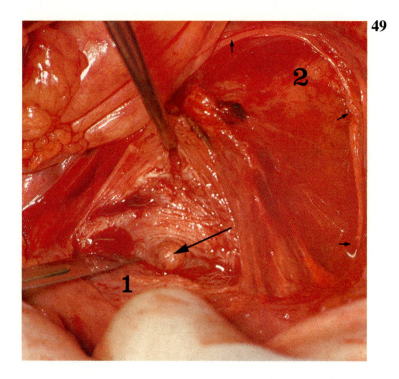

50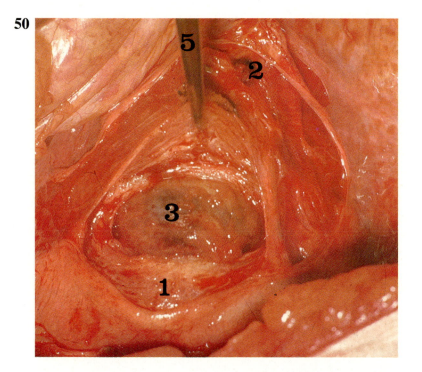

51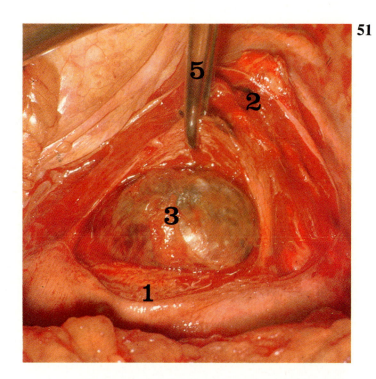

52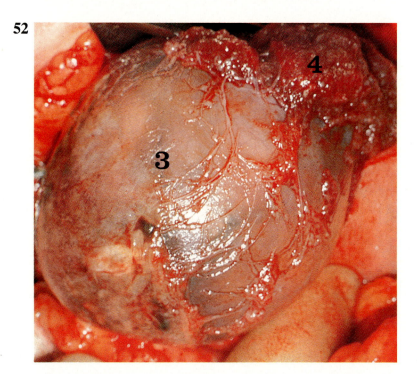

53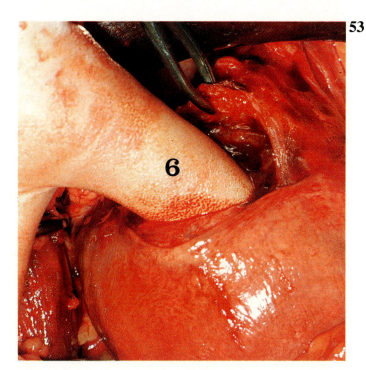

50 to 53 Expulsion of complete embryo sac by uterine contraction

The uterus is stimulated to contract at this stage by an I.V. injection of 0.5 mg of ergometrine, or preferably by speeding up a syntocinon drip of 20 units in 500 ml of Ringer-lactate solution which is already *in situ*. The uterus contracts strongly within one minute of giving the drug and the intact sac with the embryo within it is expelled through the uterine incision. The latter enlarges to the required size in its uncut softer endometrial layer. Three stages of the expulsion are seen in **Figures 50**, **51** and **52** and in the last photograph the placenta is clearly seen (4). The sac is numbered (3) and the lower uterus and bladder (1) and (2) as before. The lower leaf of the uterine incision is supported by tissue forceps numbered (5) in all the photographs. In **Figure 53** the surgeon explores the uterine cavity with his forefinger (6) to ensure that it is quite empty. The soft uterine decidual surface is not disturbed.

54

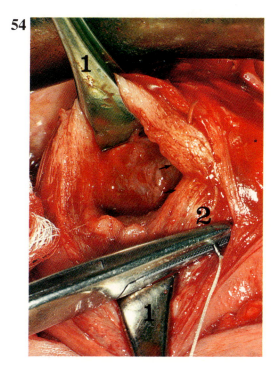

55

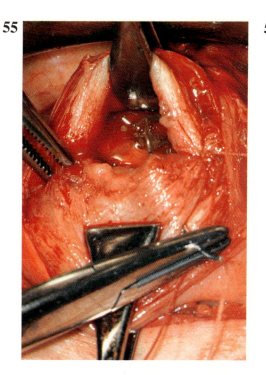

56

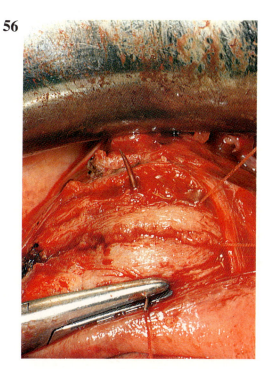

57

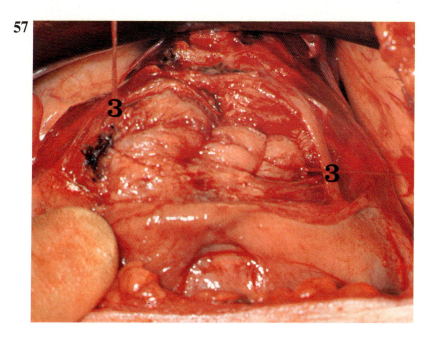

54 to 57 Closure of uterine muscle incision – first layer

A round-bodied needle carrying a No. 0 PGA suture is used to make the first of a double layer closure of the lower segment. In **Figure 54** the edges of the wound are held everted by Green-Armytage forceps (1) and (1) while the stitch (2) picks up both edges of the incision but does not include the endometrial layer (fine arrows), and so that stitches do not obtrude on the uterine cavity. In **Figures 55** and **56** a second stitch is being placed and in **Figure 57** closure is complete with the lateral sutures uncut and retained as holders (3).

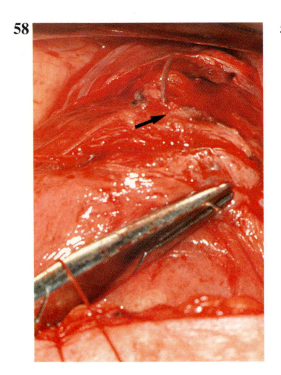

59

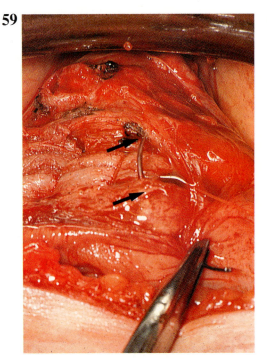

60

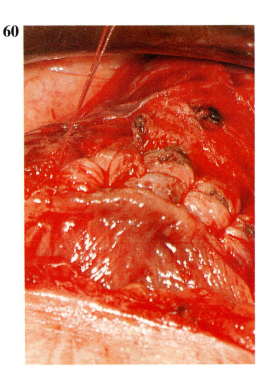

58 to 60 Closure of uterine muscle incision – second layer

An inverting type of stitch using the same suture material and needle is used to close the second muscle layer. The needle picks up a good bite of muscle from the lower edge in **Figure 58** (arrowed), does the same on the upper edge in **Figure 59** (arrowed) and a series of such stitches are completed across the incision. In **Figure 60** the final stitch is being tied and the wound is seen to be dry and firmly closed.

61 and 62 Closure of pelvic peritoneum

Transverse closure of the peritoneal layer commences in **Figure 61** and is completed in **Figure 62**. A 000 PGA suture on a round-bodied needle is used. Note that in going from one peritoneal edge to another the needle takes a bite of the uterine muscle on the line of the incision (arrowed), so that there is no loose space to give the opportunity of haematoma formation.

61

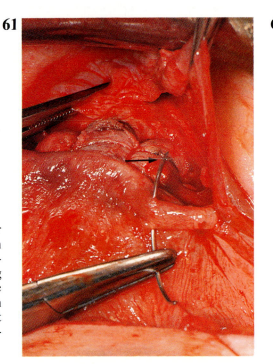

62

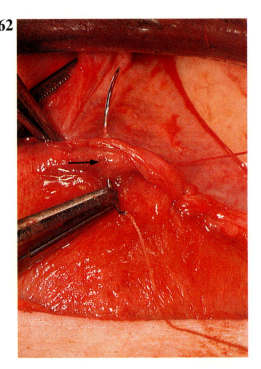

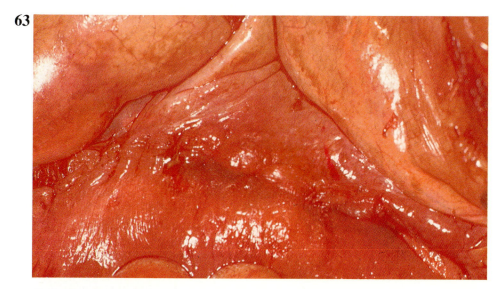

63 Peritoneum closed
The peritoneum is now closed and the utero-vesical pouch reconstituted. The line of incision is neat and dry.

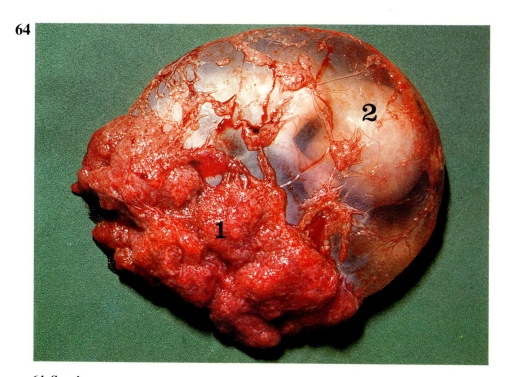

64 Specimen
The complete sac with the placenta (1) on the left side and the embryo visible through the membranes on the right side (2).

3: Spontaneous abortion

There has been a dramatic fall in the death rate from abortion in the United Kingdom over the past 15 years, much of which can undoubtedly be attributed to the implementation of the Abortion Act in 1968. **Figure 1** is taken from the Report on Confidential Enquiries into Maternal Deaths in England and Wales 1973–75 (1979)[1] and sets out in graph form the essential figures. There were a further 5 deaths from abortion which were not included because they had not been reported. While the deaths from illegal abortion have fallen steeply to a low level, mortality from spontaneous abortion shows only a slow fall with a flattening of the curve, and there is a disturbing rise in the number of deaths from legal abortion. It is clear that there is no room for complacency in the management of abortion cases of whatever type, and an attempt is made to emphasise the chief pitfalls in this chapter.

The first requirement is that the importance of the condition should not be underestimated. So many cases of abortion have to be dealt with in busy gynaecological departments that their management tends to be delegated to the junior staff. In relation to legal abortions it is noteworthy that the Confidential Report found that virtually all the deaths with avoidable factors occurred because of the inexperience of the clinicians concerned.

Abortion cases are classified as threatened, complete, inevitable, incomplete, missed and septic. The use of surgery in the treatment of threatened abortion is limited and is referred to on page 54. The vast majority of complete miscarriages require no treatment at all and may indeed not even have been reported to the doctor. All the others are likely to require surgical attention of some kind and the patient's general condition during or following abortion may range from slight indisposition to being desperately ill.

1. Inevitable and incomplete abortion

Abortion is inevitable when detachment of the ovum has reached a stage where nothing will prevent its expulsion; it is incomplete when the ovum has been expelled but parts of the fetus, membranes or placenta are still retained within the uterus. Treatment of the two conditions is similar. The clinician has the option of employing medical means initially and in perhaps a third of cases ergometrine injections or other oxytocic drugs will make expulsion complete. The authors, however, do not favour such management because it is both time consuming and uncertain. All too often, and although the abortus appears complete, bleeding recommences and surgical evacuation becomes necessary. The patient is already distressed by the miscarriage and intolerant of anything other than successfully completing the unhappy episode.

The most satisfactory treatment is prompt evacuation of the uterus under a short general anaesthetic as described below. Suction curette evacuation as used in termination of pregnancy is sometimes recommended for routine use in these cases and while it may occasionally be suitable there are several disadvantages and the authors believe that the traditional methods are superior. Except in very recent abortions, retained products frequently take the form of a rubbery piece of placenta/decidua too large to enter a suction curette and likely to occlude its end. In the presence of continuing uterine haemorrhage it is also preferable to see the amount of blood loss at first hand rather than suddenly realise that a suction bottle is already half full of blood. There is also more likelihood of damaging the endometrial surface with the sharp edge of the plastic curette than with sponge forceps or a carefully introduced blunt metal one. Such considerations apart, the cervix is nearly always soft and open so that little or any dilatation is required to allow digital exploration and separation of retained products, so that the uterus is known with certainty to be empty.

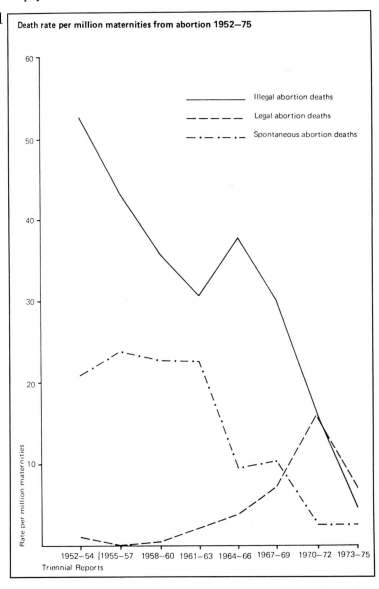

1 Death rate per million maternities from abortion 1952–75

From the *Report On Confidential Enquiries Into Maternal Deaths In England And Wales 1973–1975*, published by Her Majesty's Stationery Office.

Clinicians constantly encounter the problem of whether or not an abortion is complete. Very frequently it appears to be so, yet bleeding may recommence after the patient has gone home or even later when she has resumed her employment. One cannot generalise, but in the light of experience and the possible risk of uterine infection from retained tissue, it is sound policy to do a surgical evacuation of the uterus if there is any element of doubt. The procedure is described on pages 46–48.

2. Missed abortion

The term 'missed abortion' is used up to the 20th week of pregnancy when the ovum has been retained *in utero* for 8 weeks or more after the death of the fetus. Its management has always been difficult because the ovum tends to remain stubbornly *in situ* despite all therapy. The traditional treatment has been to await spontaneous expulsion of the uterine contents and thus avoid the danger of introducing infection into dead tissue. Not surprisingly the patient does not relish the thought of carrying around a dead fetus in her uterus and in a proportion of cases blood fibrinogen levels may fall to dangerously low levels after a month of non-treatment. Fortunately the advent of the prostaglandins has eased the situation and methods of administration are discussed in Chapter 2 of this volume. In a recent review of the subject[2] the conclusion is reached that while the uterus may be emptied in cases of missed abortion by intra-venous infusion or extra-amniotic injection of prostaglandins, equally good results follow simple vaginal administration of PGE_2 in gels or pessaries[3]. High dosage can cause gastro-intestinal irritation[4] but if the dose is related to gestation and the size of the uterus side effects are not troublesome.

Once the conceptus has been expelled there may still be retained products of conception and the treatment is then essentially that for an incomplete abortion. There are some features peculiar to these cases, however, and the technique illustrated and described on page 49 emphasises these points.

3. Septic abortion

An abortion is defined as septic when it is infected and there is dissemination of micro-organisms or their products into the maternal circulatory system. The clinical condition is almost always associated with the presence of retained products of conception within the uterus, and surgical evacuation is necessary once the general condition of the treated patient is such as to allow it being done with safety. Some of these patients are very ill and are in danger of developing endotoxic shock perhaps with associated anuria and general peritonitis. It is difficult to indicate or anticipate the possible combinations of circumstances that demand surgical treatment but there is one important broad

principle regarding surgical intervention. Primary antibiotic therapy in combination with general medical measures and blood replacement may well be required to save the patient's life, but a fundamental need in these cases is that the focus of infection be removed or drained. This is referred to again on page 50.

Surgical measures, however, are only part of the treatment and do not remove the need of essential general and antibiotic therapy. Clinical examination is made to discover the extent of the infection and blood cultures and cervical specimens are taken to get laboratory guidance on the type of individual bacterial organism responsible. Since treatment should be immediate an attempt is made to reach a presumptive diagnosis, so that therapy starts off in the correct direction. Thus clinical suspicion of a C. Welchii infection would indicate antibiotic therapy of a different kind from that used in a purely E. Coli infection. It is increasingly recognised[5] that in infections associated with abortion and parturition, normal vaginal flora (both aerobic and anerobic) are likely to be the agents responsible once the environment has been disturbed.

The anaerobes are predominantly members of the bacterioides species and B. Fragilis has been isolated from up to 79 per cent of cases in this group. E. Coli is the predominant aerobe. Experimental work in animals[6] showed that as far as peritoneal infection was concerned E. Coli was associated with acute peritonitis, sepicaemia and a high mortality rate, while B. Fragilis was associated with abscess formation. The day is long past when the anaerobes should be looked on as commensals, and this must be taken account of in prescribing treatment.

Broad spectrum antibiotics to cover gram negative and gram positive organisms are given in large doses and should not normally be changed before they have a chance to act, or until laboratory findings indicate that they are inappropriate. Penicillin and Kanamycin are very effective as initial agents against aerobic organisms and in a moderately severe case would be given in a dosage of Penicillin 500,000–1,000,000 units every 6 hours and Kanamycin 0.5 mg I.M. every 12 hours. Metronidazole tablets (400 mg three times daily) are added to combat the bacteriodes strains. It is rapidly bacteriocidal for anaerobes and therapeutic levels can generally be obtained by oral, rectal or if necessary intravenous administration. It is non-toxic, stable and inexpensive. Such treatment will control most infections.

1. Evacuation of the uterus for incomplete or inevitable abortion

Large numbers of these operations are done in hospital and the great majority are performed by relatively junior medical staff. Perforation of the uterus is recognised as the main danger of the procedure but fortunately its incidence is not unduly high. In other respects, however, the operation is too often done quickly and carelessly so that unnecessary and even dangerous sequelae result. This is an important matter and the authors have no compunction in calling attention to some of the more obvious shortcomings. For example, the operation is sometimes begun after only token skin preparation and without the application of adequate drapes. This shows that the risk of introducing infection to the upper genital tract is not realised. Sharp toothed or over-heavy forceps applied

to manipulate the anterior lip of the cervix causes lacerations with subsequent symptomatology while rapid dilatation of the cervix may lead to lateral splitting of the cervical and uterine muscle.

Piece-meal removal of the uterine contents with forceps without first digitally separating them from the uterine wall is accompanied by a continuous trickling of blood which can quickly reach an embarrassing amount. When the uterus is considered to be empty the operator may then do a curettage with a sharp instrument. This is seldom necessary and can only increase the risk of uterine infection. These are all examples of bad surgical practice and result from lax

Surgical techniques

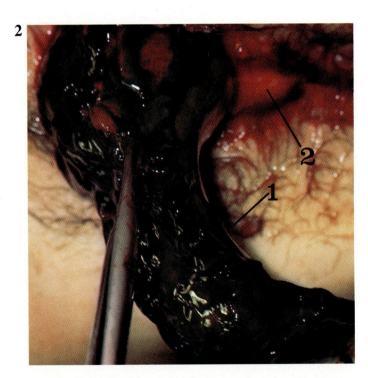

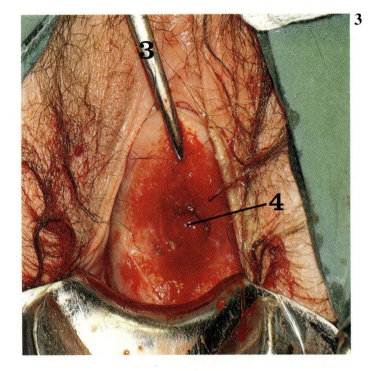

2 and 3 Typical appearances in a case of incomplete abortion
In **Figure 2** the usual extruded blood clot (1) and a trickle of fresh blood (2) are seen at the vulva. The uterus is nearly always palpable suprapubically and if pressed on, a further mass of clot escapes from the vagina. In **Figure 3** the patient is in the lithotomy position. The clot has been cleared from the vagina and the anterior lip of the cervix is held in tissue forceps (3). The cervix is obviously wide open and would easily admit the forefinger. Further clot can be seen within the uterine cavity (4).

training; it is incumbent on established staff to see that trainees do not adopt them.

The operation is properly done as a full surgical procedure with the patient under a general anaesthetic. Her general condition is checked as being satisfactory preoperatively. The haemoglobin and haematocrit levels should be above 10 grams and 30 pcv respectively – otherwise blood replacement is required. An intravenous drip is in place during the operation and intravenous oxytocin (30 u to 1 litre of 5 per cent dextrose in water) is transfused to help contract the uterus during the latter part of the operation. A decision on whether or not to insert a vaginal pack at the completion of the operation is a matter of individual preference. If the object of the operation has been achieved, it should not be necessary. On the other hand unimportant or insignificant bleeding perhaps from the anterior lip of the cervix can be disconcerting when reported after the operation, and some also feel that the uterus contracts down more satisfactorily in the presence of a firm vaginal pack. Occasionally when one knows the uterus to be empty, but a trickle of blood continues and cannot be disregarded, the insertion of a pack from a 6 inch roll of gauze with its end tucked into the cervical canal brings everything under control immediately. There is no disadvantage in the procedure and the gauze is removed in 6 hours.

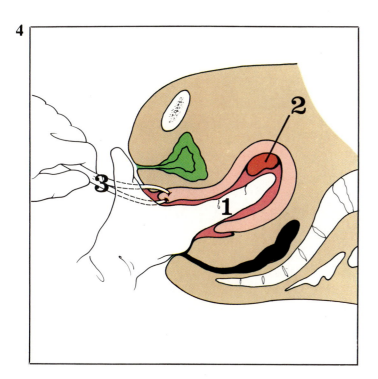

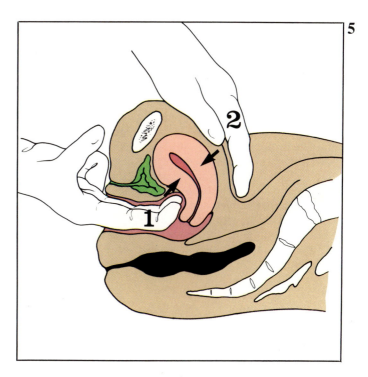

4 Digital exploration of uterine cavity – diagramatic illustration
In the circumstances seen in **Figure 3** the uterus is first compressed abdominally to expel loose blod clot into the vagina. With the anterior lip of the cervix held by the forceps (3) in the left hand, the right forefinger (1) is introduced through the open cervix till the fundus of the uterus can be reached. The fingertip is then swept around the uterine cavity in all directions to separate from its wall any adherent retained products (2). When this has been effected the loose contents are removed with sponge forceps and spoon curette (see **Figure 8**).

5 Bimanual compression of uterus – diagramatic illustration
The uterine cavity is considered to be empty, but there is still a trickle of blood and the uterus may not be contracting strongly. With the tips of two fingers in the anterior vaginal fornix, the uterus is brought into anteversion and firmly compressed between the vaginal fingers (1) and the external hand on the abdomen (2), in the direction of the arrows. This obliterates the cavity, expelling any remaining blood or debris and encouraging the uterus to contract strongly.

6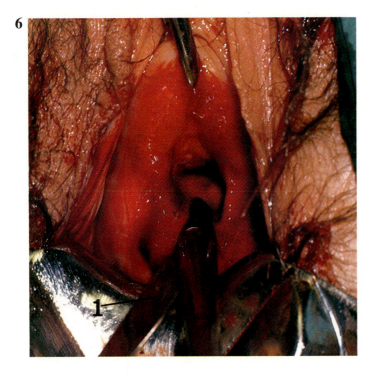

7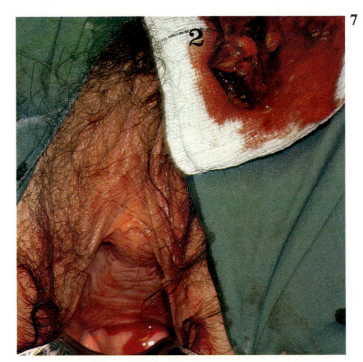

6 to 8 Important steps in evacuation of uterus

In **Figure 6** and following digital exploration of the uterine cavity, sponge forceps (1) are used to remove the mass of blood clot from the cavity and from the vagina. In **Figure 7** a firm clot or piece of debris which was evacuated is seen on the swab to the right of the photograph (2). The vagina meantime appears dry but sponge forceps cannot be expected to remove thin clot, fluid blood and debris. **Figure 8** shows the spoon curette end of a Rheinstadter's flushing curette which is ideal for use in emptying the uterus in these circumstances. No flushing attachment is used and the instrument is employed simply as a conveniently sized and blunt edged spoon with just the right angle between its head and shank to fit the uterine walls accurately. Following its use, the manoeuvre shown in **Figure 5** completes the operation.

8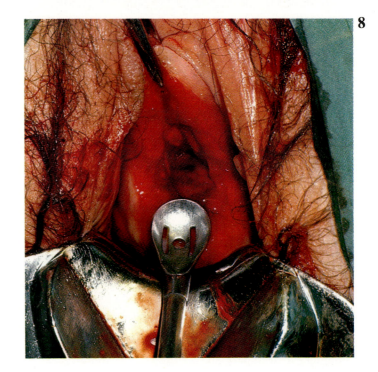

2. Evacuation of the uterus for missed abortion

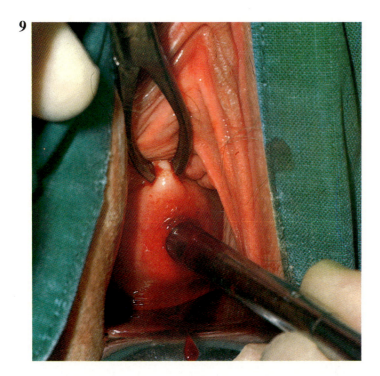

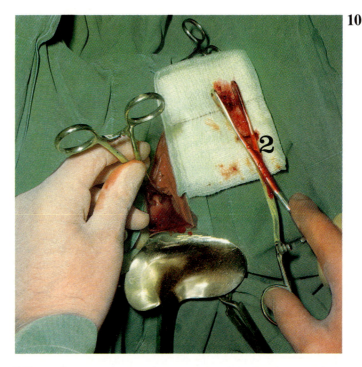

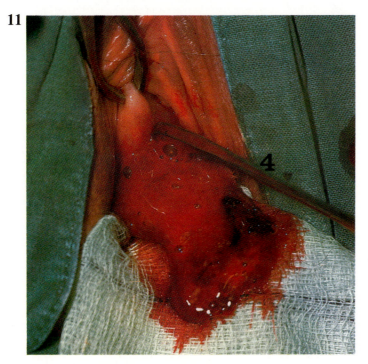

9 to 11 Evacuation of uterus in a case of missed abortion
This is a case where the embryo perished early in the second trimester, the uterus had contracted down to less than 12 weeks size, and there was periodic vaginal bleeding. With improving prostaglandin methods such cases will probably come to be treated medically: **Figure 9** shows dilatation of the cervix and **Figure 10** illustrates adherent and rather fibrous uterine contents gradually being removed with the sponge forceps (2). In **Figure 11** a sharp but wide ended curette (4) is used to sweep the uterine walls in turn.

When the uterus requires evacuation for incomplete emptying following the use of prostaglandins, it is done exactly as for incomplete abortion and has already been described. The prostaglandins produce a cervix which is soft and partially dilated and the uterus is actively contracting, so that it has probably already detached the major part of the retained and previously adherent conceptus and the procedure is usually simple and bloodless.

In other circumstances, as when the uterus has decreased to less than 10 weeks pregnancy size, it can be emptied surgically without recourse to prostaglandins but, as already mentioned, there are possible hazards and the surgeon should be aware of these. The cervix is usually closed and must therefore be dilated slowly and carefully to admit sponge or ovum forceps which are used to grasp and gently twist or peel off the adherent ovum from the uterine wall. It is easy to split the cervix during dilatation unless it is done very slowly, and care and judgement is required to keep the sponge forceps in the axis of the uterus to avoid damaging the myometrium if by chance it is caught between the blades. The operation is performed slowly and can be very tedious. Small pieces of the conceptus come away and it is clear that one has not obtained a proper grasp of the contents; suddenly the forceps achieve a better hold and the main mass of ovum peels off the uterine wall in one piece. It is unlikely to be complete and any remaining products of conception and decidual debris are detached from the uterus with the broadest ended curette that the cervical canal will admit. The material to be removed is fibrous so that a sharp curette is preferable: the important requirement is that it be broad so that there is no fear of penetrating the fundus uteri.

3. Evacuation of the uterus during management of septic abortion

It is probably a relic of pre-antibiotic practice but one constantly encounters a dangerous reluctance to tackle the source of the infection in cases of septic abortion. It is quite essential that retained products within the uterus be evacuated. This can, in fact, often be done without disturbance in an ill patient by the gentle use of a pair of sponge forceps and without anaesthesia. In cases where curettage is considered necessary, it can adequately be done under local anaesthesia; the essential requirement is to remove the bulk of the retained products without traumatising the endometrial wall.

The immediate beneficial effect of emptying the uterus in a seriously ill patient is shown on the temperature chart in **Figure 12**. Both temperature and pulse rate drop almost at once, the rigors cease and the clinical condition of the patient improves dramatically.

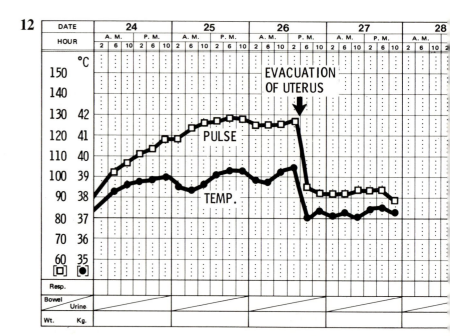

13 Septic abortion appearance of cervix
Profuse purulent discharge (1) exudes from the cervical canal (2) of the patient described in **Figure 12,** prior to uterine evacuation.

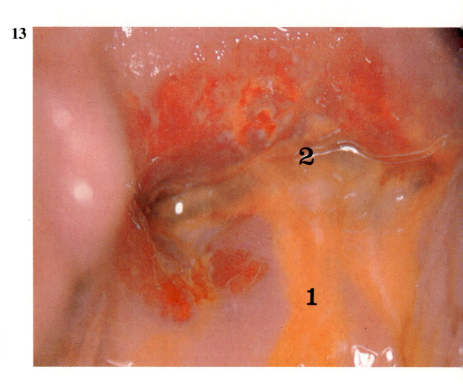

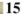

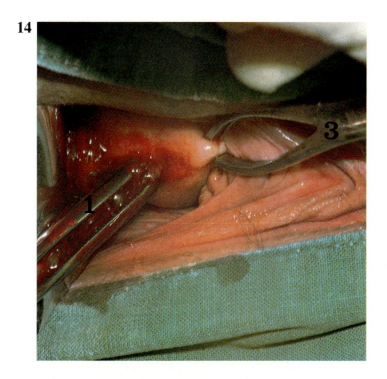

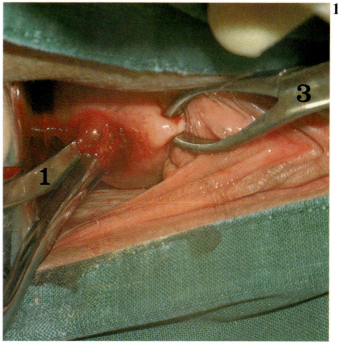

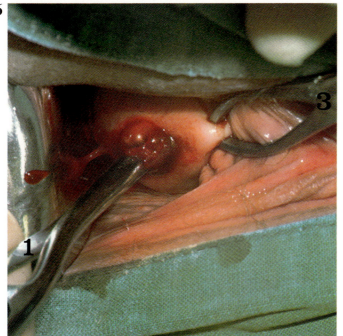

14 to 16

This patient had a severe pyrexia with rigors and had obviously lost a lot of blood. She gave a history which was suspicious of criminal interference and there was a discharge of thin blood clot from the cervix. General resuscitation and antibiotic therapy were instituted, but with no prospect of being able to give a general anaesthetic soon.

The patient was placed on her left side in bed and the cervix exposed by a speculum. In **Figure 14** the anterior lip of the cervix is shown held with tissue forceps (3) and narrow sponge forceps (1) release thin blood clot as it is introduced into the cervical canal. In **Figure 15** the uterine cavity is gently explored with the opened forceps and a hold on a sizeable piece of the contents is sought. This was obtained and in **Figure 16** it is seen being removed through the cervix.

No local anaesthetic was used and the patient was hardly disturbed by the procedure. If the tissue forceps are applied very slowly to the cervix there is practically no pain; rapid closing of the jaws always causes a sharp pain. The patient's general condition improved rapidly following the procedure (much as in the manner shown on the chart on page 50) but a later evacuation of some retained products was required. By that time she was able to have a general anaesthetic with safety.

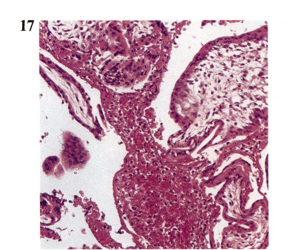

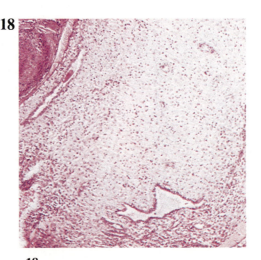

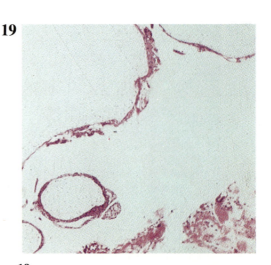

17
Histological appearances of retained products of conception from a case of incomplete abortion. (× 128)

18
Histological section of decidual endometrium with complete absence of chorionic villi. (× 64)

19
Histological picture of hydatidiform mole. (× 128)

Evacuation of the uterus for apparent incomplete abortion may on occasion provide unexpected findings. There may be evidence of something unusual at the time but such surprises generally have to await histological examination of the tissues. The possibility of unusual findings emphasises the importance of always sending a specimen of the evacuated material for histological examination.

The most frequent of such circumstances is where the bleeding has not been heavy and the retained 'products' are limited in amount. Histological examination shows decidual tissue only, with no evidence of chorionic villi; the pathologist will correctly suggest the possibility of ectopic gestation. Such a patient is immediately contacted and brought back to hospital for investigation and treatment. Another and less frequent finding is the presence of vesicles in the evacuated tissue and indicating a diagnosis of hydatidiform mole. More frequently vesicles are not recognised by the naked eye, but histological examination shows that there is hydatidiform degeneration.

Figures 17, 18 and **19** show the histological features of:
1 Retained products of an intrauterine pregnancy
2 Decidual endometrium with no evidence of chorionic villi
3 Hydatidiform mole.

Management of severely ill cases of septic abortion and septic shock

Cases of severe septic abortion have become much less common in the United Kingdom with the general availability of therapeutic abortion, but one still sees these desperately ill patients and in many parts of the world this problem is an immense one. The condition must be of concern to many readers and is therefore dealt with as a special problem requiring intensive management. A regime which embodies a simple and straightforward approach to the treatment of such cases is delineated.

All aspects of the treatment of severe infection must be considered. The primary requirements are to start antibiotic treatment and see to body fluid replacement but surgical needs should be met early since the greatest danger to the patient is the rapid onset of endotoxic shock which becomes irreversible.

Antibiotics fluid replacement and surgical measures

If the patient is severely ill massive antibiotic therapy in the form of 5 million units of penicillin i.v. every 8 hours and 0.5g of Kanamycin i.m. every 12 hours would be appropriate. Metronidazole 500mg or 600mg of Clindamycin should be given intravenously every 8 hours to combat the anaerobes. Resistance of some bacteriodes strains to Clindamycin has been reported and there is a risk of side effects which include a pseudo-membranous type of colitis.

If the response to treatment is unsatisfactory or sensitivity tests show the need for change, penicillin is usually replaced by Gentamycin which belongs to the same aminoglycoside group as Kanamycin. It is given intramuscularly 8 hourly in a dosage of 60–80mg depending on the weight of the patient. It is a powerful drug but one is reluctant to use the aminoglycosides more than necessary where there may be impaired renal function. Repeated blood cultures and organism sensitivities will indicate the need for any changes in antibiotic therapy.

Fluid replacement
Fluid requirements must be carefully assessed as patients with septic abortion have frequently lost a lot of blood and blood replacement will often do more than anything else to combat the infection. Electrolyte balance is continuously recorded and corrected as required.

Surgical treatment
The first purely surgical requirements is that a definitive diagnosis should be made on the likelihood of uterine perforation. If it is suspected laparotomy should be carried out at the earliest possible opportunity. Only when the abdomen has been opened will it be possible to decide what is required, but drainage of the pelvic peritoneal cavity will always be required and hysterectomy may be necessary.

Recognition of septic shock

It is particularly important to assess the degree of septic shock which may or may not be accompanied by renal failure. Evidence of septic shock means that the patient has a most dangerous complication of septic abortion and intensive therapy is an urgent necessity. The condition usually results from infection with gram negative organisms (E. Coli, proteus vulgaris and pseudomonas aeruginosa), the neurogenic shock being caused by an endotoxin released from the cell wall of the organism[7,8]. The anaerobic gram positive C Welchii (C perfringens) is capable of producing an even more severe condition with massive intravascular haemolysis and neurogenic shock. The shock producing agent in this case is an exotoxin. Gas gangrene affects the cardiac as well as the skeletal and smooth muscle and the resultant myocarditis causes a mortality rate of over 50 per cent. Staphylococcus aureus is also capable of producing an exotoxin with septic shock effect.

The onset of septic shock is often insidious, and it is therefore important to keep the possibility in mind, since only if it is recognised in the early stages is its treatment likely to succeed. Anxiety and disorientation may give the first warning and are soon followed by air hunger. Oliguria is usually noted at this stage. Hyperpyrexia and rigors give way to the classical picture of shock with cold perspiration and increasing mental apathy. Vomiting and diarrhoea may occur and urinary output frequently ceases completely.

A protocol for initial management

Management of such cases can only be indicated in general terms – the measures employed being dictated by the clinical condition of the individual patient and the results of laboratory examinations. Most clinicians have developed a personal regime; that used by the authors lists the principles of treatment under the following headings:

1. Rapid replacement of blood volume and repeated estimates of blood electrolyte levels.
2. Central venous pressure monitoring as a necessary guide to fluid replacement.
3. Repeated cervical smears and blood cultures with organism sensitivities to identify the infecting agent.
4. Antibiotic therapy along the lines indicated above.
5. Use of intravenously administered cortisone where indicated and preferably at an early stage.
6. Surgery. Early removal of the focus of infection and/or early establishment of uterine drainage. Hysterectomy is indicated in cases of ruptured tubo-ovarian abscess and uterine rupture. It may be indicated in cases of clostridial infection, persistent hypotension and oliguria and acidosis which do not respond to therapy.

There is no consensus of opinion on the use of vasopressor and vaso-dilator drugs and some clinicians say that it is not justifiable to use them as stimulants when the patient is in these desperate circumstances. In the authors' experience each case is so different from the last that rigidly held opinions are unwise. In appropriate circumstances they may be of help but the problem is that deleterious side effects are apt to vitate any advantage gained. With regard to hysterectomy the authors' experience is that little can be achieved if the patient is already in the degree of shock described here. It is more important at this stage to give one's full attention to correcting severe acidosis by the administration of sodium bicarbonate and supplying intermittent oxygen. A clear airway must also be ensured.

4: Surgical treatment of recurrent abortion

Recurring abortion and particularly of the type which takes place in the second trimester of pregnancy may sometimes be due to gynaecological abnormalities which can be corrected surgically. Three conditions in particular are held to be blameworthy in this respect:

1 An incompetent cervix
2 Uterine fibroids which interfere with placental implantation
3 Certain types of double uterus.

Opinion is far from unanimous on the correctness of treating any of these by surgery but there is sufficient evidence to indicate that cerclage, myomectomy and uteroplasty each have an established place in the treatment of recurrent abortion.

I: Cerclage for cervical incompetence in recurrent abortion

The general question of cervical incompetence and its implication in recurrent abortion is considered in Volume 5 of the Atlas (pages 48 to 54). While there is considerable evidence that cervical weakness is sometimes congenital in origin, most cases result from trauma during precipitate labour or in circumstances where delivery takes place before the cervix is fully dilated. It may also follow injury by too rapid dilatation at D. & C. or the effects of a cone biopsy on the cervix.

The basic indication for inserting a cervical suture is to avoid miscarriage in a patient with a history of recurrent abortion and whose cervix is considered incompetent. It may be done in response to a threat to abort, but more usually it is a planned procedure which is done about the 15th week of pregnancy. Most clinicians wish to reinforce or confirm their clinical diagnosis by adding radiological evidence of cervical weakness. In genuine cases x-ray investigations done between pregnancies show that a jelly-like radio-opaque medium injected into the uterus escapes around the cannula to outline a wide and deficient cervix (see **Figure I**).

The operation is frequently done but it is exceedingly difficult to obtain evidence of its true value. Shirodkar[1] claimed 81 per cent fetal salvage with the operation and McDonald[2] reviewing the results of 269 cases treated by his own and Shirodkar's methods had live birth rates of 86.5 and 72.9 respectively. Such high rates may be obtainable when the indications are particularly strong but there is a large group of cases where the indications are less compelling and many of these patients have cerclage operations. It is quite

1A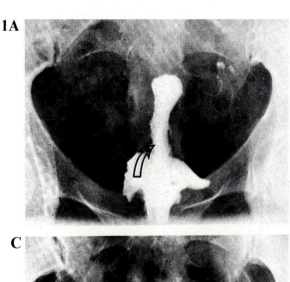

B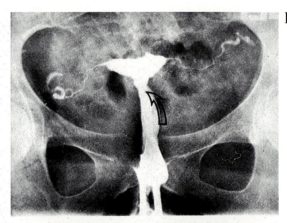

C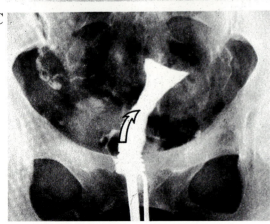

D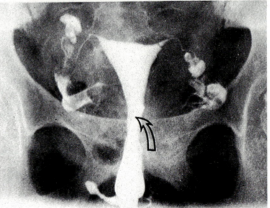

1a to d Cervico-hysterograms of the proposed incompetent cervix
Cervico-hysterograms showing extensive widening of the internal cervical os (arrowed), an appearance regarded by many clinicians as pathognomic of cervical incompetence. All these women had at least two second trimester miscarriages. Prophylactic repair of the cervix in the inter-pregnancy period was undertaken in one of them and a Shirodkar suture inserted at the 15th gestational week in two others resulted in the carriage of a live infant to term in each case. Reproduced from *The Cervix*, Jordan, J. and Singer, A. (1976), Saunders, London.

impossible in such circumstances to say whether the subsequent pregnancies went to term because of, or in spite of, the cervical suture.

Shirodkar[3] was the first to employ an encircling suture within the thickness of the cervix at the level of the internal os during pregnancy and he subsequently modified the operation[4] to the present simplified form which is so widely used. This form of cerclage done during pregnancy is generally referred to as a Shirodkar operation, although in many instances the method of inserting the suture and the nature of the suture itself makes the operation more correctly attributable to others.

The steps of a Shirodkar operation are described and illustrated on pages 56 and 57 and the general measures employed and described are applicable to other variations or methods of cerclage which may be used during pregnancy.

In all these methods the anterior vaginal wall is opened so that the bladder can be reflected off the cervix. To ensure that the encircling suture is correctly maintained in the centre of the cervical wall, it is necessary to have a 'staging post' in the form of a small incision on the posterior aspect of the cervix. The operation is not difficult, but the needle is necessarily large and round bodied and with its bulky thread requires considerable, steady and firm pressure to complete its course through the cervical muscle. The authors admit to a slight feeling of unease at applying a degree of pressure which must put a shearing strain on the attachments of the ovum at the isthmal level.

McDonald questions whether it is necessary to use methods with possible complications and makes a sound case for the use of his own operation where he inserts a simple purse-string suture of No. 4 'Mersilene' (Ethnor) around the cervix at the cervico-vaginal junction[5]. **Figures 2 and 3** illustrate the essential features of his procedure and are reproduced by kind permission of the author and the publishers. The essential steps of the operation are best described in the author's own words. 'The suture of 4 Mersilene on an atraumatic needle is inserted around the exocervix as high as possible, to approximate to the level of the internal os, care being taken to keep below the bladder edge. This is at the junction of the rugose vagina and smooth cervix (**Figure 2**). Four or five bites with the needle are made with special attention to the stitch behind the cervix. This may be difficult to insert and must be deep into the muscle of the cervix (**Figure 3**). If the ligature pulls out later, it is almost always from the posterior aspect, the Mersilene remaining attached to the anterior lip. The suture is pulled tight enough to close the internal os completely, the knot being made in front of the cervix and the ends left long enough to facilitate subsequent division. No trouble has been caused through ischaemia of the cervix, because the lateral blood vessels are external to the ligature.'

The operation has the advantage of being a closed as opposed to an open one and should involve less tissue trauma during insertion of the stitch which is readily accessible for removal later. As already mentioned, McDonald had rather better results with the method than with Shirodkar's operation.

2

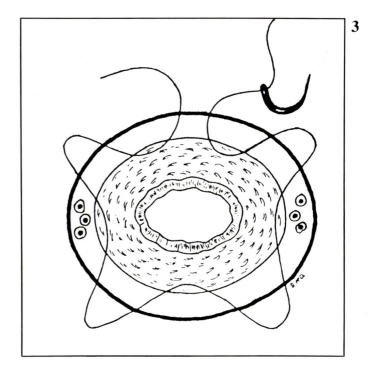

3

From *Clinics In Obstetrics And Gynaecology*, vol. 7, no. 3, 1980, *Operative Obstetrics, Problems and Perspectives*, edited by Ian Macgillivray, published by W. B. Saunders Company Ltd.

Technique of Shirodkar procedure

The operation is not done before the 12th week of pregnancy and the suture should preferably be in place before 20 weeks; the ideal time to insert it is around the 15th week. It is a planned anticipatory procedure and if the cervix has already begun to dilate, or if a bulging sac has to be pushed back into the uterus, the chances of success are minimal. The operation should be done with extreme gentleness and the supporting suture should be at the level of the internal cervical os. It is carried out under general or epidural anaesthesia and the patient is in the lithotomy position with the bladder previously emptied by catheter. The patient remains in hospital under rest for 48 hours after the operation. It is common practice to administer a beta-mimetic agent post-operatively in an attempt to prevent the onset of premature labour.

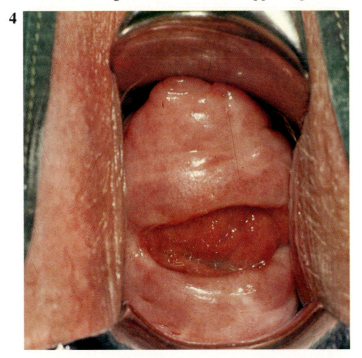

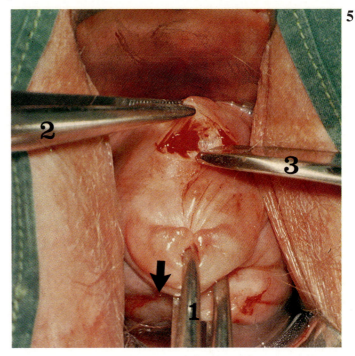

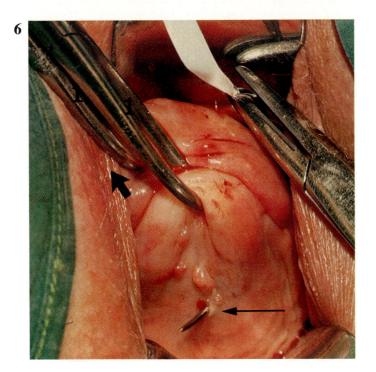

4 Clinical appearance of cervix at 14 weeks pregnancy in recurrent abortion case
The external os is slightly open but not obviously more than in many normal cases. The decision to operate is based on a history of three almost unheralded mid-trimester miscarriages and evidence of an incompetent cervix on clinical and radiological investigation carried out between pregnancies.

5 Incision of vaginal skin on anterior aspect of cervix
A tissue forceps (1) steadies the anterior lip of the cervix in the direction of the arrow and the dissecting forceps (2) elevates the skin where it becomes loose on the anterior aspect of the cervix, just about the level of the internal cervical os. Angled scissors (3) open up a 1 cm transverse incision at the estimated level of the internal os.

6 Needle traversing left side of cervix
The cervix is drawn to the right by the tissue forceps (1) and (1) in the direction of the broad arrow. The needle holder guides the needle gently and slowly through the centre of the muscular wall in a semi-circle at the estimated level of the internal os. It is aimed at the same level in the midline posteriorly and can be seen to do so (arrowed).

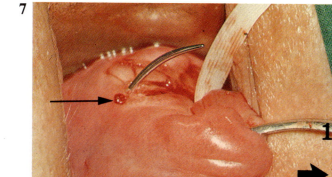

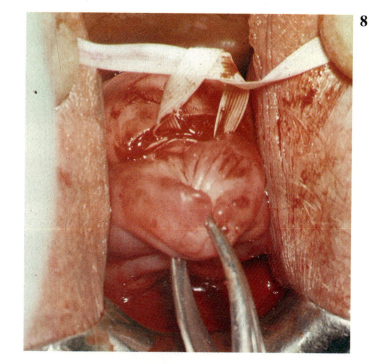

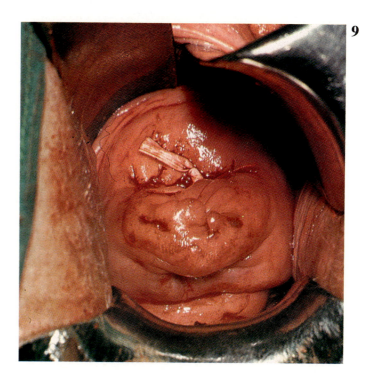

7 Needle traversing right side of cervix
The tissue forceps (1) and (1) draw the cervix to the left as arrowed and the needle traverses the right side of the cervix in a semi-circular arc from posterior to anterior. It enters at the small posterior position incision and emerges at the larger anterior one (arrowed).

8 Completion of suture
The stitch is tightened to give maximum support without endangering the blood supply to the cervix. A No. 6 Hegar's dilator is used to estimate tightness. A reef knot is then tied.

9 Appearance of cervix after insertion of Shirodkar suture
This photograph shows the suture *in situ*. It is firm but not too tight and as near the internal os as feasible. When the suture is tied it should lightly grasp a No. 6 Hegar dilator placed in the cervical canal. The stitch is buried in the cervical muscle except where tied off anteriorly; it is thus easily accessible for removal when labour ensues.

II: Myomectomy for uterine fibroids in recurrent abortion

There is no doubt that uterine fibroids can be an important factor in infertility[6,7] and the present day management of such cases is described in Volume 5 of the Atlas, page 70.

From sheer size or perhaps from its submucous location a fibroid may present an impediment to conception. It is more usual, however, for infertility to be the result of repeated second trimester abortions where the uterus is known to contain fibroids. The patient may have aborted at the same stage of pregnancy on two or more occasions.

There is certainly a place for myomectomy in the treatment of this latter group, and it is often spectacularly successful in allowing subsequent pregnancies to go to term. The surgeon is usually expected to subscribe to the patient's future hopes of success when operation is contemplated but it is always wise to make a cautious prognosis. The operation is, of course, done between pregnancies since myomectomy should never be attempted during pregnancy. A full account of the operation is given in Volume 2 of the Atlas, pages 165–181, and some of the principal technical considerations are recalled in the illustrations and attached legends on this and the facing page.

Myomectomy technique

The operation is done in the first half of the menstrual cycle under general anaesthesia or epidural block. 'Work-up' of the case should be complete so that the surgeon knows as precisely as possible what he will find and the probable best method of dealing with it. Preliminary investigations should include a careful D. & C., laparoscopy with tubal patency tests and, where available, hysteroscopy.

It is useful to keep in mind the blood supply of the uterus and this is recalled in diagrammatic form in **Figure 10**. A Bonney's myomectomy clamp applied in the region of the isthmus would be preferable for control of the uterine vessels in myomectomy because it supports and fixes the uterus in position. Plastic sheathed bulldog clamps on the infundibulo-pelvic ligaments interrupt the ovarian anastomotic arterial supply.

At operation the site of the myomectomy incision depends on the position of the fibroid but it is sometimes possible and always preferable to incise the uterus at a point adjacent to or underlying loose peritoneum so that the muscle incision can be subsequently covered with peritoneum. It is also beneficial if two or more fibroids can be removed through the same muscle incision by tunnelling laterally from the cavity of the first fibroid removed; such a procedure may sometimes be planned in advance after careful examination.

Surgical technique is obviously important and a primary principle is gentle enucleation of the fibroid or fibroids from their capsule through incisions of minimal length which cut into the substance of the fibroid to define the capsule clearly (**Figure 11**). When removing an intramural fibroid it is essential to see that the cavity of the uterus is opened, both to allow exploration for fibroids presenting into the cavity and to establish a safe drainage exit for blood oozing from the site of the fibroid (**Figures 12** and **13**). The fibroid cavities themselves are always carefully closed by building up the requisite number of muscle layers so that there is no dead space (**Figure 14**). The surface peritoneum should be approximated neatly to avoid adhesions if there is no adjacent loose peritoneum to cover the area (**Figure 15**).

Myomectomy

Stage 1. Planning haemostasis

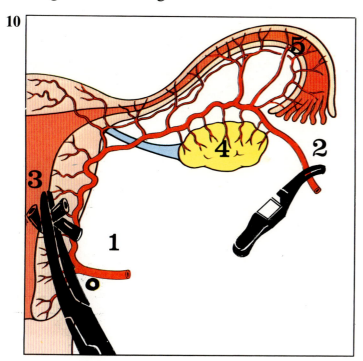

Stage 2. Enucleation of fibroids

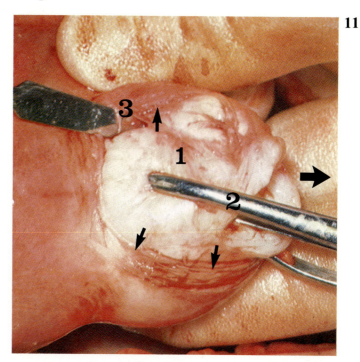

10 Plan for interruption of arterial blood supply to uterus
The tourniquet at isthmal level occludes the uterine artery (1) while the bulldog clamp on the infundibulo-pelvic ligament controls the ovarian artery (2). The uterus is numbered (3), the ovary (4) and the tube (5). A Bonney's clamp is usually preferred to the tourniquet in myomectomy; it supports the uterus in the centre of the wound during the operation.

11 Incision and enucleation of fibroid
The incision is of minimal length to remove the fibroid (1) and is made boldly into the tumour to display the capsule (arrowed). The fibroid is grasped in Littlewood's forceps (2) and drawn outwards (broad arrow) while the plane of separation between the fibroid and the capsule is defined with a dissector (3) and subsequently by the surgeon's forefinger.

Stage 3. Opening into endometrial cavity

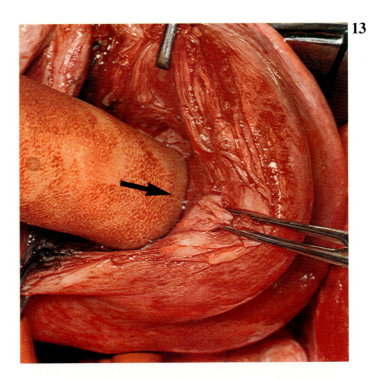

12 and 13 Opening into endometrial cavity

The authors consider it essential to open through from emptied fibroid cavities of any size into the endometrial space. This allows exploration of the uterus for submucous fibroids obtruding into it but the main reason is to allow drainage of blood from the cavity postoperatively. The blood drains through the cervix into the vagina and this safety-valve mechanism avoids the postoperative haema-tomata and abscesses which previously bedevilled the operation. In **Figure 12** the cavity of the enucleated fibroid is held open by tissue forceps (3) while the blades of the scissors (4) have opened the endometrial cavity as shown by the escape of methylene blue dye (5). In **Figure 13** the surgeon's finger explores the uterine cavity through the fibroid cavity (arrowed).

Stage 4. Closure of fibroid cavity

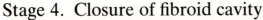
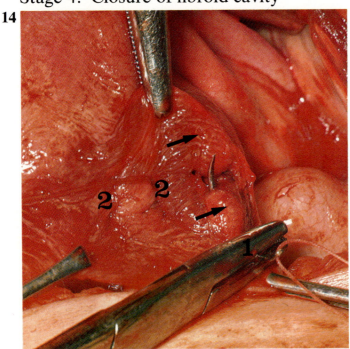

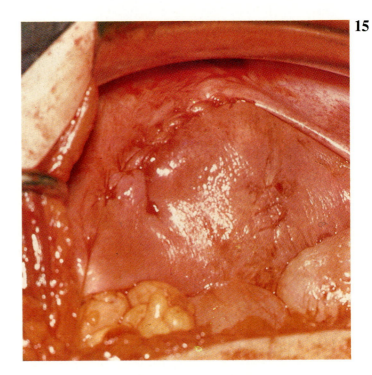

14 and 15 Closure and covering of fibroid cavity

The cavity is closed in a series of muscular layers (not usually more than 3) and then covered by loose peritoneum or by a sero-muscular stitch. In **Figure 14** the needle (1) is taking the first bite (arrowed) and will do the same on the opposing edge (arrowed) when closing the second layer of uterine muscle. The tied sutures (2) have closed off the depth of the cavity as a first layer but have not invaded the endometrial layer or cavity. In **Figure 15** the peritoneum has been closed by a continuous suture. It is in the region of the utero-vesical pouch so that there is abundant loose tissue.

III: Uteroplasty for congenital uterine abnormality in recurrent abortion

In some forms of double uterus repeated second trimester miscarriage is seen to occur, and despite a general and almost traditional reluctance to resort to surgery, experience has shown that it can overcome the problem in many of these cases. There is one reported group of 53 patients with double uterus who were studied for reproductive difficulties[8]. All of them were treated with hormones initially and 31 of them had at least one child following such therapy. The remaining 22 patients in this group had reconstructive uterine surgery; 16 of them had a history of three or more miscarriages. The 22 had collectively 86 prior pregnancies of which none had gone to term. Following operation 16 of the 22 achieved a living child (73 per cent success rate) and there were altogether a total of 37 pregnancies of which 25 went to term, 3 were born prematurely and 9 miscarried.

There are two types of double uterus suitable for such surgery. The most commonly encountered and the best prospect for success is the septate or sub-septate uterus (see **Figure 1**, page 9) and obviously the smaller the septum the better the prospect from the operation. The aim is to unify the two halves of the uterus by a plastic procedure which is essentially very simple and is indicated diagrammatically in **Figure 16** with the end result shown in **Figure 18** (page 61). The Jones operation is that most commonly used and the general principles and main technical features of the operation are shown on pages 62–63.

The other form of double uterus that is suitable for uteroplasty is the bicornate type with a single cervix (**Figure 17**). This abnormality demands a more difficult plastic procedure than the other and the operation has to some extent to be tailored to fit the requirements of the individual case. The original Strassman procedure may sometimes be suitable and such an operation is described in detail in Volume 5 of the Atlas (pages 66 to 69). A full account of the Jones operation is also given in Volume 5 (pages 57 to 65).

Technique of the Jones operation

The necessary incisions into the muscle must encounter the rich coronary arterial blood supply to the uterus and even a limited amount of blood at the operation site interferes with the precise muscle suturing which has to be done.

Application of a rubber tourniquet around the uterus at the level of the isthmus satisfactorily occludes the uterine vessels and plastic covered bulldog clamps on the infundibulo-pelvic ligaments deprive the area of its alternative blood source (**Figure 10**, page 59).

The initial steps of the operation are to fix the uterus in position and then outline a wedge-shaped excision over the fundus uteri; this is in the sagittal plane with its ends on the anterior and posterior uterine walls (**Figure 16**). It is placed centrally and includes the septum in the wedge or sector of uterine muscle to be excised. The uterine cavity is previously packed and distended with gauze soaked in methylene blue or other dye so that one cuts down on to a supporting and easily recognised cushion of gauze which delineates the uterine cavity on each side. The raw uterine muscle surfaces are bisected parallel to the serous edge by a scalpel cutting to a depth of 1.5 cm so that the com-

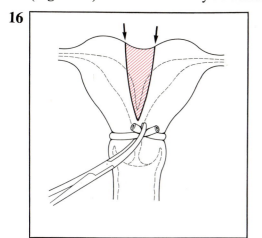 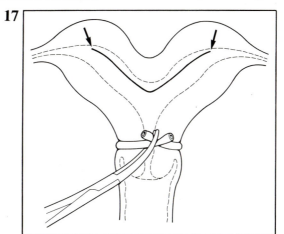 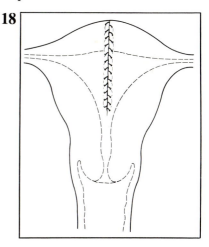

16 Diagram of plan for Jones operation

17 Diagram of plan for Strassman operation

18 Diagram of uterine appearance following operation

bined muscle and endometrial layer can be approximated before suturing the remainder of the uterine wall thickness with a muscular and then a sero-muscular layer.

The operation is straightforward but there is one hazard: it is easy to be left with insufficient muscle tissue medial to each cornu. This can result in the new fundus being two narrow and it particularly endangers the interstitial portion of the tubes which may be caught up in and occluded by the uterine muscle stitches.

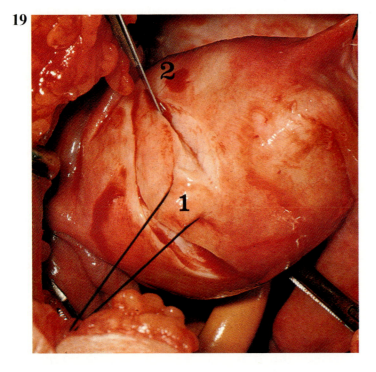

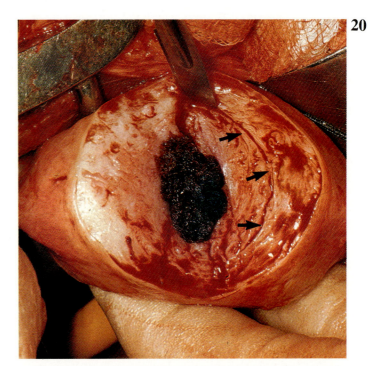

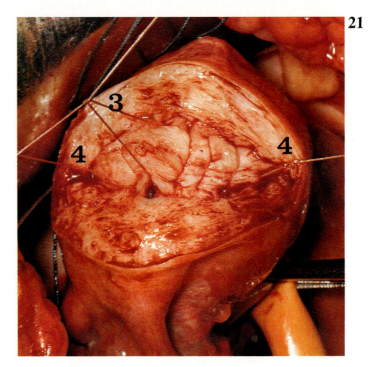

19 Fundal incision to excise uterine septum
A fundal stitch (1) holds the sector to be removed while the scalpel (2) excises a wedge of muscle towards the uterine cavity as shown.

20 Linear incision of uterine wall to allow three-layer closure
The myometrium is too thick for a single layer closure and is therefore incised (bisected) to a depth of 1.5 cm on each side in a line parallel to the serosal edge.

21 Suture of deep muscle layer
The deep layer of muscle has been closed by a continuous suture which is about to be tied off (3). An anchor stitch (4) steadies each end of the wound. The endometrium is not included within this stitch which does not therefore obtrude on the uterine cavity.

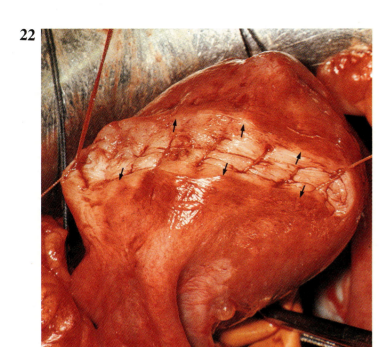

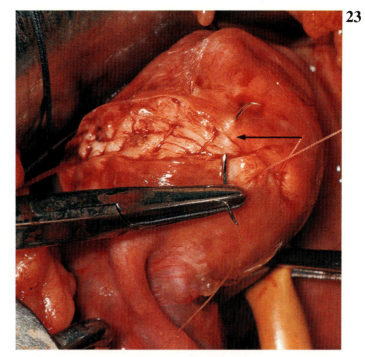

22 Suture of main muscle layer
The outer half of the bisected uterine wall has now been closed by a continuous suture. Note that the serosal edge (arrowed) has been omitted from the closure so that it can be utilised for a separate inverting peritoneal stitch.

23 and 24 Completed closure of sero-muscular layer
In **Figure 23** the needle travels from within outwards (arrowed) on each serosal edge as it progresses along the wound and this results in an inverted smooth surface which will not encourage adhesions. The end result is seen in **Figure 24**.

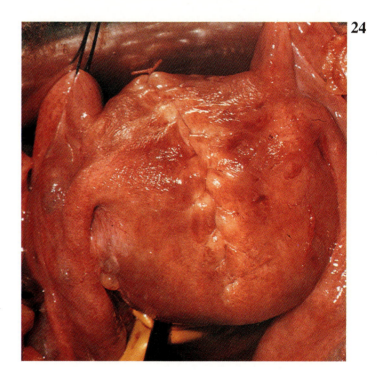

5: Ectopic pregnancy

The Atlas is primarily concerned with the operative treatment of ectopic gestation but the condition is a dangerous one which is responsible for about 10 per cent of maternal mortality in the United States[1] besides having serious effects on subsequent reproduction. A brief general survey of the clinical condition is therefore appropriate.

Aetiology and incidence

It is increasingly clear that ectopic gestation is directly related to the results of tubal infection and it is estimated that women who have had pelvic inflammatory disease have a tenfold increased risk of ectopic pregnancy[2]. There is evidence also that incomplete treatment of acute cases by antibiotics is an important factor[3]. In certain parts of the world where salpingitis is prevalent, the incidence of ectopic pregnancy is very high.

Site of ectopic pregnancy

Approximately 95 per cent of cases occur in the free part of the fallopian tube itself and the majority are ampullary. Some are isthmal and a few are fimbrial; 3 or 4 per cent are interstitial while cervical and cornual pregnancies are so rare and difficult to substantiate that they scarcely merit classification as ectopic pregnancies. Primary ovarian pregnancy is accepted as a rare happening and primary abdominal pregnancy is looked on as a doubtful clinical entity. Most, if not all, of these latter cases are secondary to an intra-tubal pregnancy where rupture of the tube wall allows the ovum to escape into the peritoneal cavity while retaining an attachment to the tube which nurtures it while it continues to grow in a nidation provided by omentum, bowel and surrounding viscera. The possible ectopic sites are shown diagrammatically in **Figure 1**. Allocation of precise percentages is not attempted since published figures vary considerably.

1 Ectopic pregnancy sites
The possible sites of ectopic pregnancy are indicated by numerals:
1. Ampullary
2. Fimbrial
3. Isthmal
4. Interstitial
5. Broad ligament (secondary to tubal)
6. Abdominal (secondary to tubal)
7. Ovarian.

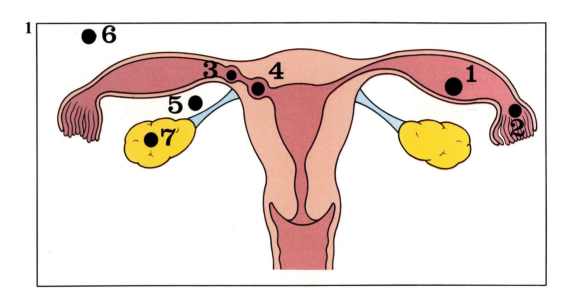

Prognosis and effects on future reproduction

In England and Wales in the years 1973–1975 21 women died from ectopic pregnancy and the principal cause was delay in diagnosis and surgical treatment, (Report on Confidential Enquiries into Maternal Deaths in England and Wales, 1973–1975)[4]. The effects on further childbearing are severe and a woman who has an ectopic pregnancy almost certainly has defective tubal or ovum pick-up function which operates bilaterally. The risks of repeated ectopic, sterility and abortion are high. Thus it was found[5] that 70 per cent of first ectopics do not produce a living child thereafter and there was an incidence of 9.2 per cent of repeat ectopics in 1330 extra-uterine pregnancies[6]. Relative figures vary greatly and in a recent symposium of 4 experienced clinicians[1] a figure of 30 per cent seemed to be accepted. It is generally agreed that 80 per cent of recurrences occur within 4 years of the first.

Diagnosis

The Confidential Report emphasises the importance of diagnosis being made early and surgical treatment instituted at once. The possibility of ectopic pregnancy is always there if a woman is at childbearing age and this should never be forgotten. The two common types of ectopic pregnancy present very differently. Frank rupture of the fallopian tube with bleeding into the peritoneal cavity gives a picture of shock and haemorrhage which with the accompanying classical symptoms and signs should provide an easy diagnosis.

A 'leaking' ectopic pregnancy can be much more difficult to diagnose especially if the patient has a history of menstrual irregularity, looks well and perhaps minimises her symptoms. In the past, experienced gynaecologists became skilled in diagnosing such conditions largely because they occurred relatively frequently and they were automatically aware of the possibility. Diagnosis was usually confirmed by posterior pouch puncture, examination under anaesthesia and curettage. Even so there was a fairly high incidence of false positive diagnoses.

There are now available several valuable new aids to early diagnosis. Sensitive early pregnancy tests detect HCG 13 or 14 days after conception in over 90 per cent of cases and at a later stage ultra-sonic scanning will detect a small extra-uterine sac or pelvic haematocele (see **Figures 2 & 3**). It may also outline an abdominal pregnancy at a later stage. The outstanding diagnostic advance, however, is laparoscopy which has completely altered the picture by giving a first hand view of the state of both tubes and thereby completely eliminating diagnostic error. Once a clinical diagnosis is seriously considered it is quite essential to make a laparoscopic examination so that the clinician can see what is happening. The method is not used in frank intra-peritoneal haemorrhage cases where the blood would make examination impossible in any case. In 'leaking' ectopic cases blood may in fact obscure the findings, and in such circumstances laparotomy would be necessary although the bleeding might have come from a corpus luteum haematoma. In the type of case being discussed laparoscopy would be done under general anaesthesia with the patient prepared for laparotomy if indicated. The laparoscopic appearance in 3 different cases is shown in **Figures 4, 5,** and **6**.

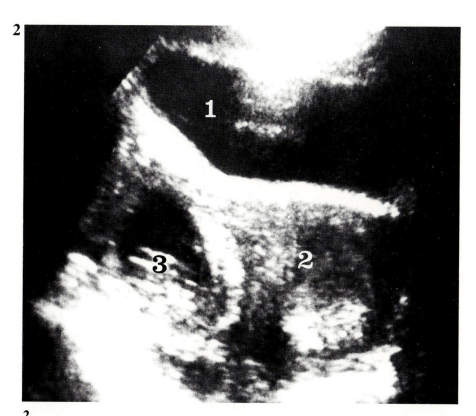

2
Ultrasonic scan showing a gestation sac containing an embryo in the region of the left fallopian tube. The bladder is numbered (1), uterus (2) and the fetal parts within the gestation sac (3).

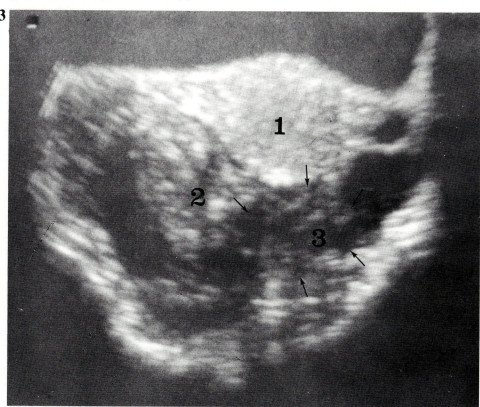

3
Ultrasonic scan showing a pelvic haematocele behind and to the left of the uterus with associated bowel distention. The relative features are numbered thus: Uterus (1), haematocele (2) and outlined with fine arrows, distended bowel and blood clot (3).

65

4

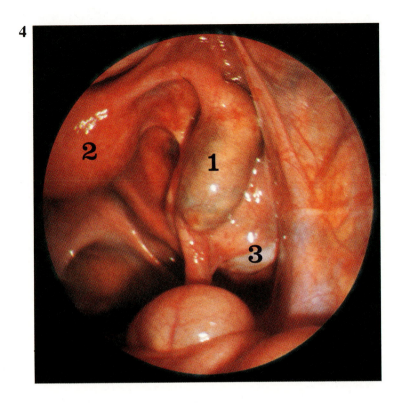

5

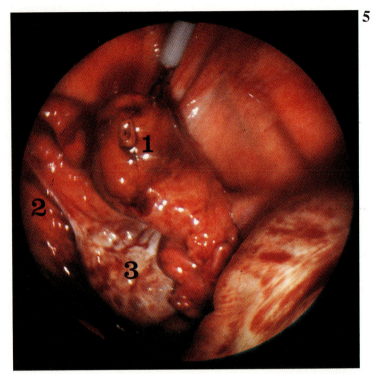

4 to 6 Ectopic pregnancy: laparoscopic appearance
Three different views of ectopic pregnancy as seen through the
laparoscope. In **Figures 4** and **5** unruptured right tubal pregnancies seen at (1); the uterus is at (2) and the ovary at (3). In
Figure 6 the tubal pregnancy in the left tube (1) has started to
bleed (2) into the peritoneal cavity.

6

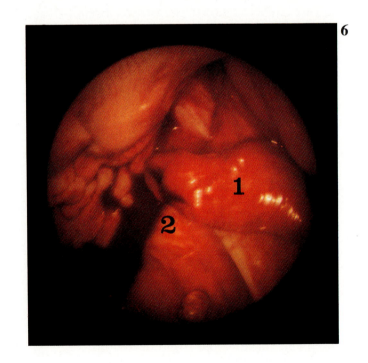

Treatment of ectopic pregnancy

A ruptured ectopic pregnancy usually presents in one of two ways and it is necessary to recognise the clinical type since the management is rather different.

I: Recent frank rupture of the fallopian tube with massive intra-peritoneal haemorrhage and accompanying shock

In the majority of such cases the tubal wall is split by the growing pregnancy and the bleeding is from an eroded medium sized artery. Any part of the tube may be involved but the isthmal and the rarer interstitial parts are associated with a severe degree of bleeding since the narrow lumen practically explodes at an early stage of pregnancy and bleeding is generally from fairly large arteries.

II: Slow recurrent bleeding from an extra-uterine pregnancy with resultant intra-abdominal collection of blood and the formation of a peritubal haematocele

These cases are sub-acute in type and there is usually no major degree of shock or haemorrhage. The condition is usually referred to in Britain as 'a leaking ectopic'.

Management of Group I cases: frank rupture of tube

The prime requirement in such circumstances is to secure the source of the intra-abdominal bleeding by immediate emergency abdominal operation. While preparations for that are being made, the blood group is obtained and at least three pints of blood cross matched and made available. Rather than delay blood replacement Group O Rhesus Negative blood may be used if it is available. Blood is rarely immediately to hand and transfusion is started with plasma or dextran through a drip apparatus suitable for giving blood subsequently.

It is important not to start dextran infusion before blood samples for grouping and/or cross matching have been taken since it can vitiate laboratory tests. It also impairs blood clotting and no more than a total of 1 litre should be given. The patient is transferred to the operating room while such procedures are in progress and there is no question of awaiting full resuscitation or return of blood pressure to normal levels before administering a general anaesthetic and commencing operation. Anaesthetists are fully aware and accept that such a policy is correct and safest for the patient. The surgeon, in fact, increasingly finds that the arrangements are already going ahead and that the anaesthetist has a central venous pressure line *in situ*; this is a great safety factor both in ensuring adequate blood replacement and in preventing pulmonary oedema.

The abdomen is usually distended, and when the peritoneal cavity is opened, blood pours out. The surgeon displaces bowel and omentum and scoops out sufficient blood clot and fluid blood to recognise the affected tube or the fundus uteri and delivers the tube into the wound. A spouting artery invariably shows itself and this is controlled by compressing it in the

mesosalpinx between the finger and thumb until a forceps can be applied (see **Figure 7**). Once the bleeding point has been controlled, the crisis is over as far as the haemorrhage is concerned, and the surgeon can clear the blood from the operative field, displace the mentum and intestine behind a gauze pack and assess the situation. The patient has meantime been having blood replacement and her condition immediately improves at this stage; the change is usually commented on by the anaesthetist.

Some experienced surgeons are of the opinion that improvement begins when the blood is released from the distended abdomen and before the bleeding has been stopped and that may well be so. The steps described and destined to stop the immediate intra-peritoneal haemorrhage are basic to the management of a ruptured ectopic pregnancy.

The use of an anti-gravity suit to arrest bleeding temporarily in such cases has been reported[1] and one can see that the method might have considerable advantage in severe cases and if the equipment were available.

Once bleeding is under control the surgeon should make a careful clinical assessment before proceeding further.

Salpingectomy is the recognised treatment for ruptured ectopic pregnancy, but the requirements of each patient are different and surgically things are not always what they seem. Thus it is prudent to be quite sure of what has occurred and what is the correct management before embarking on that particular operation. The affected fallopian tube usually shows evidence of previous inflammation and provided the other tube is healthy, it is correct to remove the affected one. It is not in the authors' opinion justifiable routinely to remove the ipselateral ovary and enough time has elapsed to show that the fashion of doing so has conferred no obvious benefit. Conservative surgery has little place in the management of this group although one occasionally sees cases with relatively severe intraperitoneal haemorrhage where it is possible to salvage the affected tube.

The following are examples of some unexpected findings and the appropriate management:

1. Both fallopian tubes may appear intact but closer examination shows that there has been a tubal abortion from one of them and bleeding from its ostium may still be in progress. Apart from the awkward problem of haemostasis, such a tube is likely to give rise to future trouble and it should be removed.

2. It may appear that there are bilateral ectopic pregnancies, a ruptured tube on one side and a distended one, full of blood clot, on the other. The condition of contralateral accompanying haematosalpinx is not uncommon and the surgeon must establish that the blood can be milked from the haematocoele to leave the tube looking reasonably normal before removing the other one.

3. Rupture of the interstitial portion of the tube carries the risk of more severe haemorrhage and

also requires special surgical management. The surgeon is confronted by an irregular crater-like hole in the uterine cornu through which the gestation sac has escaped. An artery or arteries are spouting from the irregular wall. Elaborate methods of excising that portion of the uterine wall are sometimes described, and it is claimed that hysterectomy is sometimes necessary. The authors may have been fortunate but have not found either course to be necessary. The rupture of the tube necessarily occurs at an early stage of pregnancy and there is comparatively limited invasion of uterine muscle so that the wall of the cavity is usually clean with an absence of traumatised muscle tissue. It is necessary only to insert two mattress sutures to obliterate the cavity and control bleeding and then cover the raw area with a Lembert type fine stitch. Whether or not one should remove the tube on that side is a question that could be debated; there does not seem to be any compelling reason for doing so.

4. A rare and disconcerting situation for the inexperienced presents when the pregnancy ruptures between the layers of the broad ligament. This results in formation of a large retro-peritoneal haemorrhage with much blood clot in the base of the broad ligament. Careful assessment of the findings establishes the diagnosis, and treatment consists of salpingectomy followed by opening up the broad ligament sufficiently to evacuate the blood clot and secure any bleeding vessels. The full extent of the haematoma and retro-peritoneal bleeding is noted, but evacuation is not attempted in a region of large thin-walled blood vessels and urinary structures. The peritoneal surface is reconstituted with fine stitches and suction drains are inserted beneath it.

5. When the surgeon has to admit that the diagnosis is wrong and that all the blood has come from a ruptured Graafian follicle or corpus luteum the bleeding if still continuing is controlled by one or two fine figure of eight catgut or PGA sutures.

Disposal of what may be a very large amount of intra-peritoneal blood has been the subject of changing surgical fashion over the years. It was at one time frequently retrieved from the abdomen and retransfused into an arm vein through a gauze filter. As blood transfusion services were established, stored blood was given in the requisite quantity and the peritoneal cavity sucked and swabbed as carefully as possible to avoid the development of intraperitoneal infection and adhesions. Recent trends are towards leaving the blood in the peritoneal cavity from which it is absorbed without substantially increasing the risk of infection or adhesion. Removal of blood and clots from the cavity could be said to involve some abrasion and contamination. Because of their fear of subsequent ileus the authors have not had the courage to leave the abdomen awash with the usual mixture of free blood and large purple clots. If the latter are scooped out there is, however, no need to be too assiduous in removing the former.

7

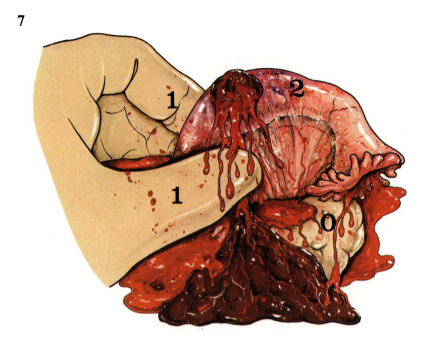

7 Establishing point of tubal rupture and controlling bleeding
The diagram shows the important initial step when opening the abdomen in a case of frank rupture with haemoperitoneum. Immediately it is obvious which tube is involved it is lifted from the pelvis between the thumb (1) and fingers (1) of the surgeon's left hand and the tube (2) is examined. Digital pressure on the adjacent mesosalpinx will control haemorrhage sufficiently to allow the surgeon to clear the main mass of surrounding clot and to decide on the method of treatment. The ovary is numbered (0).

Management of Group II cases: 'leaking' ectopic pregnancy

The circumstances surrounding operation in this case are very different from those in frank tubal rupture. The surgeon is not primarily occupied in halting and reversing the effects of haemorrhage and shock and the operation is in the nature of an exploratory laparotomy to establish the site of the ectopic pregnancy by a gently conducted operation in which the considerable amount of old blood clot in the pelvis is removed and the situation assessed before deciding on the appropriate operation. Even so it is advisable to anticipate possible rapid haemorrhage in such cases; the pre-operative haemoglobin level should be satisfactory, cross matched blood should be available and an intravenous cannula or needle should be in place and open.

Many, perhaps a majority, of these cases come to the operating room to have laparoscopy followed by laparotomy if that is required; previously they came for examination under anaesthesia and D & C and the aim in both instances is to confirm the suspected diagnosis of a leaking ectopic pregnancy. Although it occurred much more frequently under the old regime, an iatrogenic complication still occurs and should be guarded against. It is the severe intra-peritoneal bleeding which follows disturbance of the pelvic haematocoele when examining the patient digitally under anaesthesia. Before laparoscopy was in use, and by the time the surgeon and assistant had together confirmed the correctness of the diagnosis, the anaesthetist frequently noted a drop in blood pressure and on opening the peritoneal cavity the pelvis was full of old blood clot while the abdomen was rapidly filling with fresh blood from a spouting artery. Comparatively gentle examination is often sufficient to precipitate bleeding and while most clinicians naturally prefer to make some sort of examination of the pelvis before introducing the laparoscope it should be carried out with extreme gentleness. Even if the haemorrhage incurred is minimal it will invalidate the laparoscopic examination and prejudice clinical decisions.

Laparoscopic examination is also carried out with extreme gentleness and the value of the procedure is, of course, enormous. It is possible to see at once if there is an ectopic pregnancy, the side affected and perhaps the portion of the tube involved and its relationship to the surrounding haematoma.

At laparotomy the omentum and intestines are displaced upwards by an abdominal pack and any free blood clot removed from the pelvis. The most frequent finding is of an oedematous and discoloured tube surrounded by haematoma in an area bounded by the posterior aspect of the broad ligament, the pelvic floor and the posterior aspect of the uterus. Not infrequently there is minimal blood in the peritoneal cavity and the tube appears as it did at laparoscopy – free on its mesosalpinx, distended in the isthmal, ampullary or fimbrial portion, and about to rupture through the tubal wall into the peritoneal cavity or perhaps partly protruding and accompanied by leaking blood from the fimbrial ostium.

In the latter instance it may be advisable to remove the pregnancy either by milking it from the tube if it is at the fimbrial end or incising the tubal wall and in each case conserving the tube. The techniques for such procedures are illustrated below. Advice cannot be offered on the indications for and against removing a fallopian tube that in some cases is obviously distorted by old infection, and in others looks normal yet carries the risk of recurrent ectopic pregnancy in 5–10 per cent of cases. Decisions must always depend on the many factors in the individual case and it has not been our practice to become involved in such questions in the Atlas.

Where the ectopic pregnancy is walled off by old blood and haematoma in the pelvis, the first step in surgical management is to disengage the tube gently with the fingers while the hand approaches it from the lateral aspect and working medially separates the soft adhesions between the distended tube and the pelvic floor in the first place and the posterior aspect of the broad ligament thereafter. It is then possible to lift up the tube and ovary in one piece and decide on the operative procedure required. There is usually little doubt about what is best in the circumstances and salpingectomy is the rule. The operation is that described and illustrated on page 72. The occurrence of a broad ligament haematoma has already been referred to and if encountered in sub-acute or more chronic form is dealt with in the same fashion.

Abdominal pregnancy

There remains the question of surgical treatment of abdominal pregnancy, whether it be ovarian in origin or an extruded tubal pregnancy which has been able to survive. The condition of abdominal pregnancy is generally rare but may be encountered in certain circumstances and locations. Thus ovarian pregnancy is said to be on the increase in women fitted with an IUD, presumably because it prevents nidation of the ovum in the endometrium and proximal oviduct and is alleged to account for 1 in 9 of ectopics occurring in IUD users. The numbers reported in the literature are increasing[7,8,9] and many are not recorded. Abdominal pregnancy is much rarer but is encountered in large urban black communities such as New Orleans[10]. The management is surgical and is the same for all types.

Abdominal pregnancy at or near term is rare and difficult to diagnose; there may or may not be the opportunity to rescue a live fetus. Operation is mandatory but no guidelines can be set for such a procedure. The fetus is located in its sac and is then delivered, but the placenta may be attached to surrounding structures by very large vessels and removal would cause severe bleeding. It is always worth making a tentative effort to strip the amnion from the chorion and this may be possible without causing bleeding, although very often it is not. There must be no question of trying to remove the chorion and if separation between the two membranes is not feasible, no further attempt should be made to remove the placenta. The umbilical cord is cut quite short and the whole structure left to absorb.

Retroperitoneal drainage should be instituted if possible. Absorption is likely to take many weeks and the patient may run a stormy course with the possible development of hypofibrinogenaemia. Because of this one must hope to be able to remove the placenta subsequently and placental function is monitored continually by quantitative chorionic gonadotrophin titres; when it has ceased to function it should be safe to operate. Methotrexate may be used to encourage trophoblastic degeneration.

It is much more likely that an abdominal pregnancy will end with death of the fetus before it is viable. In some cases the onset of a spurious labour and the presence of definite clinical findings point to the diagnosis; more often the diagnosis is missed at the time of fetal death, and it is only later that an apparent ovarian cyst or pelvic tumour is recognised at laparotomy for what is really is – a retained and shrunken dead fetus complete in its membranes.

If the fetus is still alive laparotomy is indicated because of the considerable danger of severe abdominal bleeding, and if it has recently perished it should also be removed. In either case there is likely to be danger in separating the placenta and the procedure previously described is followed. The placenta is left *in situ* if removal is likely to be dangerous.

Where the fetus is recognised radiologically as having been dead for some time or where it is unexpectedly encountered in the removal of a pelvic 'tumour' removal of the pregnancy is generally much easier. There may be some difficulty in separating the exterior of the amniotic sac from the chorion and surrounding structure, but the placenta has nearly always degenerated and can be stripped off without injury to other viscera.

The main danger for the surgeon in these cases is becoming involved in an attempt to remove a 'live' placenta since this can lead to uncontrollable haemorrhage. To leave the placenta *in situ* with perhaps many weeks of discomfort and distress for the patient is a poor solution but it is preferable to the nightmare of uncontrollable haemorrhage which may result in her death.

Surgical techniques

Different operations are required for different types of ectopic pregnancy and varying circumstances. Practically all cases would be covered by carrying out one of the three procedures illustrated in the following pages:

1. Salpingectomy – removal of affected fallopian tube.
2. Excision of ectopic conceptus with conservation of affected fallopian tube.
3. Removal of an abdominal pregnancy.

8

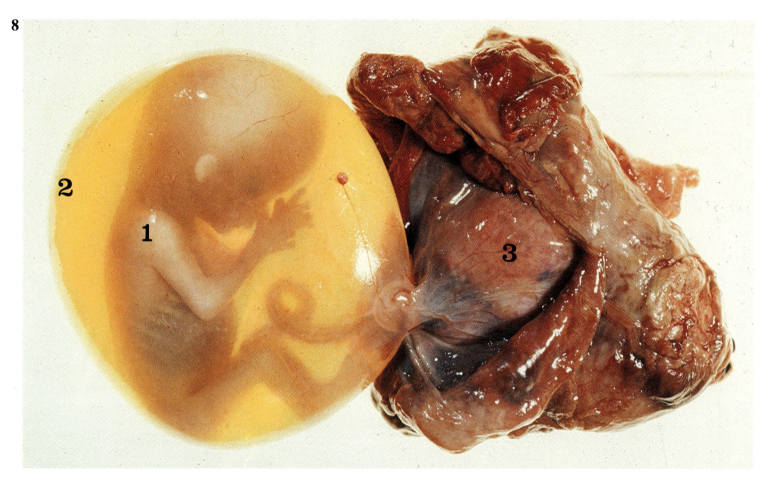

8 Specimen of abdominal pregnancy
An 18 weeks size fetus (1) within an intact membrane sac (2)
is not in the usual relationship to the placenta (3) which is
implanted on adjacent peritoneal surfaces and abdominal
visceral structures.

1. Salpingectomy – removal of affected fallopian tube

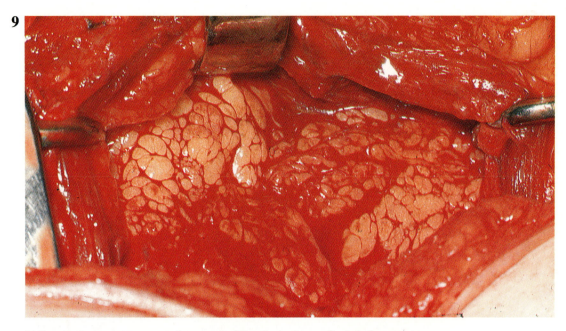

9 Laparotomy appearance in a case of frank rupture of a tubal pregnancy
The peritoneal cavity is filled with blood and as in this case the omentum is usually the only visible intra-peritoneal structure. The blood is partly fluid and partly clotted.

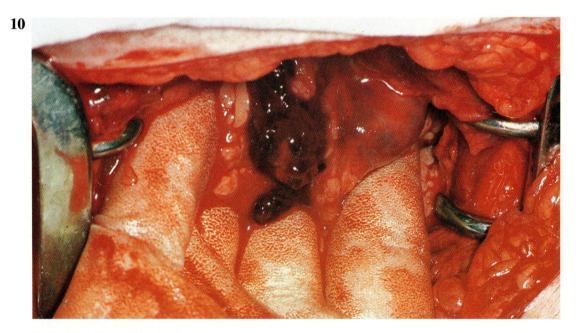

10 Exploration of the pelvis
The surgeon's hand is gently introduced into the pelvis to locate the uterine fundus and then examines each tube in turn. By palpation and sometimes vision the affected tube is recognised and is brought up gently into the wound between fingers and thumb. The method of digitally controlling bleeding has already been referred to (page 68) and time is taken to estimate the situation before deciding on the surgical procedure to adopt.

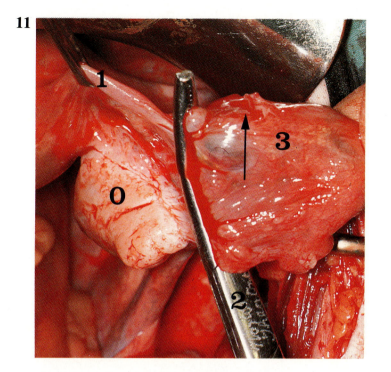

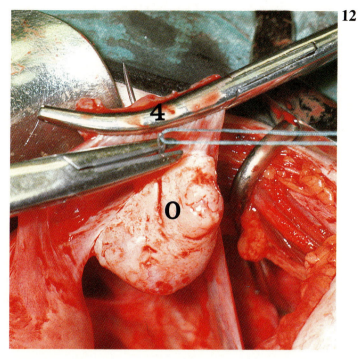

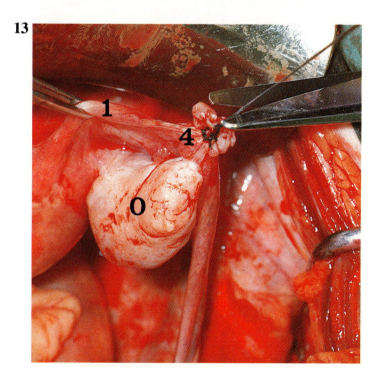

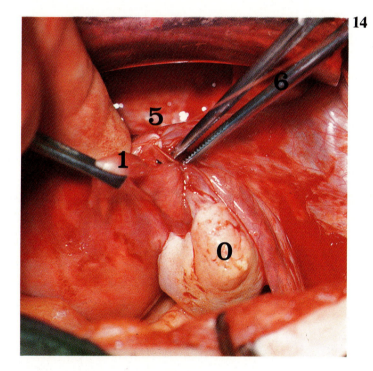

11 to 14 Right salpingectomy

In this case salpingectomy was indicated because of a grossly damaged ampullary portion of the tube. In **Figure 11** the isthmal part of the tube is steadied by a fine tissue forceps (1) while a curved Kocher forceps (2) is used to clamp off the ruptured and distorted tube (3). The site of the rupture is arrowed. In **Figure 12** the lateral part of the tube has been excised and the pedicle is transfixed with a round bodied needle carrying a No. 1 PGA suture (4). The pedicle is secured and the ligature is being cut short in **Figure 13.** In **Figure 14** the pedicle is being surrounded by a purse string suture which is in process of being tied (5) while dissecting forceps (6) invert the pedicle beneath the stitch. The right ovary is numbered (0) in all the photographs.

2. Excision of conceptus with conservation of affected fallopian tube

15 to 17 Appearance of intact right tube at laparotomy
In **Figure 15** the ampullary portion of the tube (1) is distended with blood clot which is escaping from the fimbrial end (2). The tubal integument appears intact. In **Figure 16** the uterus is supported at (3) and the right tube lifted from the pelvis. There is a mass of blood clot still issuing from the fimbrial end and the tube is seen to be free of adhesions. In **Figure 17** the forefinger and thumb (4) have been used to 'milk' the blood clot from the tube which is now largely empty. The ovary is numbered (0) when visible.

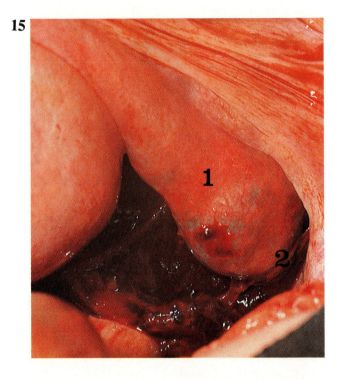

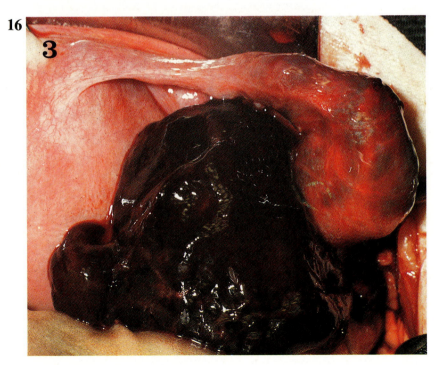

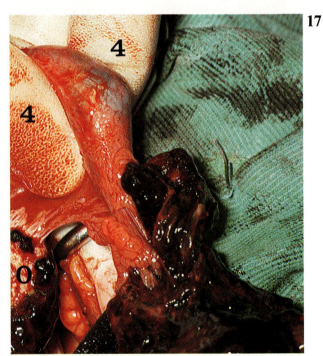

18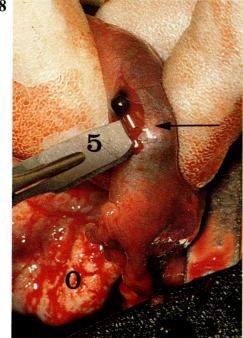

19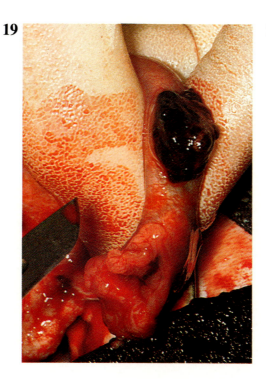

20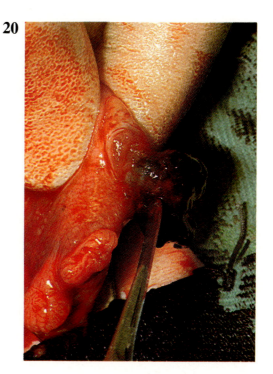

21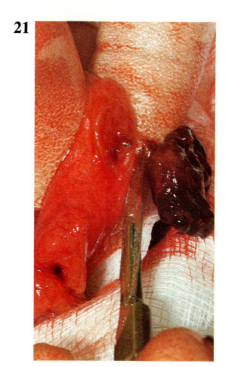

22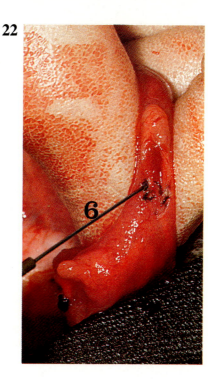

18 to 22 Excision of conceptus from ampulla of right tube

The pregnancy could be felt within the tube which had thinned and was about to rupture where arrowed in **Figure 18.** The scalpel (5) makes a short incision in the long axis of the tube at that point and the tubal mole is encouraged into the wound with the fingers in **Figure 19.** In **Figure 20** it is teased clear with curved scissors and finally detached with the point of the scalpel in **Figure 21.** There was only one small bleeding point and this is sealed with a fine diathermy needle (6) in **Figure 22.**

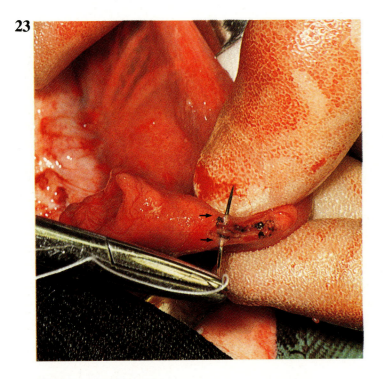

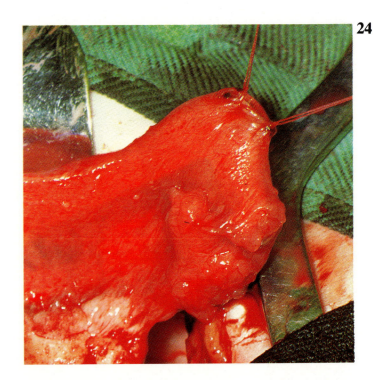

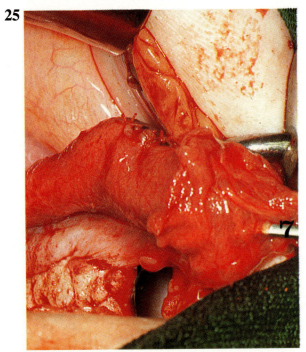

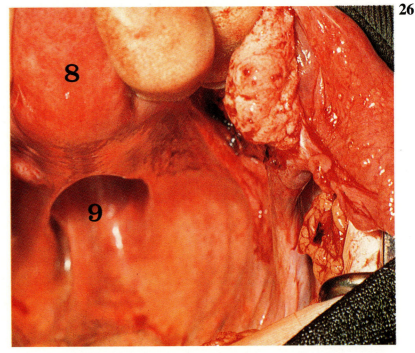

23 to 26 Suture of ampullary wall of right tube

Two interrupted sutures of 000 PGA material on a fine round bodied needle were sufficient to close the incision in **Figures 23** and **24** – the aim was to approximate without setting up tissue reaction. The wound is dry and the surface reasonably smooth but it would have been preferable to use a greater number of fine unabsorbable stitches of 4 × 0 nylon or prolene. With regard to technique, note that the needle in **Figure 23** picks up only the serosal and main muscle layers (arrowed); it does not include the endosalpinx or obtrude on the lumen of the tube. In **Figure 25** a probe (7) establishes that the lumen is open and in **Figure 26** examination of the posterior pouch establishes that it is free of blood and adhesions. The uterus is numbered (8), the pouch of Douglas (9) and the right tube is seen on the right of the photograph.

3. Removal of an abdominal pregnancy

27 Appearance on opening abdomen in abdominal pregnancy
The fetus was known to be extra-uterine and to have perished. The fundus uteri (1) is held upwards and forwards by holding sutures on the round ligaments and the remains of the abdominal pregnancy are seen to be encapsulated in the mass of tissue (2) behind and to the left of the uterus. There is a shallow sulcus between its upper surface and where it is adherent to the posterior aspect of the uterus (arrowed). Elsewhere it appears free. The ovaries are numbered 0.

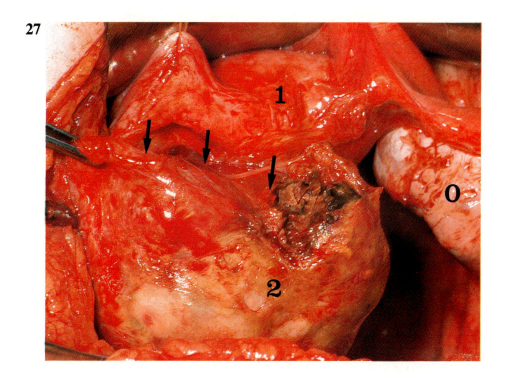

28 Abdominal pregnancy – specimen
The specimen is shown at this stage because it makes it easier to understand the abdominal appearances at operation. The embryo (1) has been retrieved from the sac of membranes which enveloped and covered the surface of the spread out placenta (3). The placental end of the umbilical cord is seen at (4). The placenta is disproportionately large by the size of the fetus and is implanted over a large area which fortunately did not include hollow viscera or vital organs. It appeared that the main contribution was from the omentum.

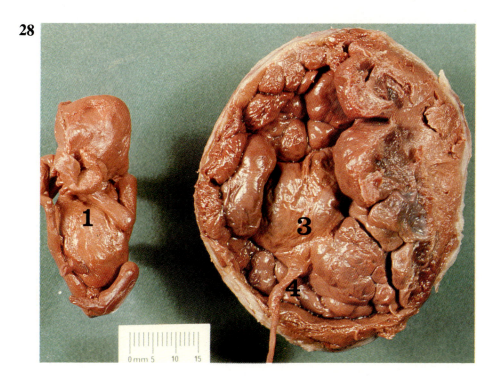

29

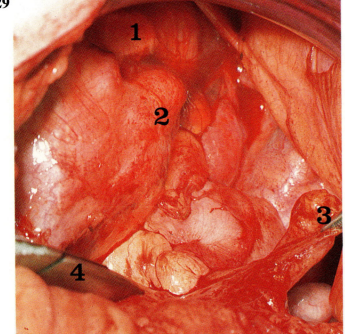

30

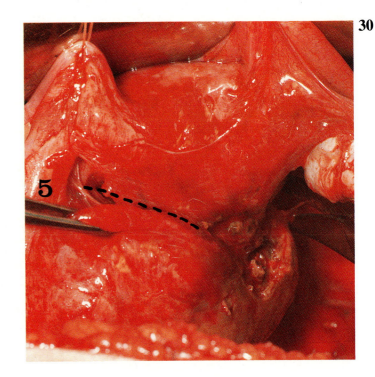

31

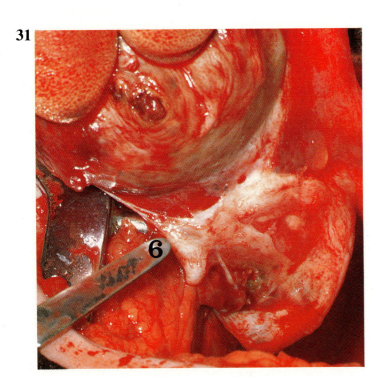

29 to 31 Mobilisation of abdominal pregnancy mass
Mobilisation commences by approaching laterally across the pelvic floor as in **Figure 29.** The uterus (1) is held forwards and carries the pregnancy mass (2) with it. Adherent bowel and omentum have been detached and are held in forceps (3) while the scissors (4) are used as blunt dissectors to encourage the pregnancy upwards off the pelvic floor. In **Figure 30** separation at the upper attachment is about to begin. Dissecting forceps (5) steady the mass while a plane of separation is found in the sulcus along the broken line. In **Figure 31** the abdominal pregnancy is largely free but still needs some separation laterally on the left side with the help of a Greville MacDonald dissector (6).

32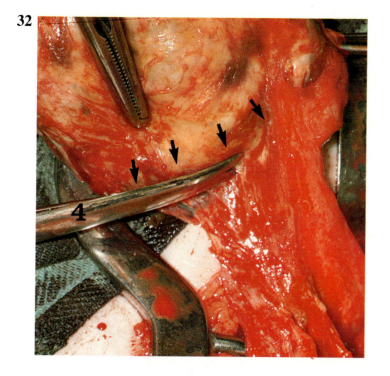

33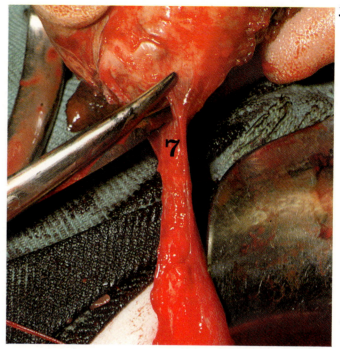

34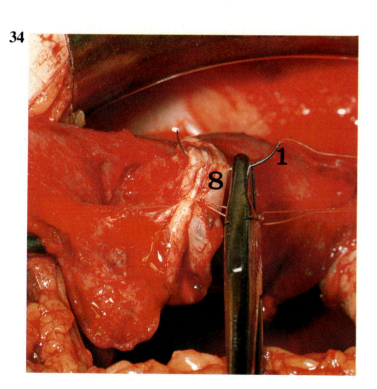

32 to 34 Removal of abdominal pregnancy mass
In **Figure 32** the mass of tissue has now been separated from the posterior aspect of the uterus and pelvic floor and dissection is being completed with curved scissors (4) along a line of cleavage (arrowed). A remaining pedicle (7) is divided in **Figure 33**. In **Figure 34** the cavity left by removal of the abdominal pregnancy is closed by a series of 00 PGA sutures (8) which pick up the peritoneal edges and include a shallow bite in the depth of the cavity to obliterate dead space. The uterine fundus is numbered (1).

6: The acute abdomen in pregnancy

The pregnant woman is no less liable to suffer an acute abdominal crisis than her non-pregnant sister, and in the face of acute abdominal symptoms, it is absolutely essential to be immediately alert and make all necessary examinations and investigations to confirm or exclude serious disease. Delay in diagnosis is the commonest mistake and can literally be fatal. Fear of upsetting the patient and even the risk of endangering the pregnancy should not deflect the clinician from obtaining all necessary laboratory and if need be, radiological help.

There are two particularly dangerous conditions – acute appendicitis and acute intestinal obstruction. An undiagnosed obstructed appendix ruptures and sets up a peritonitis which quickly becomes general in type because the infection cannot be adequately localised by the disturbed and displaced intra-peritoneal contents. Small bowel obstruction is quickly followed by a state of massive dehydration and hypotension which is exceedingly difficult to reverse in the pregnant woman. If bowel necrosis supervenes on strangulation, considerable lengths of intestine may require resection in a very ill patient. The operation is difficult and hazardous and the prognosis is always doubtful.

1. Acute appendicitis in pregnancy

The incidence of acute appendicitis in pregnancy is in the region of 0.6–0.7 per cent[1,2] and it makes up 75 per cent of acute abdominal cases seen in pregnancy. Maternal mortality is influenced by stage of pregnancy, severity of the infection and delay in diagnosis; of the sources quoted the latter[2] gives a figure of 1.0 per cent, the former[1] of 2.0 per cent. The non-pregnant mortality rate from unruptured acute appendicitis is 0.1 per cent.

The increasing size of the uterus and other bodily changes during pregnancy may confuse clinical findings. As the uterus rises into the abdomen it pivots to the left and by pulling on the right broad ligament may be responsible for the frequent pain in the right iliac fossa in early pregnancy. This may sometimes suggest appendicitis but there is no accompanying nausea or tenderness. Acute appendicitis presents the same symptoms and clinical picture in the pregnant as in the non-pregnant but the patient may not appear ill and symptoms are apt to be related to some dietary upset or indiscretion. The condition is treacherous in that pelvic vascular engorgement encourages thrombosis in the appendicular vessels and the increased amount of circulating cortico-steroids militates against the containment of the inflammation. The site of tenderness in the right lower quadrant often seems too high, even allowing for upward displacement of the caecum, and the white blood count is perhaps little higher than the normal pregnancy figure. A suspected or even previously confirmed urinary tract infection may further confuse the issue.

When acute appendicitis is seen as a possibility, all possible active steps are taken to confirm the diagnosis. If that cannot be done, but the possibility of its presence cannot be excluded, an operation must be performed. The surgeon should not be inhibited by the thought of possibly removing a normal appendix as the risks of delay in treatment are too serious to admit of such considerations. One standard text[3] takes the view that a diagnostic error is more acceptable than the effects of rupture of the appendix with a current maternal mortality rate of 5–10 per cent. Another authoritative opinion[4] notes that the usual rate of normal appendices removed from the non-pregnant is 20 per cent compared with 30 per cent in pregnancy; he does not think the additional 10 per cent unreasonable.

The operation itself is done with extreme gentleness and minimal disturbance of the uterus and the peritoneum. The approach is through an oblique muscle splitting incision of the McBurney type but the skin incision is much more horizontal and lies in the line of the skin crease. The level at which it is made depends on the stage of the pregnancy but is always higher and more lateral than in the non-pregnant patient. **Figure 1** recalls the surface marking of the appendix at the various stages of pregnancy. The surface position of the base of the appendix is shown as the requirement is that the mid-point of the incision overlies it. The appropriate incision for each stage of pregnancy has been drawn in and its relationship to the umbilicus, the anterior superior iliac spine and the iliac crest are seen. Because of the increased amount of superficial fascia in pregnancy the skin incisions are rather longer than in a non-pregnant patient.

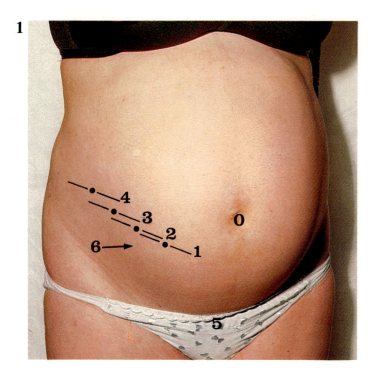

1 Level and extent of skin incision for appendicectomy
The central dots on the overlays represent the surface markings of junction of appendix and caecum at the various stages of pregnancy. – (1) at 3 months, (2) at 5 months, (3) at 7 months and (4) at term. The linear extensions at each level indicate the direction and length of the oblique skin incision required. The umbilicus is numbered (0), the symphysis pubis (5) and the anterior superior iliac spine (6).

Appendicectomy – surgical technique

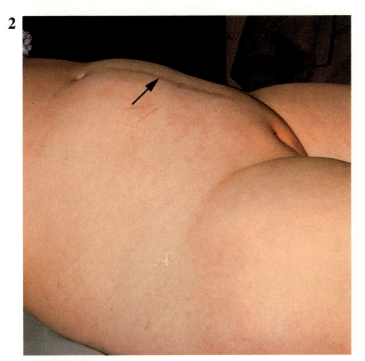

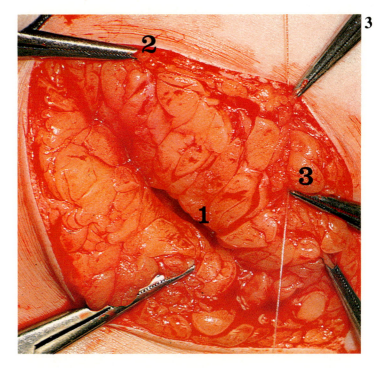

2 Planning skin incision
The patient is 22 weeks pregnant so that the incision is placed just above the level of the anterior superior iliac spine with one-third of its 10 cm length lateral and two-thirds medial to the spine. Note that the patient has a midline abdominal scar; there is however no question of excising it and using that approach. Access would be impossible and there may well be uterine or even bowel adhesions.

3 Skin incision
The incision is made boldly through skin and superficial fascia to the depth of the external oblique aponeurosis in the middle of the wound (1). There is always some bleeding from skin (2) and branches of the superficial epigastric vessels (3) and these have to be secured with forceps and ligated.

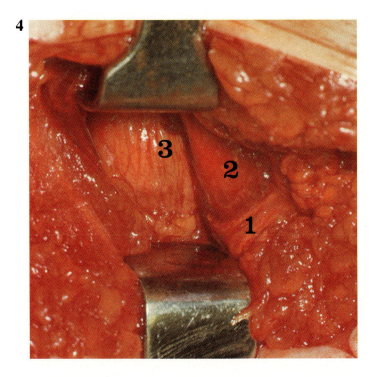

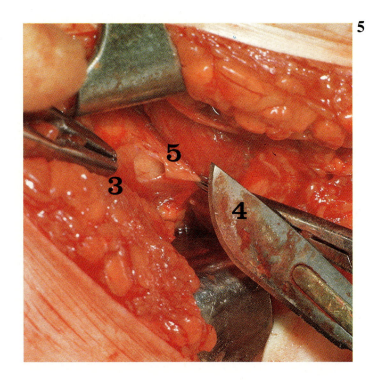

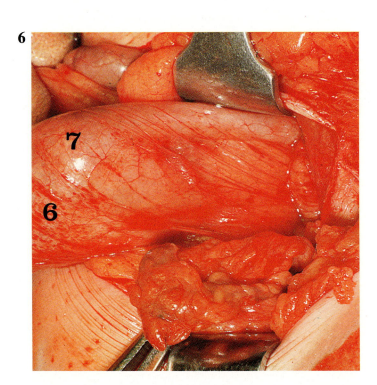

4 to 6 Opening the abdomen

There is little need to recall the steps of every surgeon's first abdominal operation. **Figure 4** shows the external oblique aponeurosis (1) split in the line of its fibres to expose the internal oblique muscle (2) which with the underlying transversus muscle is retracted to expose the peritoneum (3). This has just been incised using the scalpel (4) in **Figure 5** and a loop of bowel is pouting into the opening (5). In **Figure 6** the caecum (6) has been hooked out by the surgeon's forefinger and the base of the appendix (7) is seen being delivered into the abdomen.

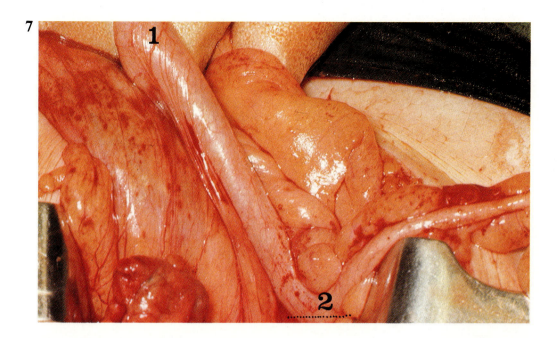

7

1

2

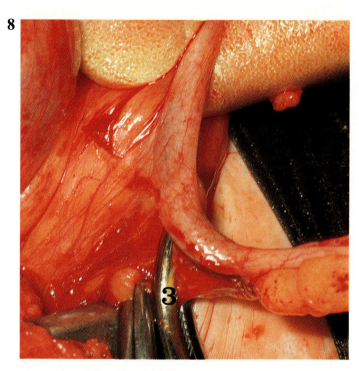

8

3

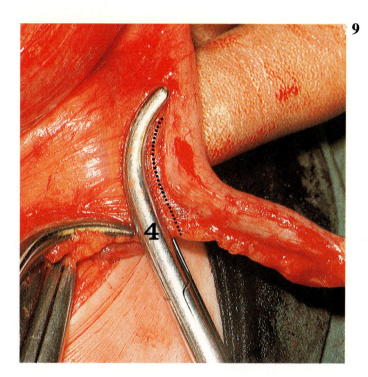

9

4

7 to 9 Freeing the appendix and detaching it from meso-appendix

In **Figure 7** the appendix is held between the surgeon's fingers at its base (1) and is seen to be long with a kink due to fine adhesions at about its mid point (2). These are divided with a gentle stroke of the scalpel (dotted line) so that the appendix can be straightened out as seen in **Figure 8** and the first forceps (3) placed on the free edge of the meso-

appendix where it secures the terminal part of the stem of the appendicular artery. The forceps on the left is merely keeping the peritoneal edge everted. In **Figure 9** the meso-appendix is further clamped by a second forceps (4) and the appendix will be detached along the dotted line to leave a cuff of tissue beyond the forceps for safe ligature (as with forceps 3).

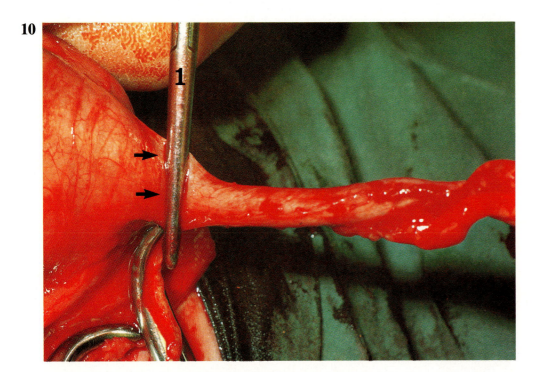

10 Clamping appendix at its base
The appendix is clamped off at its base
with forceps (1) after crushing the tissues
proximally to provide a narrow sulcus or
placement for the stump ligature in due
course. The crushed area is indicated by
arrows.

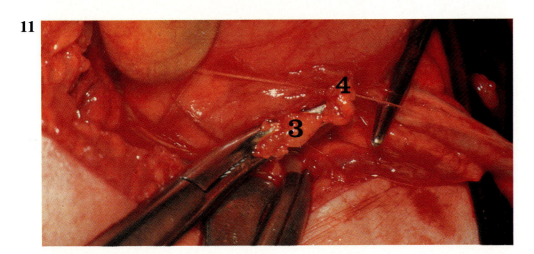

11 Ligation of pedicles of meso-appendix
The pedicle previously held in forceps (4)
is in process of being tied off and will be
repeated in that held by forceps (3). The
clamped base of the appendix is on the
right.

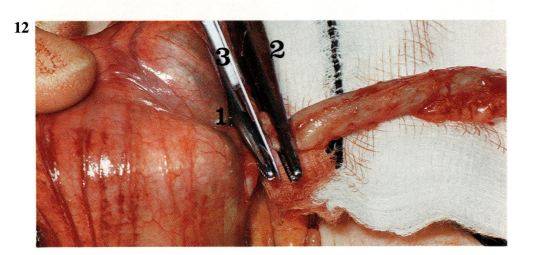

12 Removal of appendix
A second occluding forceps (2) has been
placed on the base of the appendix distal
to the first (1) and the scalpel (3) divides
the appendix between them by sliding
along the first forceps to cut it off flush and
avoid contamination of the wound from
the bowel lumen.

13

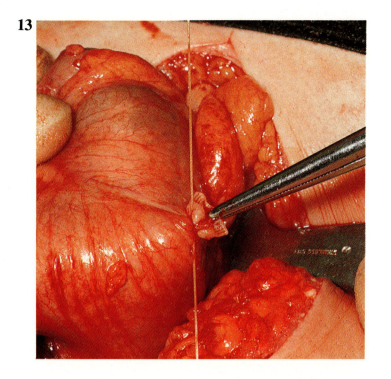

14

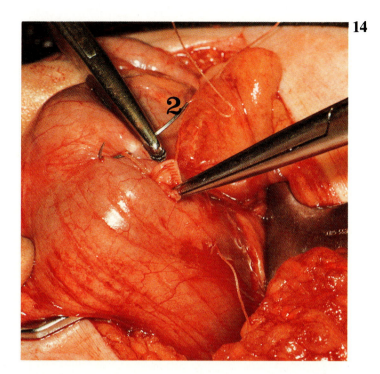

15

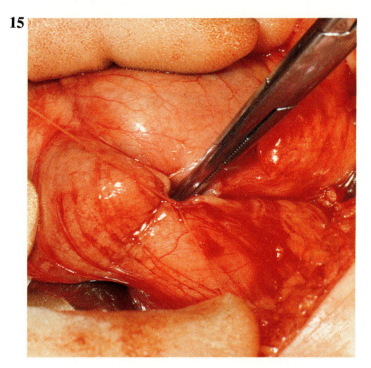

16

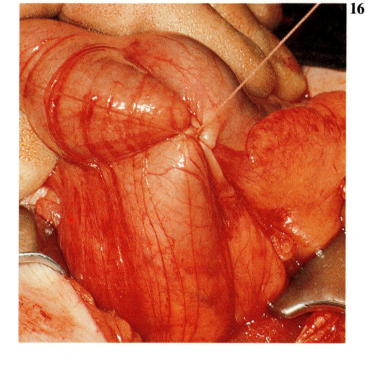

13 to 16 Ligation and inversion of appendix stump

In **Figure 13** the stump of the appendix is tied off with No. 0 PGA suture. In **Figure 14** a round bodied needle carrying a 000 PGA suture (2) encircles the ligated stump. In

Figure 15 the purse string is tightened while the stump is inverted beneath it and in **Figure 16** the purse string is tied off.

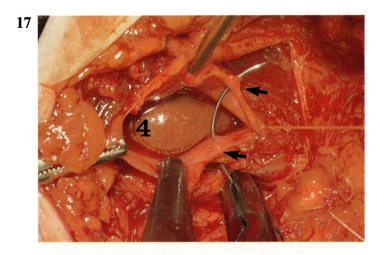

17

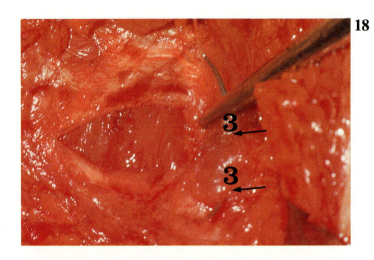

18

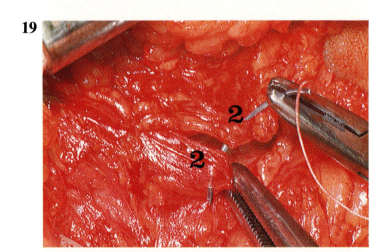

19

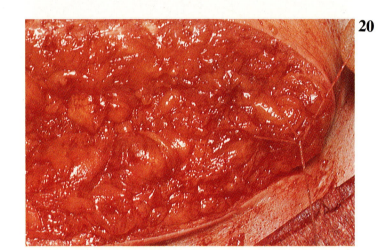

20

17 to 20 Closure of abdomen
In **Figure 17** the peritoneum (4) is seen being closed and is reinforced by including in addition a bite of the transversalis fascia (fine arrows). The needle picks up the edge of the internal oblique muscle (3) when approximating the split fibres in **Figure 18,** the leaves of the external oblique aponeurosis (2) are approximated in **Figure 19** and the fat layer is neatly closed by a few fine stitches of 000 PGA material to eliminate dead space in **Figure 20.**

21 Specimen
The diagnosis of acute appendicitis is confirmed. The lumen is about to obstruct at (1) and there is evidence of old infection and fibrotic narrowing at two points (arrowed).

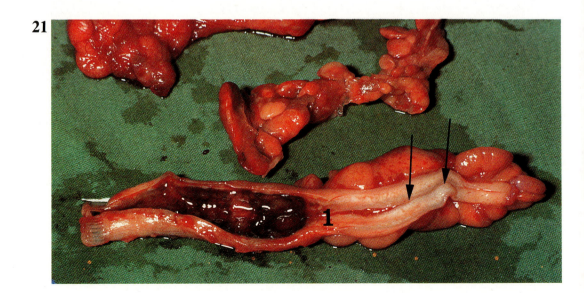

21

2. Acute intestinal obstruction in pregnancy

Occasional vomiting is a relatively common symptom of early pregnancy and of this degree and type is comparatively harmless. Subsequent to the earliest weeks or if at any time it is recurrent or persistent and especially if accompanied by abdominal pain the possibility of bowel obstruction should be questioned.

Small intestine obstruction

The small intestine is gradually displaced into the upper abdomen during pregnancy and if there are adhesions in the pelvis or lower abdomen it is liable to kinking or rotation with subsequent direct or loop obstruction. The rapidly developing loss of fluid and plasma into the bowel lumen leads to severe dehydration and toxaemia while the affected loop of intestine can quickly become necrotic with mesenteric thrombosis and spreading peritonitis. Deterioration of the patient's general condition is rapid, and it is even more essential than in the non-pregnant patient that the diagnosis be established and treatment begun as soon as possible. Perinatal death may result from hypoxia secondary to maternal hypovolaemia or to premature labour because of peritonitis so that the fetus as well as the mother is in danger unless the condition is recognised.

Large intestine obstruction

Large bowel obstruction during pregnancy is less common and less dramatic in onset but it should be kept in mind epecially if the patient has ventral or umbilical herniation. The large intestine is displaced laterally and anteriorly by the growing uterus and is liable to find any abdominal wall hiatus. The develop-

ment to a dangerous degree of obstruction is slower than in the small intestine and is preceded by constipation and abdominal distention but the obstructed loop of bowel may at any time become strangulated and peritonitis ensue. There can be occasions where even the most experienced clinicians are uncertain whether the obstruction is in the large or small bowel but at least the immediate management is the same in both cases.

In the investigation of these cases a clinical history is of great importance and physical examination may reveal abdominal scars to suggest previous peritonitis or adhesion formation. Areas of tenderness are defined by palpation, distention is percussed, peristalsis auscultated and the relative baseline studies completed. **Figure 23** is shown to recall the severe distention which rapidly develops in established intestinal obstruction.

Radiological examination

Such an examination would not be made unless intestinal obstruction were a serious possibility and the fact is that straight antero-posterior abdominal x-rays give help which the clinician can scarcely afford to do without. Air-fluid levels if present (**Figure 22**) clinch the diagnosis of intestinal obstruction and the risks of radiation to the fetus from a single exposure are far outweighed by the benefits obtainable. Early diagnosis may be necessary to save the life of the mother; it is also essential if the fetus is to have a chance of surviving the gross hypoxia which accompanies established intestinal obstruction. Every effort is made to confirm the diagnosis so that treatment can be initiated without delay. Where confirmation cannot be obtained but reasonable doubt remains, the case is treated surgically.

Treatment
Surgical treatment of the condition is by laparotomy at the earliest possible opportunity and with adequate pre-operative fluid replacement. The surgical procedure required will depend on the findings and for those with limited experience of bowel surgery a general surgical colleague should be present or readily available. If resection of intestine is required these are circumstances for the expert. The reward for early diagnosis and bold exploration is the satisfaction of dividing an adhesion and/or undoing a twisted loop of distended but viable intestine. The penalty for delay is the appalling sight and prospect of necrotic gut and mesenteric thrombus (see **Figure 25**). Where laparotomy is undertaken on evidence of possible obstruction but no abnormality is found the surgeon need not be too self-critical and above all should not be influenced against acting similarly in the future where there are indications that acute intestinal obstruction is a real possibility.

22
X-ray showing fluid levels and gas distention in large bowel obstruction.

23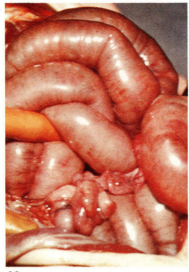

24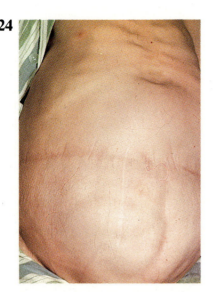

25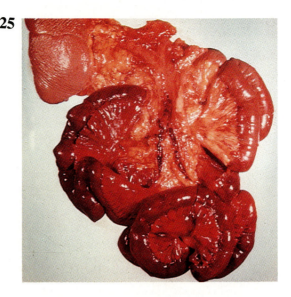

23
Typical appearances of abdominal distension in acute small intestine obstruction.

24
Distended coils of small intestine in a case of post-appendectomy obstruction.

25
Acute mesenteric vascular occlusion consequent on acute intestinal obstruction.

Differential diagnosis in the puerperium

In the special circumstances where the patient has recently been delivered either vaginally, or more particularly by caesarean section, the question of differential diagnosis has to be considered. In these circumstances the patient could be suffering from paralytic ileus or volvulus of the sigmoid colon. Ileus and obstruction ought to be clinically distinguishable from each other but unfortunately they have a habit of occurring together as when bowel obstruction is complicated by a secondary ileus. This is most likely to happen in the presence of severe pelvic inflammatory disease. A diagnosis of paralytic ileus on its own must be substantiated since the penalty for delay in treating obstruction is so severe.

Fortunately radiological examination can resolve most of the difficulties and since the patient has been delivered there is no reason why all necessary x-rays should not be taken to aid diagnosis. The principal differentiating factor is that in paralytic ileus both the small and large intestines are distended although there are other features; in intestinal obstruction a single loop or several loops of small intestine are greatly distended and show definite fluid levels. The large intestine presents a much less well defined appearance. Most surgeons have in their minds a short list of distinguishing factors which they use in differentiating the two conditions. Table I represents that used by the authors and which has at least the merit of extreme simplicity.

TABLE 1

Symptom or Sign	Diagnosis	
	Paralytic Ileus	Intestinal Obstruction
1. Abdominal pain	Discomfort only	Cramp-like and recurring – becoming worse
2. Onset	Within 72 hrs. post-operatively or post-delivery	Generally after 72 hrs.
3. Nausea and vomiting	Yes	Yes
4. Pyrexia	Yes (if peritonitis)	No
5. Tachycardia	Yes +	Yes + +
6. Distention	Yes	Yes
7. Bowel Sounds	No	Yes, peristaltic. Borborygmi and metallic tinkling
8. x-ray	Distention of small and particularly large intestine. No other features.	Loop or loops of distended small intestine. Fluid levels obvious.

Ileus is treated conservatively by nasogastric suction and maintenance of fluid requirements and electrolyte balance by intravenous infusion. Obstruction is treated surgically.

The condition of volvulus of the sigmoid colon is not too uncommon in the immediate post-delivery phase and can be detected from flat and upright antero-posterior x-rays of the abdomen. Treatment of the condition is non-operative in the first instance; by intubating the rectum. The patient is in the knee chest position and the uterus is pushed forward clear of the bowel to allow of the tube being introduced. This often allows the escape of a large amount of gas which relieves the distention and allows the bowel to resume its normal position. Such cases, however, do sometimes require surgical operation.

3. Other acute abdominal crises in pregnancy

Pregnant patients have no immunity to the various acute abdominal conditions to which all are liable. It is important therefore that the medical attendant keeps an open mind to all symptoms and does not narrow the differential diagnosis to pregnancy and pregnancy-related conditions. The need for such a broad outlook has already been seen in relation to acute appendicitis and acute intestinal obstruction.

There are, however, some pregnancy-related conditions which should be kept in mind:

1. Acute pyelitis or acute pyelonephritis

The symptoms of acute renal tract inflammation may closely resemble those of acute surgical emergencies. Severe attacks of pyelitis or pyelonephritis around the 20th week of pregnancy are far from uncommon and are accompanied by acute right-sided abdominal pain, pyrexia, vomiting and restricted breathing. Bladder symptoms may be entirely absent initially but frequency and dysuria usually follow later. On examination the diagnosis is usually suggested by extreme tenderness on compression of the kidney between the hands in the costo-vertebral angle and by tenderness in the line of the ureter. Rigidity is unusual. Urine output is reduced and is very acid: microscopic examination reveals pus and organisms to establish the diagnosis. The importance of obtaining a urine specimen and making a *hanging drop* microscopic examination cannot be over-emphasised.

2. Rupture of the splenic artery

Just why this disaster should occur in late pregnancy is not clear but it is a relatively rare possibility which should be kept in mind. The clinical picture is one of generalised abdominal pain and the development of an intra-abdominal collection of blood without findings to relate it to the uterus, the adnexae or the alimentary tract. Blood replacement and laparotomy are seen to be mandatory and the peritoneal cavity is found to be full of blood. It is usually possible to establish that the source of the bleeding is in the region of the splenic artery although the advanced state of pregnancy makes it difficult to locate the precise point. Clinicians who have had to deal with the condition agree with us that they also were thankful to find that the active source of bleeding had ceased by the time of laparotomy and apart from removing the free blood no specific surgical operation was required. The spleen and its blood supply are so friable that in cases of continuing bleeding from spontaneous or traumatic rupture, splenectomy is the only treatment.

3. Torsion of the adnexae

Apart from tubo-ovarian torsion initiated by the presence of a sizeable and possibly 'known' ovarian cyst the elevated free lateral aspect of the fallopian tube may undergo torsion especially when the ovary is on a longish pedicle. In a more limited degree the free fimbrial end of the tube may undergo torsion and this may be encouraged by the presence of a laterally placed cyst of Morgani. The whole fimbrial end of the tube may become necrotic in such circumstances.

In either case acute abdominal pain and peritoneal irritation with rebound tenderness result and a localised mass may be recognised. It is unlikely that a definitive diagnosis of such conditions would be made preoperatively but it is helpful to know of the various possibilities when doing the obligatory laparotomy.

4. Red degeneration in fibroids

This is referred to elsewhere (page 103). The symptoms and findings may be misleading and suggest the need for exploration but the history and the localisation of the tenderness to the uterus itself should indicate the diagnosis.

7: Ovarian cysts and uterine fibroids complicating pregnancy: incarcerated retroverted gravid uterus

1. Ovarian cysts and tumours

Ovarian enlargement is frequently noted at the first antenatal examination and in the majority of cases it is due to a corpus luteum or follicular type ovarian cyst. Most of these enlargements decrease in size and are not recognisable when the patient is examined again at 16 weeks. There is, however, a group of early pregnancy cysts or ovarian enlargements which are recognised as dangerous or potentially dangerous, and despite the inauspicious circumstances of pregnancy, they require immediate surgical attention. There is a further group of large cysts or ovarian tumours which have been recognised during the pregnancy and are believed to be benign. When there are indications that they may obstruct vaginal delivery or themselves suffer complications during labour they require surgical treatment at term. Table I lists the two groups of cases which require operation:

Cases for surgical treatment during pregnancy

In the Table it will be seen that apart from emergency treatment of a twisted, necrotic, haemorrhagic or ruptured cyst the indications in Group I are all governed by the need for early recognition of malignancy and anticipation of its spread.

There is evidence that carcinoma of the ovary is greatly on the increase. Thus it is estimated[1] that it has doubled in incidence in the United States in the last 30 years with the incidence of malignancy of tumours during pregnancy between 2.5 and 5 per cent; it is more common in the over 30 group. If diagnosed early and treated surgically the survival rate exceeds 60 per cent, but if there is delay the prognosis is very poor. The disease is particularly dangerous because it gives no warning of its presence and its development is even more insidious and rapid in pregnancy.

TABLE 1

1. CYSTS WHICH DEMAND LAPAROTOMY DURING PREGNANCY

(i)   The cyst has undergone torsion, has ruptured, or bleeding has taken place into its cavity.

(ii) The cyst was diagnosed as probably follicular but it increases in size after the 16th week of pregnancy.

(iii) Circumstances as in (ii) and especially when the cyst contains solid elements or is fixed in the pelvis.

(iv) Bilateral cysts which increase in size and are immobilised by adhesions.

(v)   Cysts or enlargements where there is evidence of possible ovarian malignancy, e.g. solid growth, fixation, hardness, palpable omentum, malignancy found elsewhere in the body.

2. CYSTS WHICH DEMAND SURGICAL TREATMENT AT TERM

(i)   Large cysts which lie below the presenting part and obstruct labour.

(ii) Large cysts which do not directly obstruct labour but are likely to be traumatised during delivery.

(iii) Cysts which are unlikely to interfere with delivery but their nature is in doubt and malignancy cannot be excluded with certainty.

The particular clinical features which might raise suspicion are mentioned in the Table. Clearly this is an area where the surgeon must keep alert to the possibilities and just as surgical exploration is essential in acute abdominal conditions of pregnancy even when complete confirmation is lacking, so also is laparotomy necessary for ovarian tumours if there is any doubt about their safety. Even if the ovary contains a corpus luteum it can be removed without risk of disturbing the pregnancy since its endocrine functions will have been taken over by the placenta by 14–16 weeks of pregnancy. Operations on this group should be done with the utmost care and the main consideration is to avoid peritoneal trauma by gentle handling and the avoidance of pulling on the peritoneal edges with forceps.

Cases for surgical treatment at term

Ovarian cysts necessitating surgical treatment at term are generally less sinister and the problems are primarily obstetrical. Nevertheless a proportion of such tumours prove to be malignant and even when benign their blood supply at this stage tends to be precarious so that they are particularly liable to necrosis, rupture and internal haemorrhage[2].

When it is estimated that the cyst or tumour will inevitably obstruct vaginal delivery, operation is done a week before the estimated date of delivery and a lower uterine segment caesarean section is followed by excision of the cyst or oophorectomy as required. Before finally arranging operation in such a case the surgeon should make a last careful check on the relationship of the cyst to the uterus and particularly the presenting part of the fetus. An opportunity for clinical error is seen by studying the drawings in **Figures 1** and **2**. In **Figure 1** the cyst is firmly trapped in the pelvic pouch below the presenting part and abdominal delivery is required. In **Figure 2**, however, the cyst which lay below the presenting part until the final weeks of pregnancy has now been pulled upwards by the broad ligament through its attachment to the fundus uteri, and has escaped from the pelvis. While still displacing the fetal head anteriorly it is unlikely to obstruct labour and the head will enter the pelvis immediately contractions begin.

If there is no obstruction to labour and the operation is done solely to remove the cyst, the ideal is to deliver the patient vaginally and remove the tumour abdominally after 48 hours. It is important to check carefully that torsion does not occur in the interval between delivery and operation. Torsion is particularly liable to occur when the uterus is rapidly enlarging in early pregnancy or rapidly involuting following delivery; the latter accounts for 40 per cent of cases. If in the absence of obstruction by the tumour the patient experiences severe pain and peritoneal tenderness during labour or immediately post partum, the possibility of torsion or rupture indicates the need for immediate surgical intervention. When first recognised during the puerperium cysts or tumours should be removed as soon as possible.

Diagnosis in late pregnancy

Clinical estimation of ovarian tumours in late pregnancy is limited to feeling their lower pole vaginally or preferably rectally and there is a need for supportive diagnostic aids. Radiographic examination is out of the question and laparoscopy would cause peritoneal irritation and the enlarged uterus make intra-peritoneal visualisation almost impossible, so that the method has no application in these cases. Thus it has come to be accepted that one can only satisfactorily assess the situation at laparotomy when the ovary can be seen with the naked eye and its consistency and nature actually felt with the fingers. Ultrasonic scanning by modern methods can, however, give a considerable amount of information on such ovarian enlargements and this non-invasive and harmless method is increasingly used in such cases. **Figures 3** and **4** clearly show the size and position of large ovarian cysts in pregnancy. By demonstrating the general composition and regularity or otherwise of the tumour matrix the method can give aid in clinical diagnosis.

Operations: Technique

The following procedures are the most frequently required:–

1 Ovarian cystectomy for large cyst in early pregnancy

2 Salpingo-oophorectomy for torsion of ovarian cyst

3 Ovariotomy following caesarean section in obstructed labour

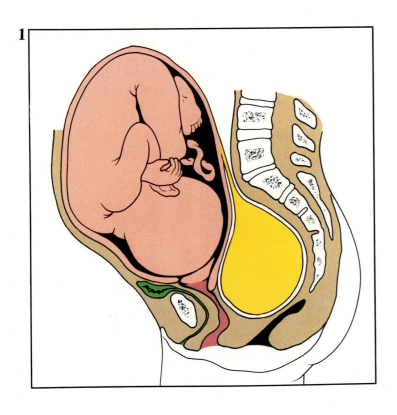

1 Ovarian cyst in late pregnancy
Ovarian cyst firmly fixed in pelvis; it will undoubtedly obstruct labour.

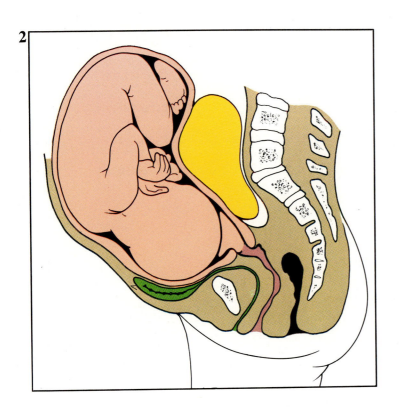

2 Ovarian cyst in late pregnancy
An ovarian cyst which is displacing the fetal head in similar fashion but without itself being trapped in the pelvis. It will probably permit vaginal delivery.

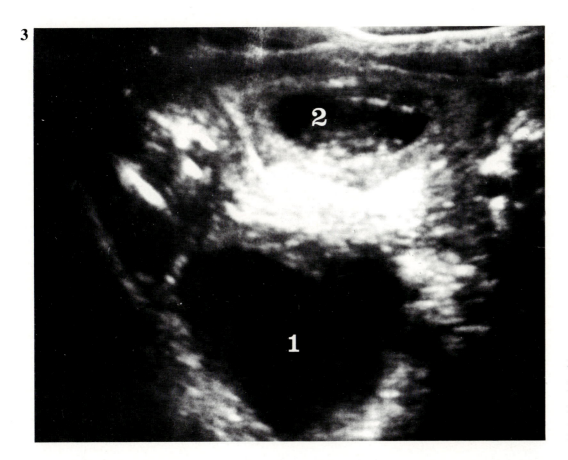

3
A transverse ultrasonic scan taken in early pregnancy revealing a large ovarian cyst (1) lying almost directly behind the pregnant uterus (2).

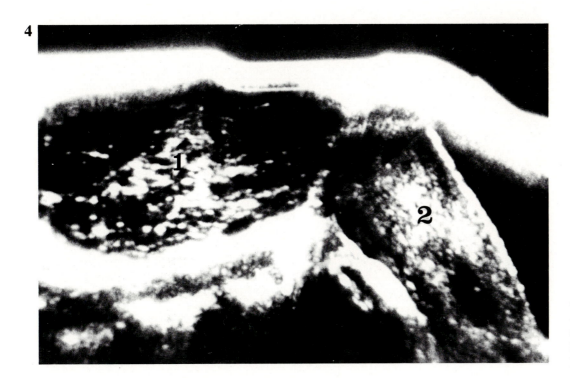

4
A longitudinal ultrasonic scan showing the presence of a pseudomucinous cyst (1) lying behind a puerperal uterus (2).

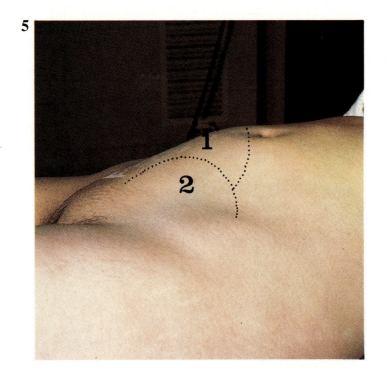

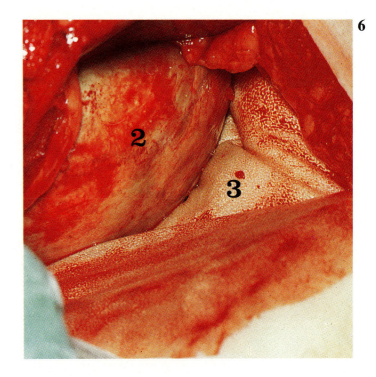

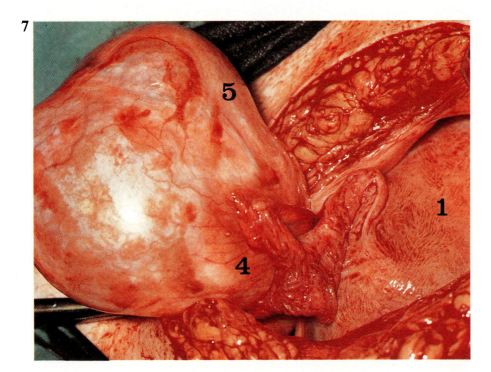

5 Surface outline of ovarian cyst
The patient is 18 weeks pregnant and the uterus (1) is displaced to the right by a cystic mobile swelling of approximately 15 cm diameter (2).

6 Exploration of abdomen at laparotomy
The surgeon's right hand (3) introduced into the abdomen behind the cyst (2) establishes that it is mobile and smooth and is displacing the uterus downwards and to the right. It is rather smaller than was estimated.

7 Cyst delivered from abdomen
The cyst has been delivered from the abdomen and is displaced forwards towards the symphysis pubis to expose its pedicle (4). There are no adhesions, no free fluid in the peritoneal cavity, and the cyst has no solid areas. It is therefore considered probably benign. The uterus is numbered (1) and the left tube (5).

8

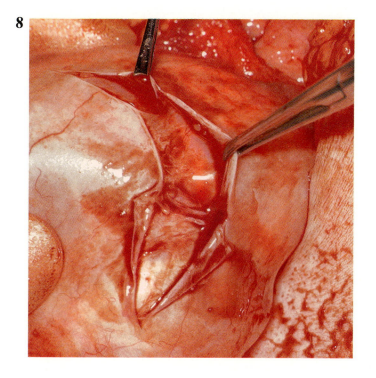

9

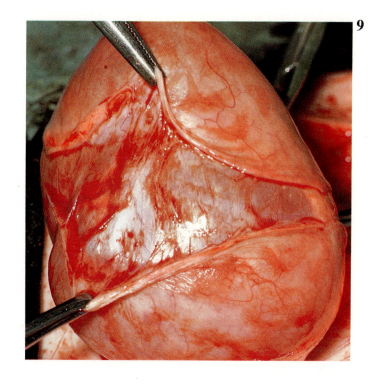

10

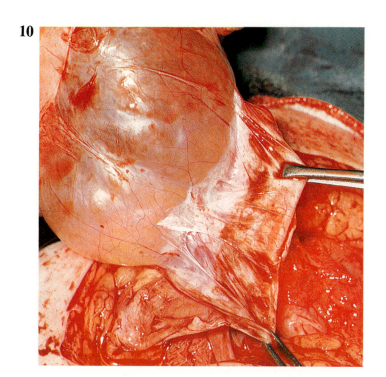

8 to 10 Ovarian cystectomy
Three stages in enucleation of the cyst are shown and are self explanatory. The thin capsule of ovarian tissue is divided well away from the main mass of the ovary to expose the cyst without perforating it. The thin layer is then dissected off with great care. This has almost been completed in **Figure 10.**

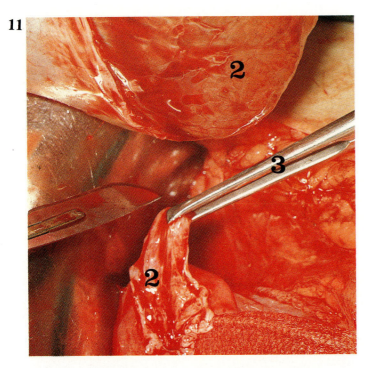

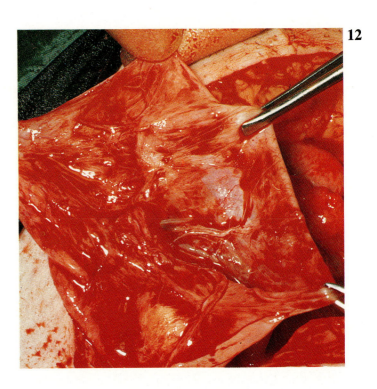

11 and 12 Displaying the ovarian base of the cyst
The cyst (2) is finally detached with the scalpel in **Figure 11** and the remaining ovarian tissue (2) is held in tissue forceps

(3). In **Figure 12** the ovarian raw surface is held open by tissue forceps and is approximately 7 cm square.

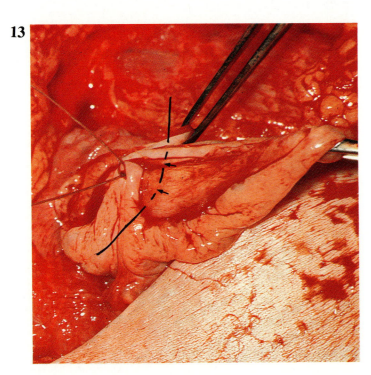

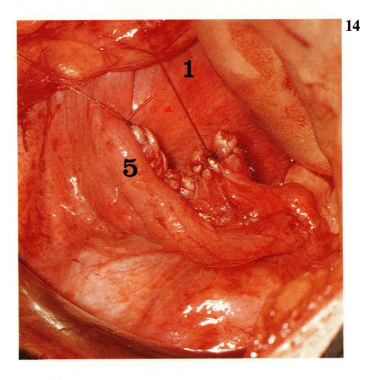

13 and 14 Reconstitution of ovary
The open surface of the ovary is closed in two layers with 00 PGA continuous sutures. The first is seen in **Figure 13.** The needle enters and leaves the cavity near the edges and takes a series of bites of the surface to eliminate dead space (arrowed). The ovary is thereby bunched up to resemble its

normal shape and the second suture closes the edges in X fashion to complete haemostasis and leave a smooth wound. (See Volume 2, pages 184–5). The reconstructed ovary is seen returned to its normal position in **Figure 14.** The uterus is numbered (1) and the left fallopian tube (5).

II Salpingo-oophorectomy for torsion of ovarian cyst

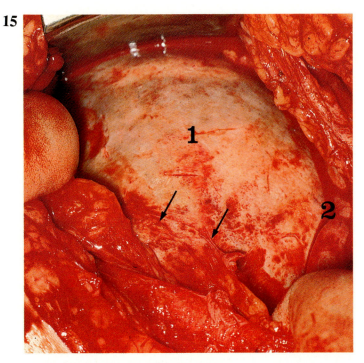

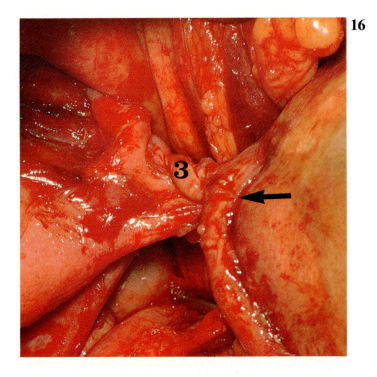

15 and 16 Appearance at laparotomy
The dull congested surface of the cyst (1) presents in the wound in **Figure 15.** There is a small amount of free fluid in the peritoneal cavity (2) and the omentum is lightly adherent to the cyst surface where arrowed. In **Figure 16** the site of torsion (arrowed) is displayed and the fallopian tube (3) is seen to be involved. Torsion has extended to 2½ turns and the blood supply has been completely cut off. Salpingo-oophorectomy is the correct treatment.

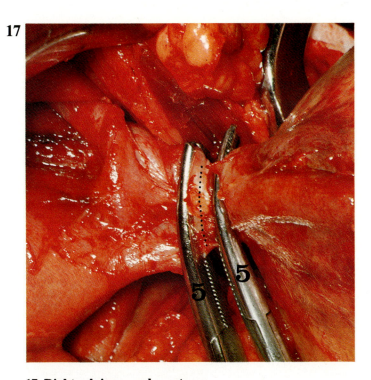

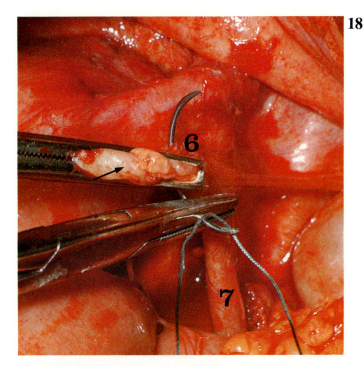

17 Right salpingo-oophorectomy
The twisted pedicle is undone and is clamped just medial to the site of interruption of the blood supply by heavy curved forceps (5) and (5). The twisted cyst is then removed by cutting between the forceps along the dotted line. A cuff of tissue is retained distal to the medial clamp.

18 Transfixing tubo-ovarian pedicle
The forceps holds the pedicle of the ovary and the lumen of the fallopian tube is indicated by the arrow. A No. 1 PGA suture (6) transfixes the pedicle in preparation for ligation. The infundibulo-pelvic ligament is seen at (7).

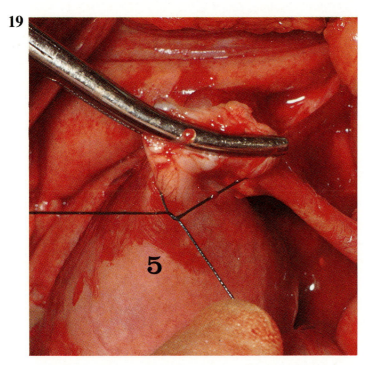

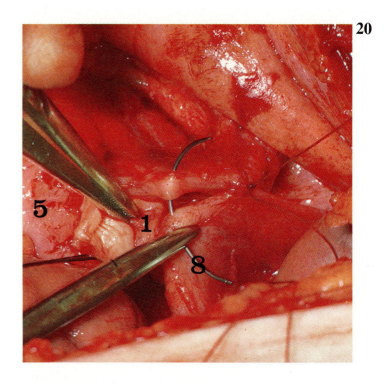

19 to 21 Ligation and inversion of tubo-ovarian pedicle
In **Figure 19** the ligature, which has already been tied under the point of the forceps, takes a firm hold of the whole pedicle under the heel of the forceps. In **Figure 20** a 000 PGA suture on a round-bodied needle (8) picks up the peritoneum to encircle the pedicle (1) preparatory to burying it. This has been completed in **Figure 21** where the suture is being cut short (arrowed). The uterus is numbered (5) where visible on the photographs.

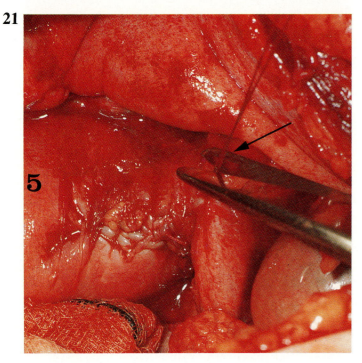

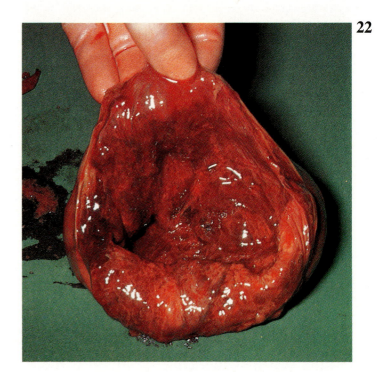

22 Specimen
A collapsed cyst with congested wall which is already undergoing necrosis.

III Ovariotomy following caesarean section in obstructed labour

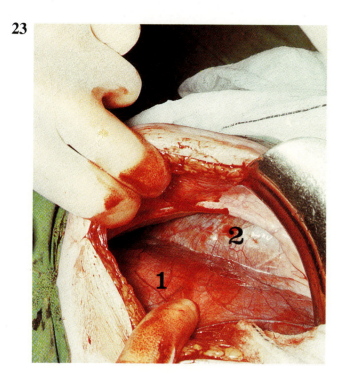

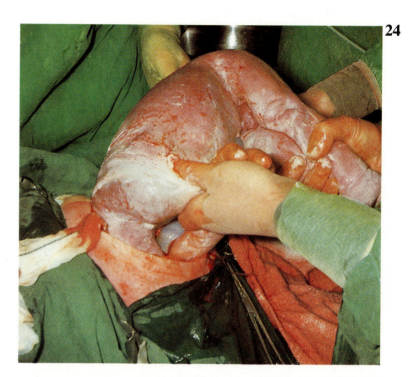

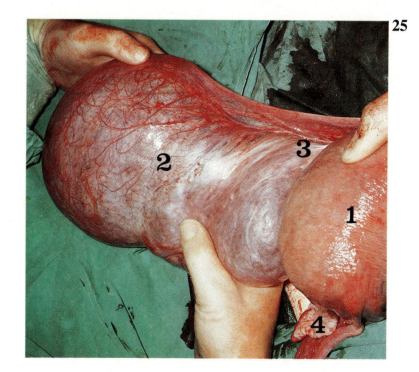

23 Appearance on opening abdomen
The uterus (1) is pushed forwards by the cyst and has to be retracted by the surgeon's finger to expose the bladder (2) and the utero-vesical pouch. Note that a midline incision has been used in this case.

24 Caesarean section
The fetus is seen being delivered through a transverse lower uterine segment incision and the uterus is subsequently sutured and the utero-vesical peritoneum closed.

25 Cyst and uterus displayed in wound
The relative size of the cyst (2) and the post-delivery uterus (1) is seen. It is held up to show the broad pedicle (3); the right ovary (4) is of normal size and consistency.

26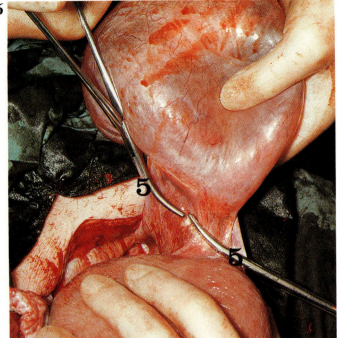

27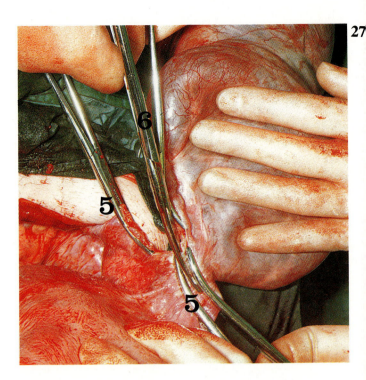

26 and 27 Ovariotomy
In **Figure 26** the broad pedicle is spanned by two long curved forceps (5) and (5) and in **Figure 27** these have been matched by similar forceps and the scissors (6) cut between to detach the cyst.

28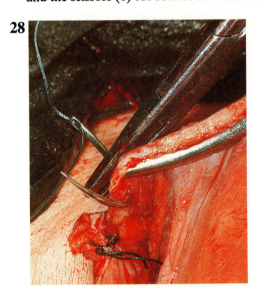

29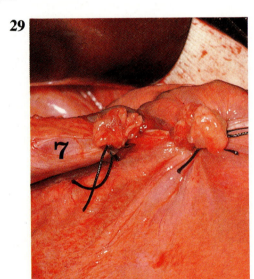

30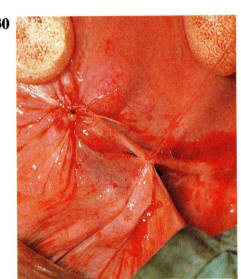

28 to 30 Ligation and covering of ovarian pedicle
In **Figure 28** one-half of the pedicle has been secured with a No. 1 PGA ligature and the other is being transfixed with the needle. In **Figure 29** both have been tied and await inversion or covering. There is very little loose peritoneum in this vascular area but the left round ligament (7) is adjacent and is always useful to cover such an area. In **Figure 30** it is being used for this purpose and the ovarian pedicle is already completely covered.

2. Uterine fibroids

Management during pregnancy

Fibroids of a size likely to cause complications are usually obvious at the beginning of pregnancy and the obstetrician should discuss their significance with the patient explaining that they are very unlikely to cause miscarriage. They may cause pain in middle pregnancy but there is no question of surgical treatment being necessary. If labour is obstructed by the fibroids surgical delivery might, however, be required.

The enormous increase in vascularity of the pregnant uterus and the very rapid rise in the level of the uterine fundus were referred to in Chapter 1 (page 15) and it is not surprising that fibroids which normally enlarge at a rate proportionate to that of the uterus cause problems in later pregnancy. **Figure 31** shows a typical case of fibroids in pregnancy and the ultrasonic scan on **Figures 32** and **33** indicate the value of that method in establishing the relative position of the fibroid or fibroids in relation to the amniotic sac and the fetus. The speed with which fibroids grow and the size they may attain can be disconcerting and patients generally need a good deal of reassurance. Treatment during pregnancy is always non-surgical.

Management at term

As term approaches contingency plans may be made to deliver by caesarean section but with the development of the lower uterine segment and retraction of the fundus in late pregnancy and early labour, the fibroid may be drawn up from the pelvis and allow the presenting part to replace it there so that operative delivery is not eventually required. If it is required, as for example when the pelvis is completely occupied by a large fibroid, it is advisable to obtain maximum information on the position of the fetus in relation to the fibroids and this may be aided by the use of sonar.

A straightforward lower uterine segment caesarean section through transverse abdominal and uterine incisions may be possible, but with large fibroids it is generally preferable to make a midline abdominal incision, since that allows of a more complete reconnaissance when the abdomen has been opened, and the site and direction of the uterine incision can be chosen to suit the position of the fetus. It can be difficult sometimes to see where one ought to make the incision and it is wise to take plenty of time in trying to make the correct choice. It is obvious that a transverse lower segment uterine incision will frequently be out of the question and the surgeon will have to accept what is the obvious approach even if it is in the upper segment. When the fetus and placenta have been delivered, the uterine incision is closed as in a routine caesarean section and no attempt is made to do myomectomy. The only two exceptions are a fibroid encountered in the line of the incision and a subserous fibroid on a well defined and relatively narrow pedicle.

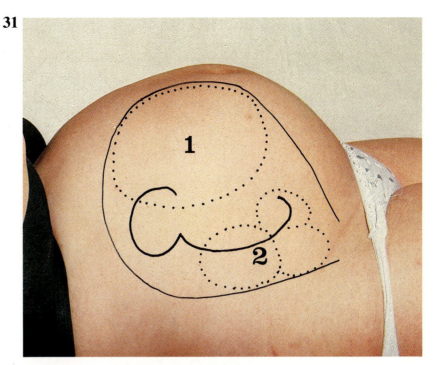

31 Abdomen enlarged by uterine fibroids
The patient is only 28 weeks pregnant but the uterus is already enormous. There is one large fibroid at the fundus which is surface marked (1) and several smaller ones on the right side (2). The general position of the fetus is indicated by the overlay.

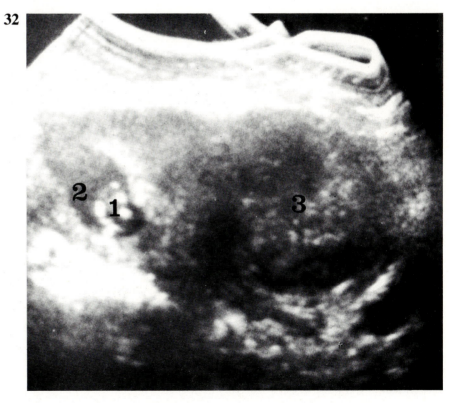

32
Transverse ultrasonic scan of a large fibroid complicating a case of early pregnancy. The fetal parts (1) are visible within the gestation sac (2) and the fibroid which has undergone some degeneration is numbered (3).

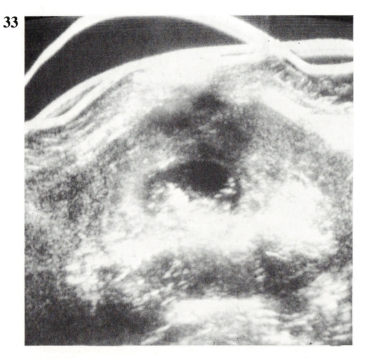

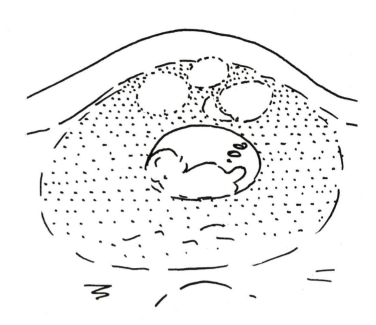

33 and 34
Longitudinal ultrasonic scan of a uterus in early pregnancy containing multiple fibroids. A trace of this scan is shown beside the photograph.

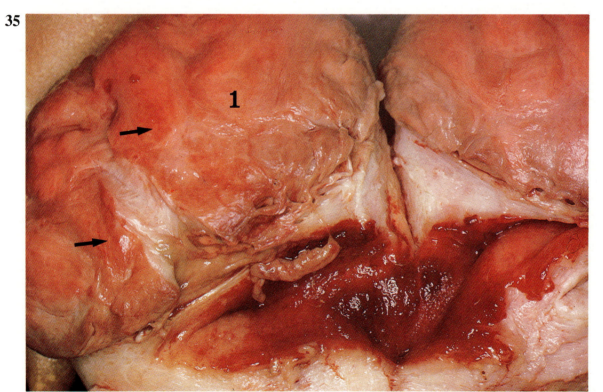

35 Red degeneration in a fibroid
The clinical history is an involved one but the uterus removed at 22 weeks pregnancy contained a fibroid which was undergoing red degeneration. Note the greasy appearance of the fibro-myomatous tissue (1) which is stained red by haemoglobin breakdown products where arrowed. The cavity of the uterus has been opened and is congested.

Red degeneration

Red degeneration in fibroids is characterised by the type of tissue reaction shown in **Figure 35.** Increasing oedema in the fibroid is followed by ischaemia with partial necrosis and the red staining resulting from haemoglobin breakdown. The complication can at times be a very painful one.

The treatment is always expectant and surgery has no place in its management. Analgesics and reassurance will be required but the symptoms gradually settle although they may recur from time to time. In the third trimester the symptoms usually abate.

Subsequent hysterectomy for fibroids

Many such cases require hysterectomy and one is always surprised by the decrease in size and harmless appearance of the fibroids a few months after delivery. **Figure 36** is shown as an example of preconceived diagnosis that was wildly astray. Throughout later pregnancy the patient was reckoned to have an irreducible transverse lie and was only saved from elective caesarean section by unexpectedly and quickly completing labour. The hysterectomy specimen shows that the transverse lie was, in fact, the enlarged sausage shaped fibroid on the left of the photograph. Ultrasonic scanning would probably have shown the true state of affairs.

36

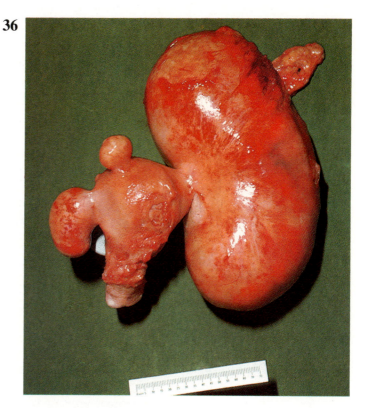

36 Hysterectomy specimen of large fibroid referred to in text.

3. Incarcerated retroverted gravid uterus

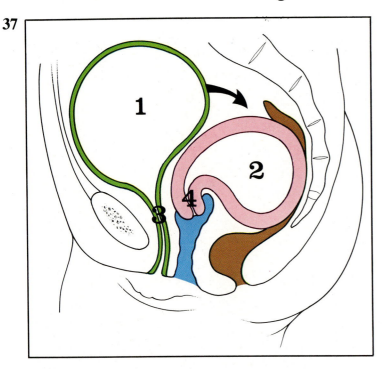

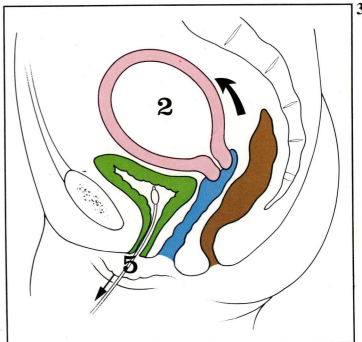

This condition is introduced in the general context of large abdominal swellings in pregnancy because it can give rise to rapid abdominal enlargement around 14–16 weeks gestation. It is not always immediately recognised that a greatly distended bladder is responsible and that a simple and non-surgical procedure will always succeed in correcting it.

Rapid uterine growth can pose problems when the uterus is retroverted and the progress of events in these circumstances is generally agreed. A uterus which is retroverted at the beginning of pregnancy will increase simultaneously in height and forward projection so that in the normal course of events the fundus will lie anterior to the sacral promontary by about the twelfth week. Even if the uterus is firmly tethered in retroversion and retroflexion it will grow forward by a process of sacculation whereby a regional thinning and forward extension of the anterior uterine wall will allow the fetus to negotiate the promontary of the sacrum towards its future abdominal location.

The factor which may upset nature's allowance for correction is a persistently full or partially full bladder, since it displaces the uterus into the posterior pelvis where it is unable either to anteflex or sacculate. As it continues to grow in its retroverted and trapped position it pushes the bladder base higher into the abdomen with consequent elongation of the urethra which becomes more easily compressed and occluded by surrounding structures. The problem is thereby compounded, the bladder becomes distended and overflow incontinence is apt to be diagnosed as 'frequency' associated with acute cystitis. The distended bladder meantime has the appearance and feel of a 12–14 weeks uterus until catheterisation reveals the true state of affairs.

37 and 38
The diagrams illustrate the mechanics of incarceration and its relief by bladder decompression. In **Figure 37** the full bladder (1) prevents the body of the uterus (2) from coming into anteversion and by pulling on the urethra (3) and elevating the cervix (4) actually increases the retroversion in the direction of the curved arrow. In **Figure 38** the catheter (5) has emptied the bladder, the urethra shortens and the cervix drops so that the uterine body is free to enter the lower abdomen in the direction of the curved arrow.

Treatment is non-surgical and is both simple and effective. A Foley catheter is introduced and the bladder is decompressed slowly over a few hours if it is very distended. Thereafter the catheter is left in place with closed drainage into a bag for 48 or at the most 72 hours during which time the uterine fundus invariably escapes into the abdomen and once there it cannot re-enter the pelvis.

There may be merit in trying to anticipate events and prevent the incarceration. When one recognises that the retroversion is more than the innocuous mobile type the patient may be advised (with suitable reassurance) to encourage the uterus into anteversion by keeping the bladder relatively empty and adopting the supine position when resting. Many patients say that they frequently rest in this way in any case. Any urinary symptoms should naturally be reported to the doctor. The incidence of the complication may be decreasing but since adopting the measures mentioned here the authors cannot remember seeing a single case of incarceration.

8: The control of haemorrhage in operative obstetrics

The changes in the cardiovascular and haematological systems described in Chapter 1 and the preponderant role of haemorrhage in most obstetric emergencies makes this a matter for special consideration. Methods of controlling bleeding during particular operations are described and the technical aspects of blood replacement are dealt with in Chapter 15 but there are some general observations on clinical approach and surgical technique which should be taken into account. The clinical picture is easily recalled. The patient is pale, cyanosed and restless with rapid respiration, tachycardia and a systolic blood pressure of under 100 mmHg. She may in fact be semi-comotose or even completely comotose. Since the pregnant woman can tolerate a greater than normal blood loss such findings indicate the effects of a severe haemorrhage. Severe bleeding may occur during pregnancy, in the course of an operation or in the immediate post-partum period; it is always frightening and it is important that the surgeon in charge maintains a calm exterior and controls events in a logical, and incisive manner. The usual requirements of blood replacement, anaesthesia, operative assistance and fetal care necessitate an obstetrical team and it is in the best interests of the patient if the surgeon can delegate the various responsibilities to those concerned. At tissue level the pregnant patient's blood vessels are dilated and thin so that hurried or rough handling will quickly give rise to even more bleeding when it is essential that the operative field be kept quite clear. Technique should be adapted to the circumstances as for example in defining arteries or veins before securing and dividing them, and since use of the diathermy is usually contraindicated bleeding points have to be secured and ligated individually. Actively bleeding vessels are secured as they are encountered, otherwise the total blood loss is added to as the operation proceeds. These points may seem self evident but the usual surgical routine may be threatened when the fetus is known to be in immediate danger or massive haemorrhage gives rise to a natural impatience and tendency to cut corners in finding the source of the bleeding.

Treatment protocol in cases of severe emergency haemorrhage and hypovolaemic shock

An outline management for cases of severe bleeding is essential and that set out here is of standard pattern.

The prime requirement is to halt the process while it is still reversible and before acidosis and cell damage lead to cardiac and vital organ failure.

The following measures are implemented very much in the order in which they are set out:

1. Pain, anxiety and restlessness are relieved by the administration of analgesic drugs of the pethedine and morphine groups as required and indicated.

2. An intravenous infusion is set up and blood is obtained for cross-matching and grouping if that is required. Five per cent dextrose or Hartmann's solution may be given initially; in desperate circumstances Group 0 Rhesus Negative blood may be used. The intravenous drip apparatus is subsequently used for the giving of blood and is the only satisfactory route for the administration of sedatives and cardiac supportive drugs in such circumstances.

3. An airway must be established and oxygen administered by mask or endotracheal tube to maintain oxygenation of the vital centres.

4. Once a supply of blood has been assured a central venous pressure catheter (see Chapter 15, page 192) is introduced since only thus can one obtain accurate information on the amount of blood replacement required.

5. The surgeon meantime prepares to seek the cause and source of the haemorrhage. This may be possible without anaesthesia but it is generally required and it is essential that the patient's general condition and degree of shock allow it to be given with safety. The circulating blood volume must be adequate to sustain body function and in the case of continuing haemorrhage, blood replacement must be adequate to compensate for it until the surgeon can bring the bleeding under control. Such decisions and the timing of surgical intervention are very dependent on blood pressure and CVP readings.

6. Blood coagulation factors have to be taken into account when giving large volume blood transfusions. The anti-coagulant citric acid – dextrose component in transfused blood can quickly cause citric intoxication in a shocked patient and 10 per cent calcium gluconate is normally added to each litre of blood after the initial 2 litres.

7. Some degree of acidosis is almost inevitable in the circumstances of severe haemorrhage and blood replacement. Biochemical confirmation should not be awaited if there is clinical evidence of its development and sodium bicarbonate 100 M.Eq. is given intravenously as indicated.

8. Following immediate emergency treatment, continuous monitoring of the patient's general condition is carried out by all parameters available. This is obtained systemically from the following sources:
   (i) cardiovascular – arterial BP recording, CVP recording, ECG.
   (ii) respiratory – respiratory rate, blood gas analysis – pH, etc.
   (iii) renal – urinary output and specific gravity, presence of casts.
   (iv) haematological – Hb & PCV estimations, coagulation factor estimates.

9. Corrective management at a later stage may be required in the light of monitored findings:
   (i) Administration of anti-coagulants in the case of disseminated intravascular coagulation.
   (ii) Administration of cortico-steroids for cardiac support in cases of severe and persistent hypovolaemic shock. The routine dosage of hydrocortisone is 1g per kilo of body weight, given intravenously.
   (iii) Few clinicians are prepared to commit themselves on the use of vaso-constrictor and vaso-dilatory drugs. They can be of benefit in a strictly limited area; outside of that sector both groups can produce unwanted and dangerous side effects. Their definitive role is beyond the scope of discussion in a summary of treatment such as this.

I. Control of haemorrhage in certain specific situations

1. From a torn cervix (post delivery)

When severe vaginal bleeding occurs at this time the first requirement is to establish its source and find whether it is possible to control it per vaginam. The cervix is exposed by a speculum and examined with the anterior and posterior lips held apart by tissue forceps. It may be apparent that the bleeding is coming from the cavity of the uterus and cannot be controlled vaginally but in a proportion of cases there is a deeply torn cervix or an extensive vaginal laceration with spouting arteries. The uterus is well contracted in such cases and the surgical management is to control any actively bleeding vessels by underrunning them with a stitch and then proceeding to a careful repair of the torn tissues. **Figure 1** indicates the method of dealing with a deeply torn cervix and repair of vaginal laceration presents no problems.

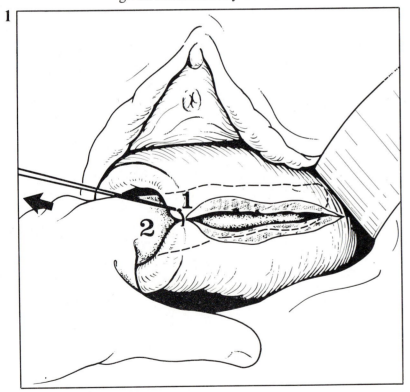

1 Repair of torn cervix
Non-viable traumatised tissue is trimmed from the torn edges and a full thickness holding suture (1) is inserted to make a precise approximation at the junction of ecto- and endo-cervix. With the uncut ends drawn in the direction of the arrow, the left forefinger (2) is introduced into the cervical canal and used as a support while the requisite number of through-and-through No. 0 PGA sutures are placed to give smooth approximation both within the canal and on the ecto-cervix.

In this context the question of *packing the uterus* should be mentioned. When bleeding continues despite an apparently contracting uterus, firmly packing it with gauze might appear a reasonable answer to a frightening situation, and it is a method which is still mentioned in some textbooks. This is a pity because the procedure is now quite discredited and the fact is that the pressure of a gauze pack within the uterus will not arrest arterial bleeding. Blood soon begins to drip from the end of the gauze and precious time and a good deal of additional blood has been lost in a mistaken and useless exercise.

2. After uterine evacuation

Evacuation of the uterus following abortion may result in serious blood loss unless it is done with care. Too rapid dilatation of the cervix can, of course, result in splitting of the circular muscle at the internal os with bleeding from a cervical artery. In recent cases of incomplete abortion the cervix is open and it is advantageous to introduce the finger into the uterus to separate the retained products. The cervix, however, becomes closed and firm remarkably soon and it is then both unrealistic and dangerous to dilate it to finger size. Intravenous ergometrine given during evacuation of the uterus cuts down blood loss considerably and should normally be used in post abortion cases. Compression of the uterus between the fingers of one hand in the vagina and the flat of the other on the lower abdomen is a useful method of expressing blood clot from the cavity and preventing further haemorrhage (see **Figure 2**).

3. Haemostasis at caesarean section

    (i)   during incision of the lower segment
    (ii) during placental separation
    (iii) in cases of placenta praevia
    (iv) in the presence of an undeveloped lower uterine segment.

    These very important aspects of haemostasis are integral to the performance of caesarean section and are fully dealt with in Chapter 9 of this volume.

4. Haemostasis during treatment of ruptured uterus

The necessary steps to control severe bleeding in such circumstances are dealt with in Chapter 10.

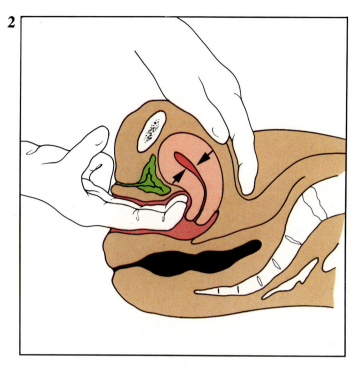

2 Compression of uterine cavity to express blood clot and encourage muscular contraction
The uterus will only contract satisfactorily if empty and when the retained products have been separated from the uterine wall and the bulkier pieces removed with forceps, this is the best method of controlling bleeding.

II. Ligation of internal iliac artery

Ligation of the internal iliac artery is a recognised method of controlling severe and continuing pelvic haemorrhage. It is particularly applicable to obstetric cases where there is tearing into the lower uterine segment or base of the broad ligament during difficult caesarean sections or as the result of a ruptured or traumatised uterus. Uncontrollable bleeding when the uterine wall seems little more substantial than the blood clot is alarming and demands positive action.

The operation is not difficult as long as one identifies the artery clearly before passing the ligature around the trunk. It is generally said that the anterior branch only should be ligated but in the emergency situation envisaged, it is dangerous and time consuming to seek to isolate the anterior branch since it is very easy to tear the accompanying internal iliac vein. Such a happening vitiates the purpose of the operation. The aim should be to secure the presenting trunk once it has been clearly defined. The posterior branch comes off posteriorly at an oblique angle and is therefore unlikely to be included in the ligature. Even if it is, the collateral circulation in its distribution is excellent. Ligation of one or both internal iliac arteries is most unlikely to have any detrimental effect on blood supply in the circumstances of pregnancy.

Surgical technique

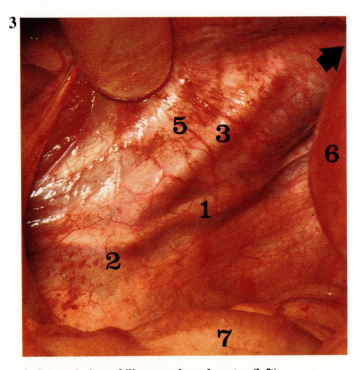

3 General view of iliac vessels and ureter (left)
The abdominal contents are held back by the fingers to demonstrate the anatomy at the pelvic brim. Through the peritoneum the outline of the ureter (1) is seen crossing the common iliac artery (2). The external iliac artery (3) is easily visible with the psoas muscle (5) lateral to it. The uterus is medial (6) and the rectum is in the foreground (7). The broad arrow points towards the symphysis pubis in these photographs.

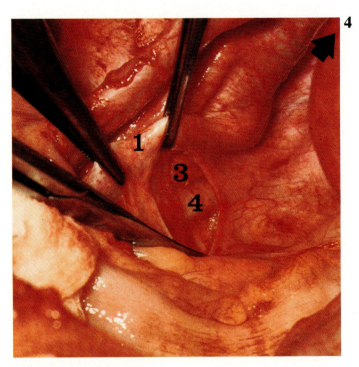

4 Exposure of left ureter
The peritoneum has been opened with scissors and the ureter (1) is lifted up to give a view of the external (3) and internal (4) iliac arteries.

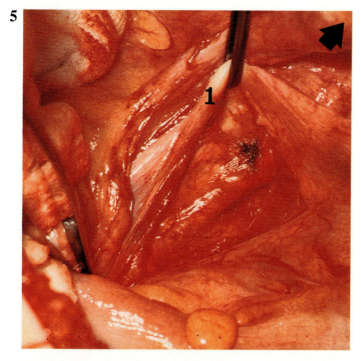

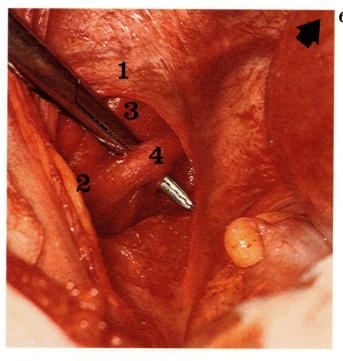

5 Retraction and safeguarding of ureter
Dissection has progressed a stage further and the ureter (1) is lifted up by an encircling tissue forceps and kept clear of the large vessels at the proposed site of ligation.

6 Exposure of internal iliac artery
The internal iliac artery (4) and the external iliac artery (3) are seen clearly just at the bifurcation of the common iliac artery (2). The forceps displays the internal iliac artery.

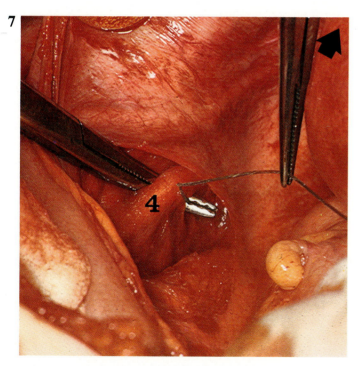

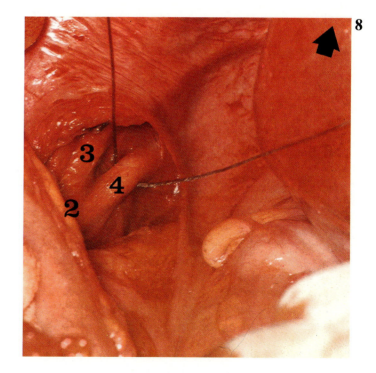

7 and 8 Ligation of internal iliac artery
In **Figure 7** the ligature is picked up by the forceps to under-run the anterior branch of the artery and in **Figure 8** encircles it ready for ligation.

III. Prophylactic exposure of internal iliac arteries prior to hysterectomy for chorio-carcinoma

In certain cases of chorio-carcinoma where hysterectomy is required it is realised from the outset that there must be a danger of severe bleeding during the operation. It may be prudent to define and encircle the internal iliac vessels with tapes as a preliminary step in the operation and this is illustrated in **Figure 9.** With the tapes in place, the surgeon is able to control or limit bleeding from the uterine arteries if mobilisation and detachment of the uterus is accompanied by severe blood loss.

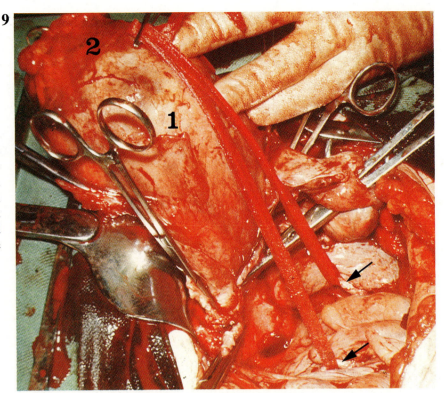

9 Exposure of internal iliac vessels
The tapes have been placed around the internal iliac arteries in the manner described in the text (arrowed). The uterus (1) is held forward and can be seen to be bulky and very vascular with omental adhesion to an area of extension of the tumour through the serosal surface at (2).

IV. Therapeutic arterial embolisation to control pelvic haemorrhage

The use of a transcatheter embolisation to control pelvic haemorrhage from various causes has been reported from several centres in the United States[1,2,3]. The method is attractive in that only local anaesthesia is required and the operation can be done when technical difficulties or the state of the patient preclude surgical management of the condition. Absorbable emboli of gelatin sponge (Gelfoam) may be used but there is a wide choice of non-absorbable materials which includes silicone microspheres, fluid mixtures and balloons[4].

Further promising experience with the method has been reported[5,6]. The authors have no personal experience of the method but bring it to the notice of readers since it is not difficult to imagine circumstances where it could be applicable.

V. Management of disseminated intravascular coagulation

This condition is happily rare but can at times be responsible for massive haemorrhage during the treatment of obstetric complications. The cause of such bleeding is not always immediately obvious. A short summary explaining the correct procedure to follow and the blood elements to have available is given in Chapter 15 (page 196).

The authors are fully aware that very many readers in various parts of the world neither have adequate laboratory facilities for blood coagulation studies nor would they be able to obtain them in an emergency. To meet essential practical requirements and clarify the central role of heparin a management protocol is presented as Appendix A on page 198. It has been prepared by a French colleague Dr Pierre Cotteel who has considerable practical experience of the condition and its successful treatment; he refers to it as an acute defibrination syndrome. We believe that it is a helpful summary of management in a difficult and dangerous clinical area.

9: Caesarean section

Historical

The origin of the term caesarean section has always aroused both medical and lay interest. There is no evidence that Julius Caesar was born by this method and the fact that his mother Aurelia was alive in Rome when he was campaigning in Britain would seem to corroborate that. Shakespeare with his incomparable knowledge of history and events is so intrigued by the novel form of birth that he weaves it into the plot of Macbeth, yet makes no reference to the method of Caesar's birth in the tragedy of that name. It is now

were carried out among the early races and particularly the Jews.

In Europe attempts at caesarean section in the living were reported from about 1500 AD onwards. The Swiss pig farmer Nufer delivered his wife who survived the procedure and he is generally credited with the first successful operation in Europe. The case report was included much later in an addendum to what might be called the first series of cases – 15 cases of caesarean

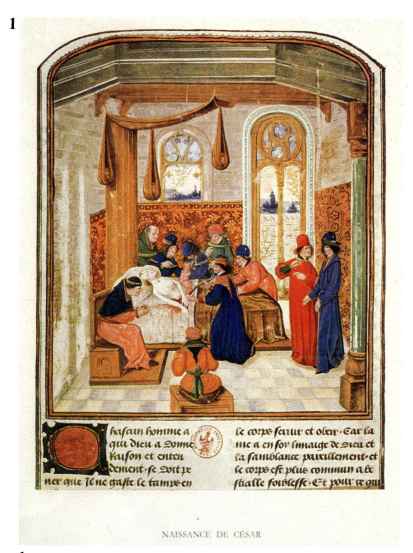

NAISSANCE DE CÉSAR

1
This beautiful miniature is from an early French manuscript and is believed to have been painted in Flanders in the second half of the 15th Century.

generally agreed that the term has no more romantic associations than its derivation from the Latin verb *caedere,* to cut.

Post-mortem caesarean sections with recovery of a live child have been reported from as early a 508 BC and there is evidence that operations on living mothers

section – reported by Francisco Rousseto and Casparo Bauhino and published in 1591.

The development of the operation makes fascinating reading and those who wish to study it further will find useful references in a recent article by Harley[1].

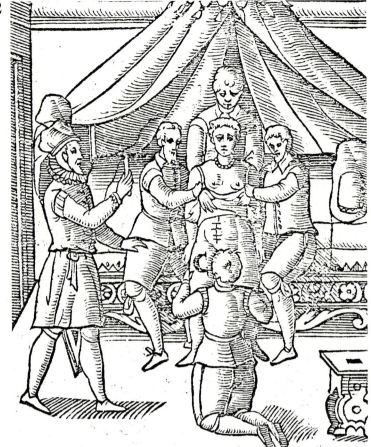

2 Preparations for operation on unanaesthetised patient

This figure is taken from an Italian publication of 1691 and shows how the problems of positioning and restraining the patient were overcome. The patient is held firmly in a semi-sitting position and would seem to have little chance of escaping her ordeal. From the surgeon's point of view access is excellent.

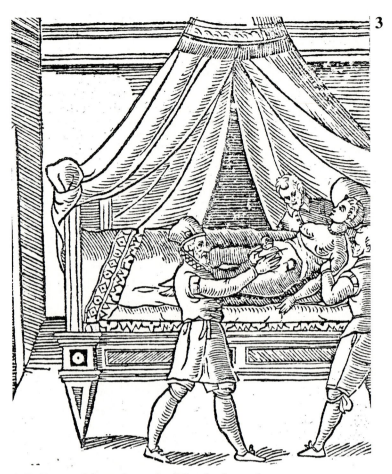

3 Delivery of fetus through abdominal opening

This figure is taken from the same source and shows the subsequent stage of the operation. With the abdomen and uterus open, the patient is laid on the bed and clearly no longer requires restraint. Relaxation of the abdominal musculature, for whatever reason, would facilitate delivery of the fetus.

Indications for operation

The specialist obstetrician has certain firm or absolute indications for caesarean section and also a large number of relative indications for the operation. These latter are largely concerned with fetal safety and therefore involve the associated problems of uterine dysfunction and delay in labour. The subject is a large one and is fully dealt with in obstetric textbooks.

Many of our readers are gynaecological surgeons who are at most occasional obstetricians and are likely to be primarily concerned with the surgical technique and short term management of the case when called upon to do the operation. Such circumstances would include late pregnancy emergencies due to haemorrhage and the many indications for elective caesarean section at term. Obstructed labour may demand operation and planned repeat caesarean sections are no respectors of time or place.

Dangers of caesarean section

It is unfortunate that caesarean section has come to be thought of as an easy and quick method of delivery. A study of the Report on Confidential Enquiries into Maternal Deaths in England and Wales 1973–1975[2] reveals 81 deaths connected with but not necessarily due to caesarean section. Sixty-one were *true* deaths; 20 were from associated diseases. A further 6 were known to have occurred but reports had not been submitted – 2 of these were from pulmonary emboli, 1 from anaesthesia and 3 from associated diseases. The fatality rate of the operation was 0.8 per 1000 caesarean sections compared with a rate of 1.1 in the previous 1970–72 report. The principal immediate causes of death continues to be haemorrhage, pulmonary embolus, sepsis, paralytic ileus, consequences of hypertensive diseases of pregnancy and anaesthesia.

There was some improvement on the previous 3 years figures but not in the case of haemorrhage or anaesthesia. One or more avoidable factor was present in all but one of the anaesthetic deaths. In 4 cases there was failure to intubate the trachea; in 11 patients death was caused by the aspiration of gastric contents.

The final paragraph of the summary and conclusions

of the chapter on caesarean section reads as follows:

> 'The percentage of one or more avoidable factors considered to be present in all the deaths connected with caesarean section was the highest ever recorded since 1952, at 60.5 per cent indicating a lack of care and inappropriate delegation of supervision of the operation.'

Everyone must be saddened by the need for such strictures but the lesson must be absorbed that caesarean section is always potentially dangerous and at times can stretch the ability of the most experienced surgeon.

The problem is not peculiar to any one country and very similar findings but with varying emphasis on individual items comes from the United States. A task force took part in a conference sponsored by the National Institute of Child Health and Human Development, The National Center for Health and Care Technology and the Office for Medical Applications for Research, NIH in September 1980 and published a consensus statement. The summary[3] makes thoughtful reading; the full report is available on request[4].

In the light of these two national reports it must be obvious that certain basic requirements should be satisfied before caesarean section is commenced. Those normally engaged in this field will be well aware of them but for others and as revision a list of the more important items is set out in Appendix B (page 199).

General surgical principles during caesarean section

The routine steps of lower segment caesarean section are described and illustrated in subsequent pages, but there are some general points which merit discussion and circumstances sometimes arise which may make alternative methods more suitable.

1. Avoidance of the inferior vena cava (IVC) syndrome
The operation is done with the patient in 15° head-down tilt with the operation table tilted to the left by 30° or a sorbo rubber wedge inserted under the patient's right buttock to give the same effect. This relieves the inferior vena cava from the pressure of the heavy pregnant uterus and avoids the supine hypotension syndrome with its possible dangers to the patient and to the fetus.

2. Choice of abdominal incision
A lower abdominal transverse incision is preferable for caesarean section. The wound is immeasurably stronger and the patient can be ambulant and without restriction of breathing immediately after the operation. Details of making the incision are described and illustrated in Volume 2 of the Atlas, pages 16–24. Transverse incisions, however, have disadvantages such as the tendency to haematoma formation and many gynaecologists still prefer and use the vertical incision. The abdomen can then be opened very quickly especially by the less experienced and this can sometimes be important as in the case of a prolapsed cord where delivery of the baby is urgent. The vertical incision also gives a better view of the peritoneal cavity and allows the fetus to be more easily extracted from the abdomen. Some[1] say it should always be used if there is the possibility of a classical caesarean section or caesarean hysterectomy being necessary. The technique of the method is referred to on page 118.

3. Avoiding the bladder when opening the peritoneal cavity
It must always be remembered that the bladder may be drawn up to an exceptionally high level in cases of prolonged or obstructed labour. The peritoneum should always, therefore, be opened cautiously and at as high a level as possible, otherwise one may open into the bladder. With a low transverse incision this is particularly important.

4. Possible indications for a vertical (De Lee) lower uterine segment incision
It has become standard practice in the United Kingdom to use a transverse incision; the uterus being incised low down on the lower segment to ensure that the main muscle layer at that level is split rather than cut, and that edges of equal thickness are thus available for a double layer closure that gives a very strong scar. There is little bleeding if the lower segment has developed and the absence of uterine contractions in that part of the uterus allows healing to proceed undisturbed and rapidly with a virtual absence of haematomata and sepsis. The wound can always be adequately covered by loose peritoneum. There are, however, occasions where it is preferable to use a vertical incision into the lower segment:
  (i)   In the case of a transverse lie with a prolapsed arm in the vagina,
  (ii) Where a constriction ring will not respond to the administration of amyl nitrate,
  (iii) Where a thin and distended lower uterine segment results from an obstructed labour and there is danger of lateral tearing[6] (the difficulty can usually be overcome by using a transverse incision with rather sharply upcurved ends to avoid the large vessels),
  (iv) The increasing modern tendency to use caesarean section to safeguard the fetus means that the lower uterine segment is frequently very poorly developed and the surgeon finds to his dismay that there is a very narrow undeveloped lower segment which is frequently covered by a plexus of large veins.

In all these circumstances the possible advantages of a vertical incision should be considered before incising the uterus. Compromise in the form of an inverted T-shaped incision with the stem of the T running up into the upper segment of the uterus is very unsatisfactory. The wound is difficult to close accurately and heals badly. The De Lee incision is safe and efficient and it must be added that many obstetricians, especially in the United States, employ it routinely at caesarean section. While the authors do not recommend its routine use, it is clearly the method of choice in the type of case under discussion. With a well developed lower segment the technique presents no problems; where there is a narrow underdeveloped lower segment, special care is required and the most satisfactory method is described and illustrated on page 129.

5. Disempaction from the pelvis of a firmly fixed fetal head

The fetal head may be very firmly fixed in the pelvis in the case of a long or obstructed labour and if one incises the lower segment transversely at the level of the fetal neck there may be a danger of tearing the lower segment laterally and involving the uterine vessels during delivery of the fetal head. The anterior shoulder is apt to prolapse into the wound and with increasing uterine retraction its replacement is almost impossible. It is at this stage that the inverted T incision is so often resorted to.

If such difficulties are likely to be encountered in the circumstances described, it is wise to anticipate trouble by having the assistant disempact the fetal head from the pelvis by vaginal pressure – before the uterus is incised. In the circumstances of a thin distended lower segment which is unlikely to bleed, the scissors are used to make sure that any lateral extension is carried upwards and does not extend laterally to involve the uterine vessels.

6. Prevention of blood loss during the operation
Caesarean section can become a very vascular operation even in skilled hands and precautions should be taken to prevent undue blood loss. If the patient has already suffered a haemorrhage, it is even more important to do so. Much can be done to preserve maternal blood volume at certain stages of the operation and in the presence of a potential source of haemorrhage:–

(i) *Incision of the lower uterine segment*
Having decided on the line of incision the surgeon makes a short transverse midline cut of no more than 2 cm long and to a depth which will expose the membranes without incising them. They then bulge into the wound but no harm is done if the sac is pierced and some amniotic fluid escapes. The forefinger of each hand is inserted at each end of the short incision and pulled apart laterally to split the circular muscle wall towards the lateral aspect on each side (**Figure 4**, page 114). Some of the vessels are torn and bleed but the thicker walled arteries, especially the larger of these which lie laterally, are displaced instead of divided or torn, and bleeding is correspondingly reduced. When the membranes are ruptured and as liquor escapes, bleeding takes place until the presenting part and body of the fetus controls it by direct pressure on the wound edge during delivery. Immediately the fetus is delivered the edges of the two leaves of the incision can be secured by Green Armytage forceps which effect haemostasis until the first layer of sutures is complete.

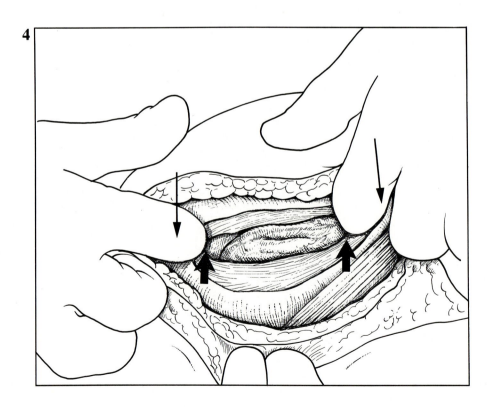

4 Incision into lower uterine segment
A short initial transverse incision of about 5 cm length has been made between the broad arrows and reveals the fetal head behind the intact membranes. The forefinger of each hand is inserted into each angle of the wound and drawn apart to split the uterine wall to the extent indicated by the thin arrows.

(ii) *Management of placental separation*

It has been routine practice in many centres to inject 0.5 mgm of Ergometrine i.v. when the presenting part is being delivered and within a minute the uterus will have contracted down strongly with complete or near-complete separation of the placenta which then presents in the uterine wound (**Figure 5**). The method is well-tried and effective but not without danger (Chapter 15, page 181). Syntocinon, 20 units in 500 ml, of Hartmann's solution, is the preferred alternative; administration of the infusion being speeded up while the placenta separates. No attempt is made to assist manually the process and the time is occupied in securing the wound edges and angles.

In some cases the uterus seems to respond only temporarily to oxytocin and may relax in varying degree with renewed bleeding from the placental site. The correct procedure in the circumstances is first to make sure that there is no retained lobe or piece of placenta within the uterus and that the cervix is sufficiently open to allow blood to escape to the vagina. Suture of the uterine incision is then completed without delay. It was discovered in relation to classical caesarean section that the uterus was incapable of contracting satisfactorily until it had been sutured and this applies no less to lower segment operations.

(iii) *Operative approach in placenta praevia*

The first question in such circumstances is whether the operation should be of lower segment or classical type. The matter has been under debate for many years and it is generally agreed that there is no longer any indication for using an upper segment incision in these cases even when the placenta is anteriorly placed beneath the line of incision on the lower segment. There is little fear of causing further haemorrhage by such an approach and once the uterine wall has been incised it is almost always possible to displace the placenta downwards towards the pelvis and gain access to the amniotic cavity over its upper border (**Figure 6**). On occasion it may be necessary to cut through a part of the placenta but even then the attendant loss of blood is much less than one would expect. Following delivery of the fetus, and if the placenta is delivered

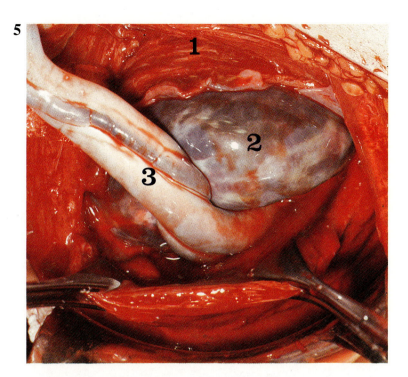

5 Separation of the placenta
During delivery of the fetus the uterus (1) has been stimulated by oxytocins and within 60 seconds it contracts firmly. The placenta (2) usually separates as a result and lies in the uterine wound ready for delivery. If gentle pulling on the umbilical cord (3) indicates that separation is not complete, it is best to wait, meantime securing the angles of the wound with sutures. No attempt should be made to accelerate natural separation.

slowly and carefully with the aid of the oxytocin already given, bleeding is seldom a matter for anxiety. It would nonetheless be foolish to pretend that dangerous bleeding never results from lower segment implantation; the tissue can indeed be of the consistency of wet blotting paper and the whole raw area may continue to bleed. Events would obviously dictate the form of management but hysterectomy could be necessary on account of continuing bleeding. Undue time and blood should not be lost in deciding that such a step is necessary.

(iv) *Incision into an undeveloped lower uterine segment*

This circumstance has already been discussed on page 113, but it should be added that there is very often a plexus of large veins overlying the lower segment which has to be divided. The De Lee incision carried out in the manner described on page 129 is seen to be a prophylactic haemostatic procedure apart from being the optimal method of delivering the fetus.

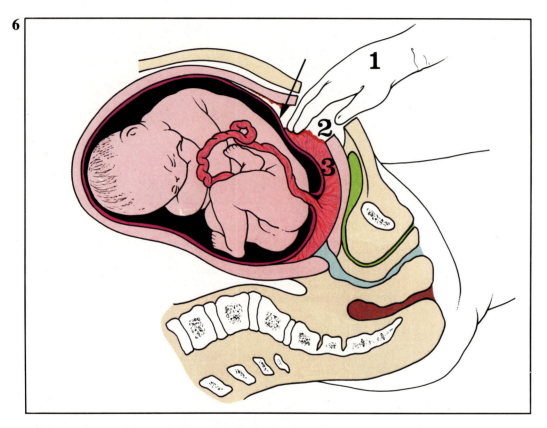

6 Lower uterine segment incision for placenta praevia

The surgeon's hand (1) is introduced through the uterine muscle incision (2) to encounter the placenta (3). The placenta is known to be low in position and the hand separates up gently between it and the uterine wall until the upper border is reached and is recognised by feeling the softer membranes beyond it. The sac is then opened where arrowed and as the liquor escapes and the uterus contracts the fetus presses on the placenta and uterine edge to control bleeding. The presentation is frequently breech which is even more advantageous for blood control and delivery.

Surgical technique – lower uterine segment caesarean section

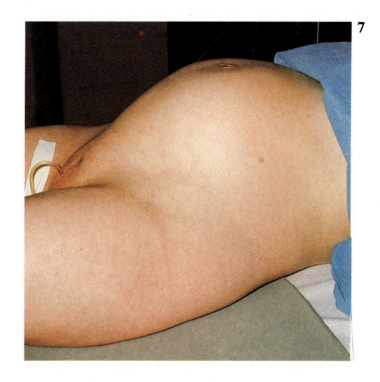

7 Patient prepared for caesarean section
The patient is having a general anesthetic and is in a 30° left lateral tilt to avoid the supine hypotension syndrome. She has been catheterised before coming to the operating room and a Foley catheter is left *in situ* during the operation attached to a free drainage system. The drapes will be applied and the surgeon ready to operate before general anaesthesia is induced.

Stage I: Opening the abdomen

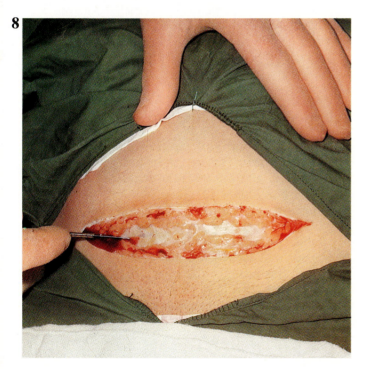

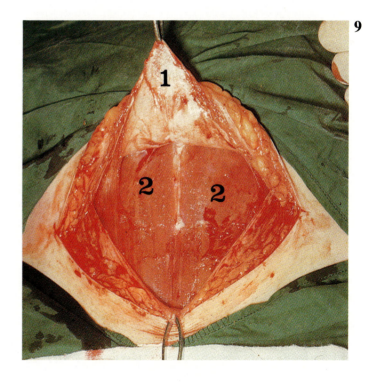

8 and 9
A transverse lower abdominal incision of 10cm length has been made through skin and superficial fascia in **Figure 8**. In **Figure 9** the rectus sheath (1) is lifted upwards to expose the recti muscles (2).

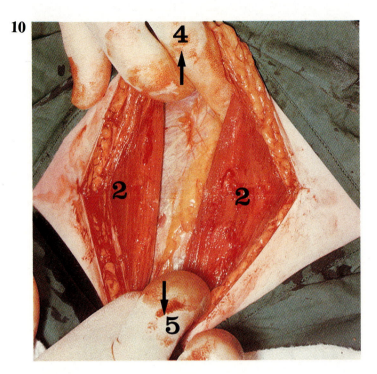

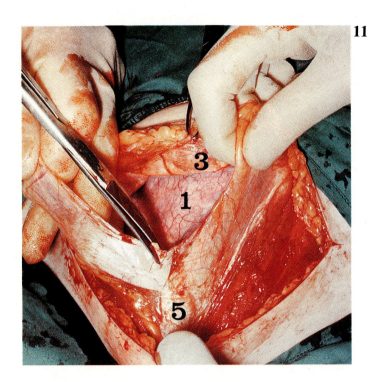

10 and 11
In **Figure 10** the surgeon separates the recti muscles (2) and exposes the peritoneum by inserting the fingers of each hand into the wound and pulling in the direction of the arrows towards the umbilicus (4) at one end and the symphysis

pubis (5) at the other. In **Figure 11** the peritoneum (3) has been opened vertically and the uterus is visible (1). The curved scissors incise the peritoneum carefully since the bladder is often at high level and could be injured.

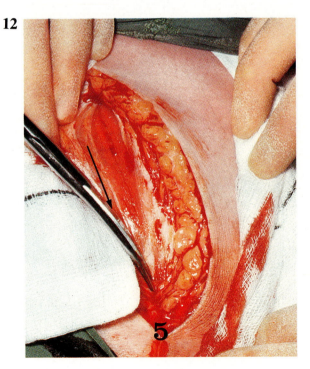

12 Opening rectus sheath in vertical incision

Alternative vertical midline incision

As explained in the introduction to this chapter circumstances may arise where a vertical incision would be preferable and the essential features of the incision are shown in **Figure 12.**

The skin incision extends from 1 cm below the umbilicus to 1.5 cm above the upper border of the symphysis pubis. As it cuts through the rectus sheath the scalpel opens into the medial side of one or other rectus sheath, in this instance the right. The opposite (left) sheath is being split in the same line (arrowed) and the two muscle bellies are separated as in the transverse incision. Incision of the peritoneum is exactly as in the transverse incision.

Stage II: Exposure of lower uterine segment

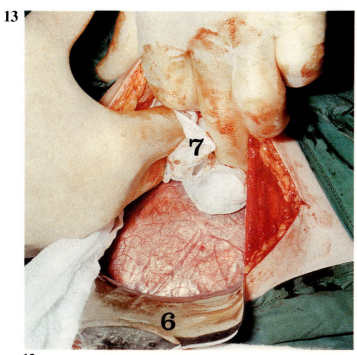

13

A Doyen's retractor (6) keeps the wound open while the surgeon inserts a continuous roll of gauze (7) to exclude omentum and loops of bowel from the operation area. Once the abdomen is opened, this roll of gauze is the only pack in use for all purposes; all others are counted, checked and removed from the operation room.

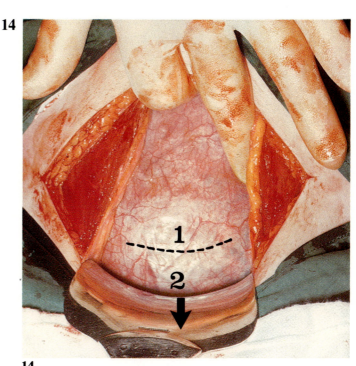

14

The lower uterine segment (1) and the bladder (2) are now exposed. The incision into the peritoneum prior to its reflection will be along the broken line.

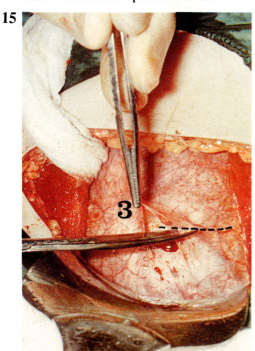

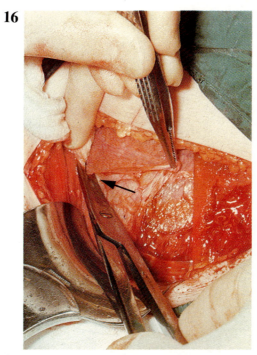

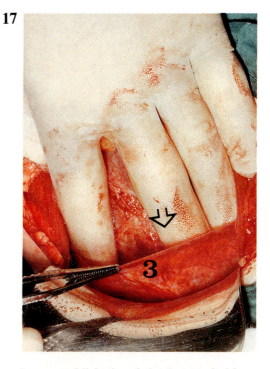

15 to 17

In **Figure 15** the peritoneum (3) is held in dissecting forceps while the fine curved scissors incise it where indicated by the broken line. In **Figure 16** the peritoneum is being separated off the upper part of the lower uterine segment with scissors where arrowed. In **Figure 17** a plane of separation between peritoneum and uterus has been established and the forceps hold the lower leaf of peritoneum (3) while the surgeon's hand carefully separates it and its underlying bladder wall from the lower uterine segment, in the direction of the arrow.

Stage III: Opening lower uterine segment

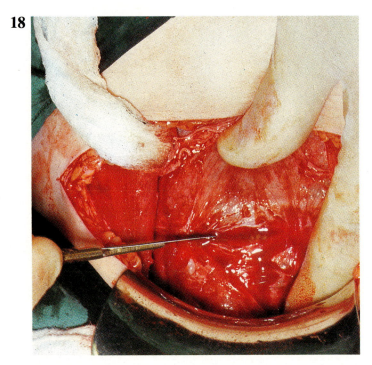

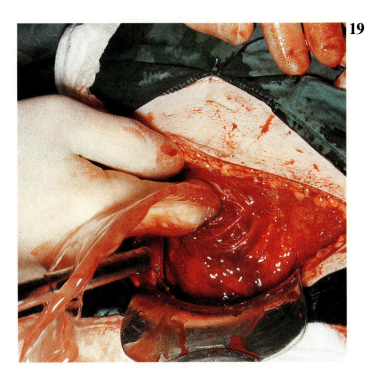

18 to 20

The lower segment is incised transversely at as low a level as is convenient for access. In **Figure 18** an initial short incision of 4–5 cm length is made centrally and it is convenient if the membranes can be left intact at this stage. It is not, however, a matter of importance and in **Figure 19** it is seen that the sac has been perforated and liquor escapes freely. The fore-

finger of each hand is now introduced into each angle of the wound as seen in **Figure 20** and drawn apart in the direction of the arrows. This splits the lower segment in the line of its main muscle fibres, but does not open the larger vessels and therefore avoids undue bleeding (see page 114).

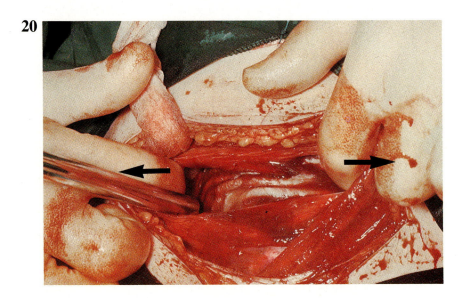

Stage IV: Delivery of the fetal head

A breech presentation provides little difficulty as it is easily delivered by extraction. With a cephalic presentation there may be problems when it is deeply fixed in the pelvis and where there is evidence of that it is wise to disempact it earlier, as has been described (page 114). Many methods of delivery of the head at caesarean section are described, but the safest way of doing so, whether it is engaged in the pelvis or free at the brim, is by the use of short obstetric forceps. Short straight Simpson's forceps as used at the Jessop Hospital for Women, Sheffield are ideal but Wrigley's forceps are also very suitable. They are applied with the leading edge of the blade directed upwards towards the abdomen in a non-engaged or floating head and downwards towards the pelvis in an engaged head. The operator first determines the position of the fetal head and then brings it into an occipito-posterior position before applying the blades if it is engaged. The authors would like to emphasise that this stage of the operation should be unhurried and controlled. There is a natural feeling that one ought to get the baby delivered expeditiously especially if there has been fetal distress but more harm than good can come from such a policy. At this stage it is essential to 'hasten slowly'.

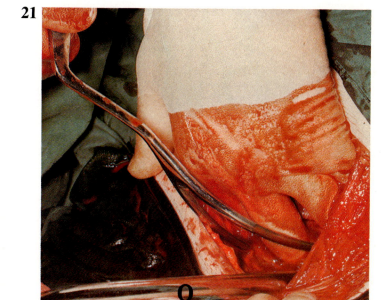

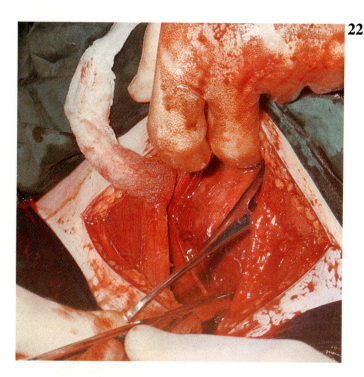

21 and 22
The head is at the brim and lying in an occipito-anterior position in this case. The Doyen's retractor has been removed, and, with the left hand steadying the fetal head, first one blade and then the other of the short forceps are applied to the side of the fetal head. There is a certain amount of bleeding from the uterine wound edge and the field is kept clear by the sucker (0) seen in the lower part of the wound.

It is at this stage that oxytocin is given. The anaesthetist is normally requested to do so and accelerates the syntocinon drip so that the uterus contracts strongly in about 60 seconds time. In less ideal conditions the alternative is to give 0.5 ml ergometrine i.v.; reasons for preferring syntocinon have been explained elsewhere (Chapter 15, page 181).

23

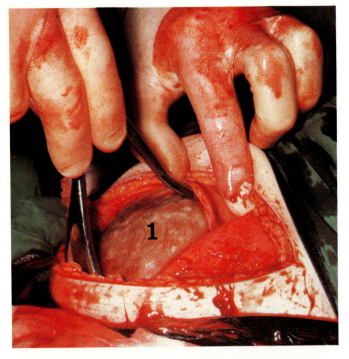

1

24

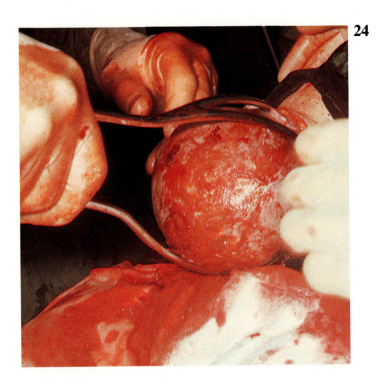

25

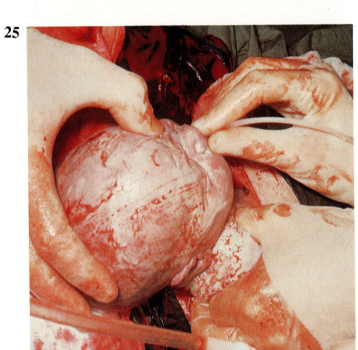

23 to 25

In **Figure 23** the forceps blades are locked on the fetal head (1) which is then delivered very slowly in the direction it wishes to take. In **Figure 24** the head has been delivered in the occipito-anterior position and in **Figure 25** the mouth and air passages are cleared of mucus with a fine neo-natal sucker.

Stage V: Completing delivery of fetus

26

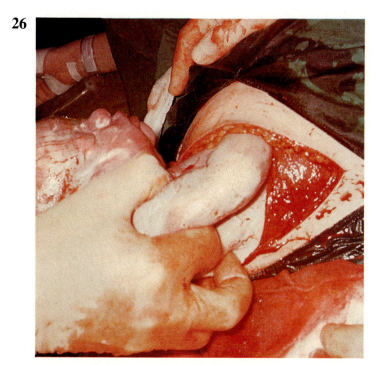

26
The surgeon gently grasps the anterior shoulder of the fetus and delivers it slowly from the uterus.

27

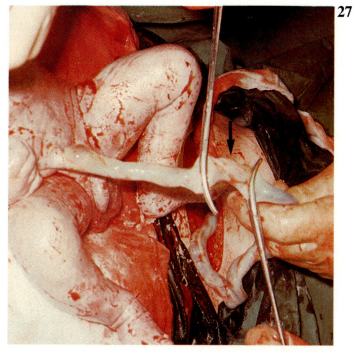

27
The umbilical cord is double clamped and about to be divided where arrowed. The rather long cord will be shortened and securely ligatured or clamped before taking the baby from the operating room.

Stage VI: Separation of the placenta

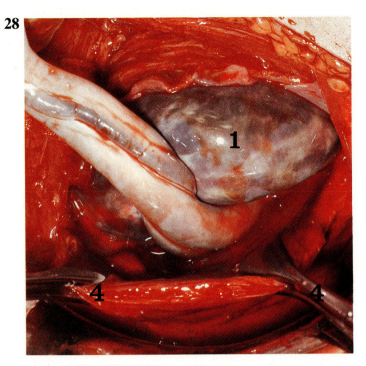

28
The uterus has contracted in response to the oxytocic drug and the placenta (1) is lying in the wound and supported on retro-placental blood which indicates that it has separated from the uterine wall. Note that a series of Green Armytage forceps (4) is applied to the uterine edge to control bleeding and define the uterine opening; two or at most three on each side are required.

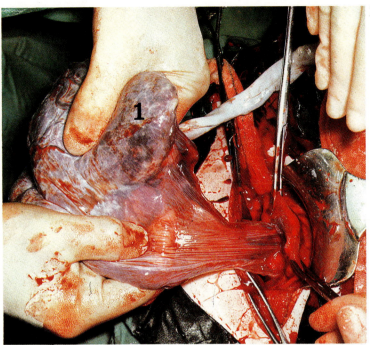

29
The placenta (1) is held in the left hand while the membranes are slowly withdrawn from the uterine cavity in the right while moving them about to encourage detachment from the uterine wall.

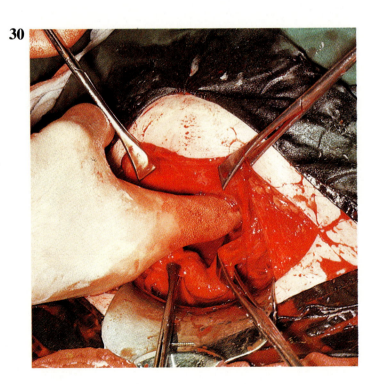

Stage VII: Exploration and manual compression of uterus

30
The uterine cavity is explored to exclude retained placental or membranous remnants and the forefinger explores the region of the internal os to ensure that drainage can take place through the cervical canal. If necessary, a large sized Hegar's dilator is passed down through the cervix into the vagina and retrieved later. The uterus is then compressed by the surgeon's hand as shown in the photograph. This expresses decidual debris and encourages contraction.

Stage VIII: Closure of uterine incision – first layer

31

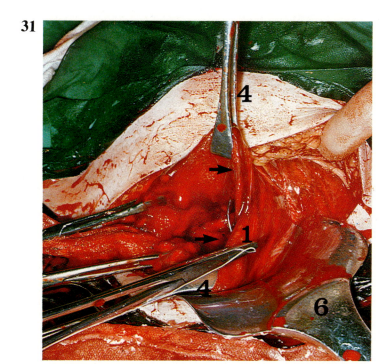

32

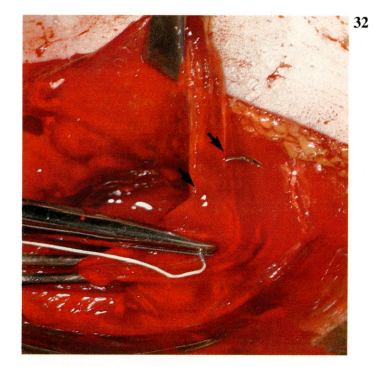

33

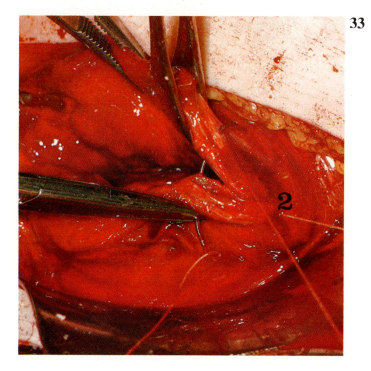

31

A round-bodied needle carrying No. 0 PGA suture (1) commences closure of the incision at the left angle of the wound. The edges are displayed on the Green Armytage forceps (4) and the bite taken by the needle excludes the endometrio-decidual layer (arrowed) so that the suture will not obtrude on the cavity. The Doyen's retractor (6) is again in place.

32

The opposing edge of the incision at the left angle is transfixed in the same fashion (arrowed). Note that there is little or no bleeding and the edges are well defined.

33

The anchor stitch has been tied at (2) and the continuous stitch proceeds along the wound to close the incision.

Stage IX: Closure of uterine incision – second layer

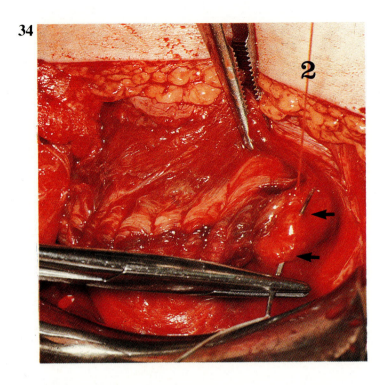

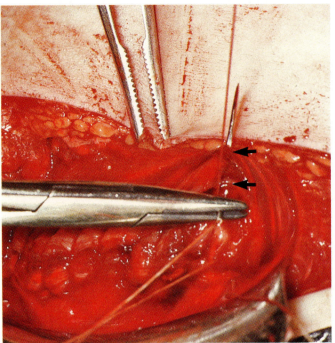

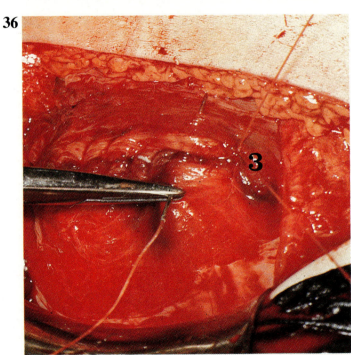

34 to 36

A similar needle and suture is used to make a Lembert type inverting second layer closure of the incision. The anchor stitch of the first layer (2) is used as a holder in **Figure 34** and the first bite of the lower edge is taken (arrowed). In **Figure 35** the needle takes in the opposite edge (arrowed) in such a way as to invert the edge when the stitch is tightened. In **Figure 36** the second layer anchor stitch is at (3) while the inverting suture progresses along the wound to cover the first layer.

Stage X: Peritoneal closure

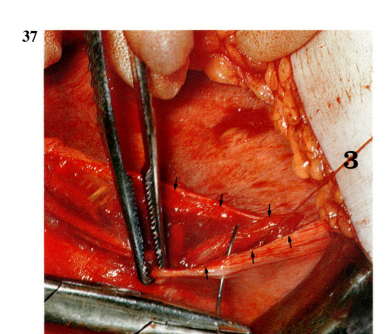

37

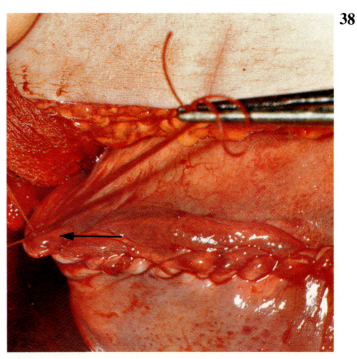

38

37
The Doyen's retractor is reapplied to release the lower peritoneal edge and the two leaves are now evident (fine arrows). The anchor stitch on the second muscle layer closure is used as a holder (3) and a round-bodied needle carrying a 00 PGA suture commences closure of the peritoneum at the left end of the wound. As it progresses across the incision it picks up a bite of the anterior surface of the uterus to help to eliminate dead space and prevent haematomata.

38
The stitch has been completed and is in process of being tied off (arrowed). The peritoneum is snugly applied to the lower segment and the wound is quite dry. It remains only to evacuate blood clot from the pelvis and retrieve the gauze roll before closing the abdomen.

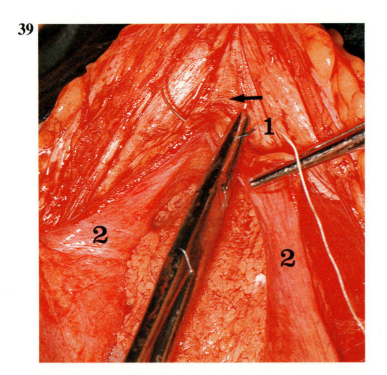

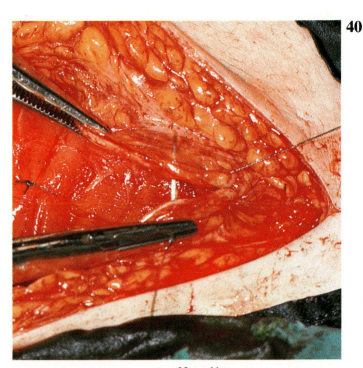

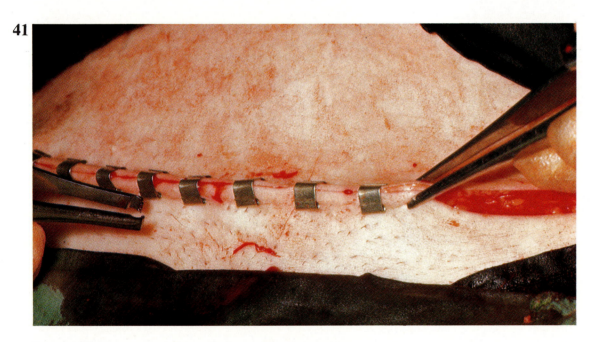

39 to 41

In **Figure 39** the round needle carrying a No. 0 PGA suture (1) commences the vertical continuous closure of the peritoneum (2) with the first stitch just below umbilical level (arrowed). In **Figure 40** the edges of the transverse incision in the rectus sheath are approximated by a continuous No. 1 PGA suture and in **Figure 41** the skin is being closed by broad clips. A few fine sutures are used for fat approximation and elimination of dead space in the superficial fascial layer.

Many surgeons routinely use a small perforated suction drain (Redivac type) inserted either beneath the rectus sheath or lying across the closed sheath and emerging through a stab incision lateral to and slightly below one end of the incision. This drain is retained for 48 hours or longer if seen to be necessary.

Immediate post-operative management

The authors believe it is the surgeon's duty to attend to certain important matters *before* the patient leaves the operating table. They are:

1. Confirmation by abdominal palpitation that the uterus is firmly contracted.
2. Expression of blood clot from the vagina and lower uterine segment by gentle uterine fundal pressure.
3. Removal of residual blood clot from the lower vagina and vulvar area by swabbing.

4. Checking that the urine in the open drainage system is not blood stained before removal of the Foley catheter.

These simple precautions ensure that any early post partum vaginal bleeding does not result from unrecognised uterine relaxation (atony) or residual (intra-operative) blood clot retention in the vagina.

The De Lee incision in cases of undeveloped lower uterine segment

Technique

The method of incision is shown diagramatically in **Figures 42, 43** and **44** and it will be seen that the procedure is a step by step controlled opening of the lower segment to an extent sufficient to deliver the fetus, and it is at the same time a prophylactic haemostatic one. It is clear that if a transverse incision were made at the level required it would be inadequate to transmit the fetus and must inevitably extend laterally to damage and tear the uterine vessels. Bleeding from large superficial veins does not ordinarily influence the choice of incision, but can be very embarrassing with a restricted opening.

The authors believe that in these particular circumstances it is correct to make a vertical or De Lee incision into the lower segment rather than the otherwise preferable transverse one. The visceral peritoneum is incised transversely in the usual way and the upper flap is reflected as high as possible off the anterior wall while the lower flap and the bladder are reflected off the cervix as deeply as possible. Once the lower segment has been displayed, the surgeon uses the forefinger and thumb of the left hand to compress and prevent bleeding from the large veins and makes a vertical incision of about 1.5 cm length in the lower segment to the depth of the membranes (**Figure 42**). Each edge of the wound is grasped with Green-Armytage forceps (**Figure 43**) and the incision is enlarged by scalpel or scissors first caudally towards the cervix and then cranially as far as is required by a series of cuts to lengthen the wound while securing the edges at the same time with Green Armytage forceps (**Figure 44**). It is usually necessary to invade the upper segment

of the uterus but this part of the incision is not more than one-third of its length. The scar cannot be as strong or comfortable as a transverse one but it is in no sense an upper segment incision and it is completely covered by peritoneum once it has been closed.

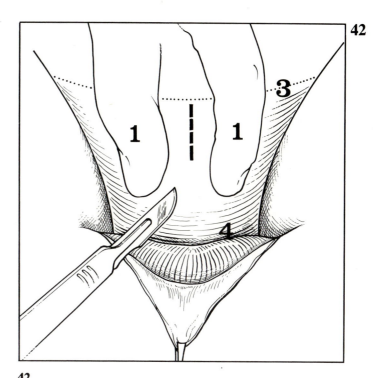

42

In this **Figure** the placing of the initial incision is indicated by the broken line. The left thumb and forefinger (1) and (1) compress the vascular uterine wall against the presenting part while the scalpel is ready to make a 3 cm long incision in the lower uterine segment. The level of peritoneal attachment to the uterus is numbered (3) and the reflected bladder (4).

43

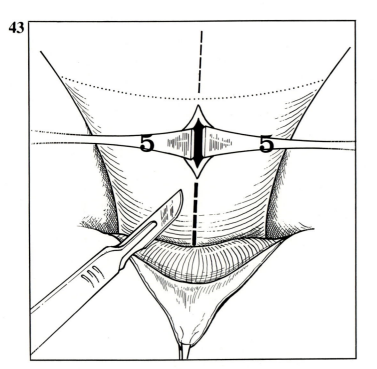

43
The incision has been made and the two edges are held in Green Armytage forceps (5). The heavy broken line of approximately 3cm length shows the space still available for incision into the lower segment. The lighter broken line indicates the site of an incision which if required will partially invade the upper uterine segment.

44

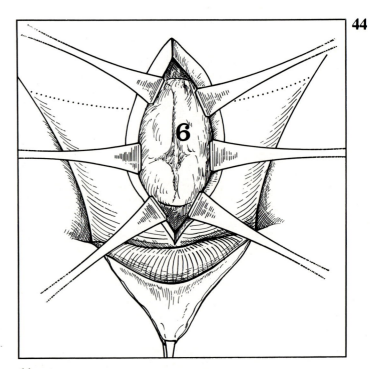

44
Here the incision is complete and has occupied the available length in the lower segment besides 2–3cm in the upper segment. The fetal head is numbered (6).

10: Hysterectomy for uterine rupture and post partum haemorrhage

Where caesarean section is done in cases of rupture of the uterus or damage to its wall by inexpert and failed attempts at vaginal delivery, it is often possible and generally preferable to repair the uterus and leave the question of hysterectomy for later and calmer consideration. Special circumstances encountered at the time of abdominal delivery, however, may make it necessary to remove the uterus and would include the following:

1. An irregular and extensive tear of the lower segment at the site of a previous scar which cannot satisfactorily be repaired.
2. Similar trauma from unsuccessful attempts at vaginal delivery.
3. Couvelaire uterus in the presence of persistent bleeding.
4. A completely atonic uterus with uncontrollable haemorrhage from the placental site.

In all these circumstances the operation becomes a serious emergency procedure with its own special problems of shock and haemorrhage and the fact that it began with caesarean delivery of the fetus is incidental. It has now become an emergency hysterectomy to arrest uterine haemorrhage and the prime requirement is to do so in the safest and most satisfactory manner possible.

A reappraisal of *caesarean hysterectomy* as a set operation is long overdue. It has traditionally been looked on as being indicated when abdominal delivery is necessary and there are indications for the removal of the uterus. The need for hysterectomy may sometimes be immediate, more often it is not, yet other factors sometimes make it seem convenient to do the two operations at the same time. When one studies the possible indications for the operation, it becomes clear that there is only a small group of desperately ill patients who require hysterectomy at the time of delivery, and the authors seriously doubt whether a planned caesarean hysterectomy operation is ever justified. The numerous 'relative' indications sometimes suggested for the joint operation such as the finding of a positive cervical smear in pregnancy or even the presence of multiple uterine fibroids are inadmissable since any advantages gained are heavily outweighed by the risks of hysterectomy on a full-term uterus in a patient who may already have lost a considerable part of her total circulating blood volume.

The authors believe it to be more helpful to dismiss the concept of *caesarean hysterectomy* altogether and concentrate on the question of the best form of hysterectomy (subtotal or total) to meet the circumstances of the individual case. The surgical and safety considerations involved are dealt with below and the optimal treatment discussed.

There are two main indications for hysterectomy at the time of delivery, namely uterine rupture and post partum haemorrhage.

1. Uterine rupture

Three particular groups of factors contribute to rupture of the uterus:

(i) Weak uterine scars as a result of –
  (a) previous caesarean section
  (b) myomectomy or uteroplasty operation
  (c) high cervical repair of a tear from a previous pregnancy.
(ii) The occurrence of powerful and sometimes uncontrolled uterine contractions when the cervix is insufficiently dilated or the uterus is prevented from expelling its contents.
(iii) Traumatic obstetrical interference or attempts at breech extraction or internal version.

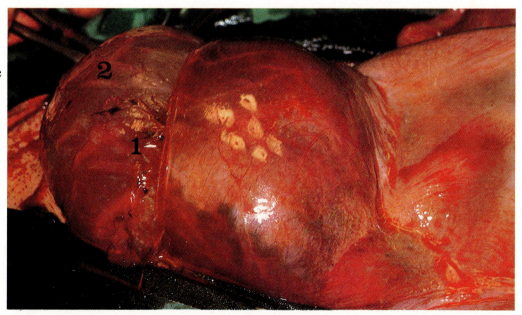

1 Ruptured uterus-appearances at laparotomy
Rupture took place through a previous lower segment caesarean section scar just prior to the onset of labour. The fetus (1) was in an intact bag of membranes (2) but had perished. There was very little bleeding.

131

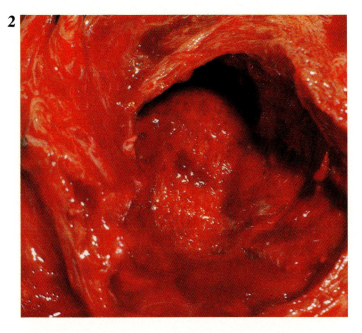

2 Ruptured uterus
The same case now with the pregnancy removed.
Removal of the uterus was clearly essential and sub-
total hysterectomy was carried out.

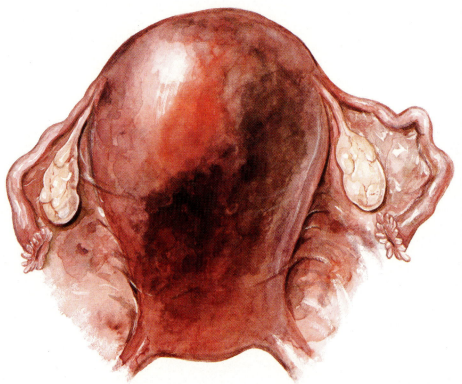

3 Couvelaire uterus
A colour drawing showing severe disruption of the uterine muscle by blood infiltration
associated with severe accidental haemorrhage. The uterus had to be removed in this
instance because of continuing haemorrhage. In most cases, even of severe muscle
disruption, the uterus contracts satisfactorily once the fetus and placenta have been
delivered.

Previous operation on the uterus is not an essential
factor and rupture may occur in obstructed labour,
during medical induction of labour in the second
trimester and from the effects of misdirected obstetrical attempts at delivery. Most cases of uterine rupture
involve scars from previous surgery and occur towards
the end of pregnancy – usually just before the estimated date of delivery. In many cases the fetus and
membranes have been expelled into the peritoneal
cavity by the time the condition is recognised (**Figure
7**). Any thoughts that uterine rupture is a rare event,
and one where recovery can confidently be expected,
are dispelled by reference to the Report On Confidential Enquiries into Maternal Deaths[1]. The 1979 Report
showed no significant reduction in deaths from this
cause in the United Kingdom since 1970. The incidence of ruptured uterus is very high in certain parts of
the world and the associated maternal mortality must
also be high.

Diagnosis during induction of mid-trimester abortion should be obvious if the patient is being
adequately monitored. Rupture in late pregnancy can
be more difficult to diagnose especially if it is of the
'silent' type and the accumulated evidence of the
patient's past obstetric history, epecially a previous
classical caesarian section, sharp lower abdominal pain
of any degree and the 'cramps' which accompany vaginal
bleeding in fully 50 per cent of cases should suggest the
diagnosis. Alterations in the smooth outline of the
uterus would strengthen such suspicions and blood in
the broad ligament on each side gives rise to a widening
of the uterine mass. Uterine contraction if present
soon ceases with some relief of pain. The presenting
part recedes while shock and signs of internal blood
loss become evident. Where diagnosis has been
delayed the classical picture is that of a moribund
patient with vaginal bleeding who complains of abdominal discomfort and distention. Ileus and vomiting
are followed by increasing shock and circulatory
collapse. Such a state of affairs should not arise and
there is little excuse for a missed or even delayed
diagnosis when a past history of uterine surgery is
available. At the present time when epidural analgesia
in labour is common, the clinician has the opportunity
of palpating the lower uterine segment via the cervix if
there is doubt about the diagnosis.

2. Post-partum haemorrhage

Persistent haemorrhage which necessitates hysterectomy may arise from one or more of the following complications:
(i)   Uterine rupture of the type already discussed (**Figures 1** and **2**).
(ii) Uterine trauma from attempts at criminal abortion.
(iii) Post-partum haemorrhage due to uterine atony.
(iv) Persistent bleeding from a Couvelaire uterus (**Figure 3**).
(v)   Bleeding from a partially detached placenta accreta (**Figure 4**).

There is seldom any difficulty in diagnosis. Bleeding from the uterus or uterine vessels continues and blood replacement can do no more than keep pace with the haemorrhage.

Surgical treatment

The uterus is traumatised in some degree or is the source of actual bleeding at the time of operation so that there are major technical problems and the procedure can be dangerous. The primary aims are to remove the products of conception and control haemorrhage. It is then necessary to repair the uterus after having excised necrotic tissue, or, in infected cases, to remove the uterus. The procedure adopted will depend on several factors and not least the condition of the mother, whose life is the first consideration. The general consensus is that less extensive tears should be repaired and some[2,3] think it is safer also to repair the uterus in very ill patients. Others[4,5] who have experience of large numbers of infected cases recommend hysterectomy and prefer the total operation. If the tear is severe and circumferential, subtotal hysterectomy is probably best and if the patient does not want more children hysterectomy is additionally indicated. Where there is infection or likely infection, then total hysterectomy is indicated and in such cases the pelvis should be drained.

Apart from the immediate problems of controlling haemorrhage and treating the torn uterus, it must be remembered that any of the recognised complications of major abdominal emergency surgery may follow such treatment. These include neurogenic shock, thromboembolism, retroperitoneal haematomata, peritonitis, intestinal ileus, pelvic abscess, bowel injury and wound infection. A high morbidity rate from such conditions is unavoidable. There is the additional danger of injury to the lower urinary tract when doing hysterectomy in these circumstances. One source[6] quotes a 3.3 per cent injury rate in 3166 cases and an 0.4 per cent fistula rate, while another[7] records a 4 per cent injury rate to the bladder recognised at the time, with a subsequent 0.7 per cent vesico-vaginal fistula rate from unrecognised trauma at the time of operation.

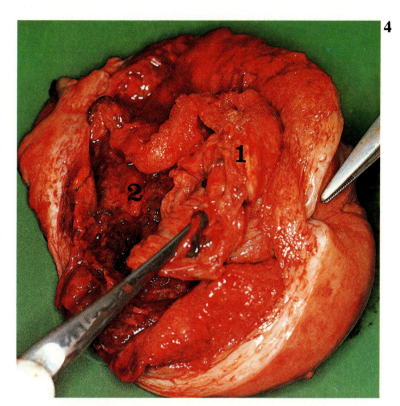

4 Placenta accreta
In this case vaginal bleeding associated with placental retention led to several unsuccessful attempts at manual removal. Hysterectomy had to be performed because of continuing haemorrhage and the removed specimen showed a morbidly adherent placenta (accreta) (1) and a lacerated uterine wall (2).

Choice of operation

A good deal has been written about whether the hysterectomy should be total or subtotal, but the authors do not believe that the decision should present much difficulty. Subtotal hysterectomy can be done easily and quickly with very little risk to the ureters or the bladder and it must be the method chosen if the patient is shocked. When the patient has not lost a lot of blood and is in reasonably good condition there may be a choice, but unless experienced in obstetrical work, the surgeon should not attempt total hysterectomy in most circumstances because of the very real dangers entailed. The one valid objection to subtotal hysterectomy is that carcinoma can develop in the remaining cervix. This is so, but the incidence of malignancy is a relatively small risk to set against the numerous serious complications which may arise from the more extensive operation. There is no doubt that total hysterectomy means an increase in operating time, increased transfusion and increased morbidity as well as mortality. This is especially true in non-elective cases and practically all urinary tract injuries reported are in the total rather than the subtotal group. There is the further pertinent point that in almost half the cases where total hysterectomy is thought to have been done, at least a part of the cervix is inadvertently left behind.

While fully convinced that in most cases subtotal hysterectomy should be done the authors have to agree that where the lower segment injury extends through the cervix into the vaginal vault or where events make subsequent infection very probable, the uterus and cervix should be removed. Quite apart from the desirability of removing the damaged and potentially infected cervix and achieving haemostasis, the opening through the vaginal vault provides for pelvic drainage.

Arrest of bleeding in cases of ruptured uterus

More immediate than the preferred type of hysterectomy is the need to control haemorrhage and that is the surgeon's first task. Early recognition of uterine damage is the single most important factor in forestalling major internal bleeding and avoiding hysterectomy. There is nearly always a history of operative or obstetric trauma to indicate the possibility of rupture of the uterus so that there is seldom reason to delay laparotomy. When the abdomen is open it takes a few minutes to establish the source and degree of bleeding and the extent of uterine damage. Each case is unique but all tend to fall into one of the following three general categories:

1. When the upper segment of the uterus has been perforated or damaged by a surgical instrument, there is an irregular tear of the uterine wall with traumatised and discoloured muscle, and probably a fair sized spouting artery. It is generally necessary only to secure the bleeding vessel, trim the damaged muscle and make a neat closure of the uterine muscle in two or three separate layers. A series of Green Armytage forceps are used to control the wound edges at all stages of the operation.

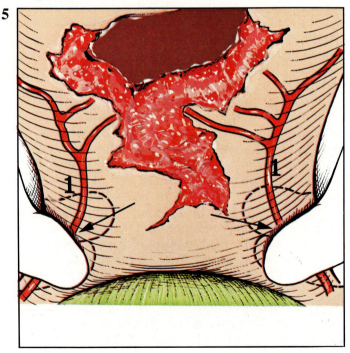

5 Diagram of a simple method of controlling uterine bleeding
The assistant can control severe uterine haemorrhage by compressing the uterine arteries (1) and (1) between fingers and thumbs (where arrowed) while lifting the uterus into the wound. The approach is over the top of the broad ligament and for simplicity the round ligaments have been omitted from the diagram.

2. Trauma below the peritoneal reflection is a more difficult problem and instead of intraperitoneal free blood there is a soft haematoma in the utero-vesical space extending laterally into the base of the broad ligament which may be greatly distended and distorted. Exposure of these areas is commenced medially by reflecting the bladder off the anterior aspect of the uterus and cervix as far as necessary and gently and gradually working laterally to evacuate blood clot from the affected broad ligament. It is often an advantage to cut the round ligament and so gain access to the broad ligament. The round ligament is easily repaired subsequently. When the source of the bleeding has been found, care must be taken to identify the vessel before clamping and ligating it because of the proximity of the ureter. Most uterine damage occurs in hospital under what should be aseptic conditions and hysterectomy should not be necessary. Cases of criminal abortion with the probability of accompanying infection are likely to require total hysterectomy.

3. Intrapartum rupture of the uterus through a previous caesarean section or operation scar may give rise to massive bleeding and a wide variety of tears and degrees of bleeding. Conservation of the uterus is often possible but a number of these cases need hysterectomy. The surgeon in either circumstance has the immediate problem of controlling bleeding and has to apply suitable haemostatic measures. Overt bleeding vessels on the torn muscle edge are temporarily controlled by Green Armytage forceps or secured by fine stitches. Major bleeding from a main trunk of the uterine artery requires prompt action and once the main part of the blood has been cleared from the operative field the vessel is secured and ligated.

   Persistent and heavy bleeding into the base of the broad ligament is approached in the manner already described but is always dangerous because there are multiple large veins in the area and the ureter is close at hand.

An unsophisticated but effective method of temporary haemostasis is shown diagramatically on **Figure 5**. The assistant carries out the manoeuvre by using the thumbs and first two fingers of each hand to compress the uterine vessels and maintain haemostasis while the surgeon identifies the bleeding point and secures it by ligation.

If control of haemorrhage by such means is unsatisfactory it may be necessary to ligate the internal iliac artery on the affected side; the technique is shown on pages 108–109. If the bleeding is thereby lessened but not fully controlled it is worth repeating it on the other side.

Truly massive haemorrhage encountered on opening the abdomen or as the by-product of one's best attempts at haemostasis can always be temporarily controlled by pressure against bony points. The lateral wall of the pelvis or the sacrum are those most immediately available but occlusive pressure on the aorta against the lumbo-sacral spine will give a short breathing space in which to examine the intrapelvic structures.

Hysterectomy

I. Sub-total hysterectomy

Sub-total hysterectomy at term does not differ in method from that performed on the non-pregnant patient and apart from the need to replace blood loss, the technique described in Volume 2 of the Atlas, Chapter 3, page 154 is appropriate. In the case described and illustrated here, the uterus had ruptured and extruded the fetus, complete in its membranes, into the peritoneal cavity. When the fetus had been removed it was seen that the lower uterine segment was so damaged and torn that hysterectomy was essential. There was no reason to believe that the case might be infected and total hysterectomy was not therefore mandatory. Only the more important steps of the operation are illustrated and described so that the reader is left with a clear impression of the main aims and requirements of what is a simple and effective procedure which is applicable to most cases. A vertical midline incision allows the abdomen to be opened quickly in such circumstances. It also gives better access and can be enlarged as required.

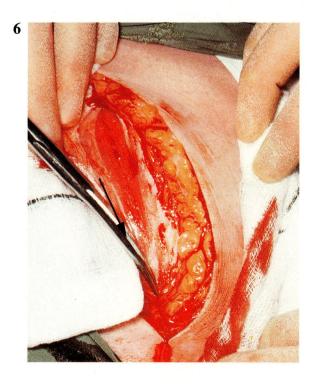

6 Vertical midline incision
The skin incision extends from 1 cm below the umbilicus to 1.5 cm above the upper border of the symphysis pubis. The rectus sheath has been opened to the right of the midline in this case and the scissors open up the left sheath (arrowed). Thereafter the muscle bellies of the recti are separated to expose the peritoneum.

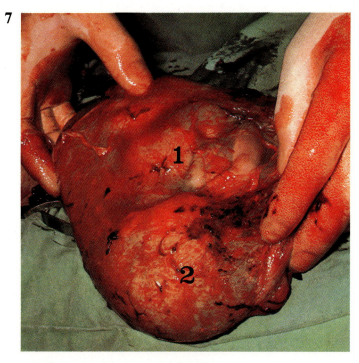

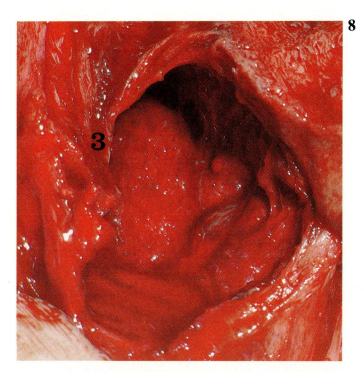

7 and 8 Appearances at laparotomy
In **Figure 7** the fetus (1) is seen in the bag of membranes which has been extruded completely into the peritoneal cavity. The placental surface is seen at (2). In **Figure 8** the rupture in the lower segment is seen and is presumed to have commenced at the very thin fibrous area (3).

Stage I: Securing upper uterine attachments

9

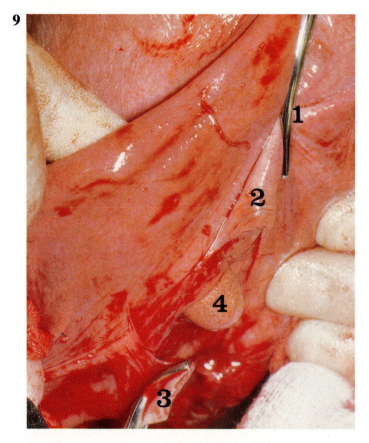

9A

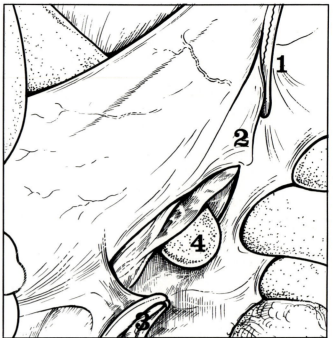

9

The broad ligament is held in the long forceps (1) and the round ligament (2) has been detached at (3). The surgeon's finger (4) is inserted through the resultant opening in the broad ligament preparatory to clamping it.

10

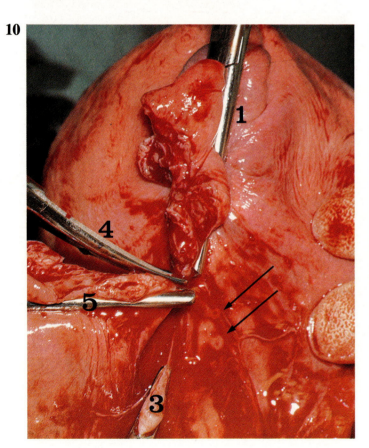

10A

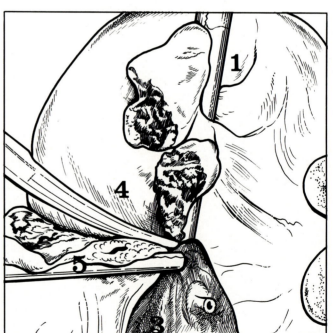

10

The broad ligament has been divided with scissors (4) between the holding forceps (1) and the newly applied forceps (5). Note that the tear in the lower segment extends into the base of the broad ligament with main branches of the uterine artery unsupported (arrowed).

Stage II: Separating bladder from ruptured uterus

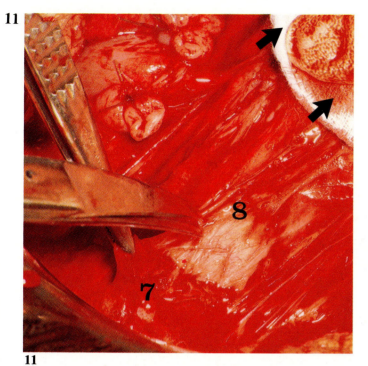

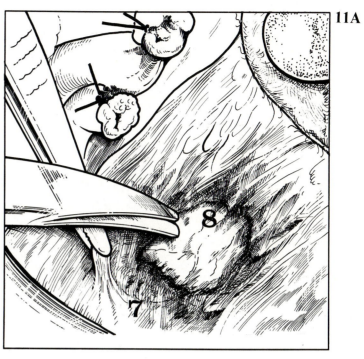

11
The torn lower segment is supported upwards in the direction of the arrows by a large swab (6) under the assistant's hand and with dissecting forceps and scissors the

bladder (7) is reflected downwards off the anterior aspect of the cervix (8).

Stage III: Securing uterine vessels

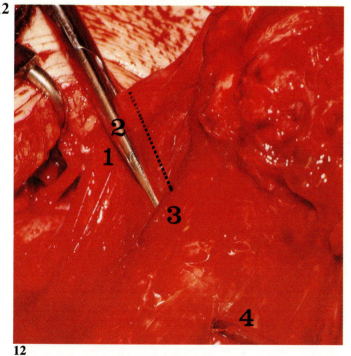

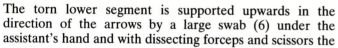

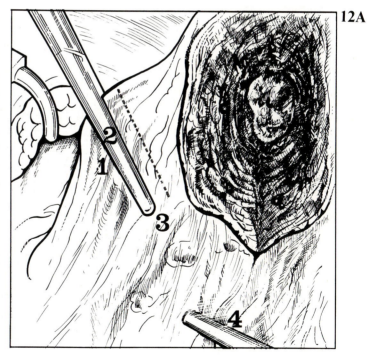

12
The right uterine vessels have been defined (1) and a long straight forceps (2) is used to clamp them at an angle of nearly 90° to the axis of the uterus. The point of the forceps is normally placed firmly against the side of the cervix (3) but

the tissues are torn and there is no landmark. The essential requirement is to include all the large vessels. The pedicle will be detached along the dotted line. The vessels on the left side are clamped by the forceps numbered (4).

Illustration of Stage III from a less vascular case

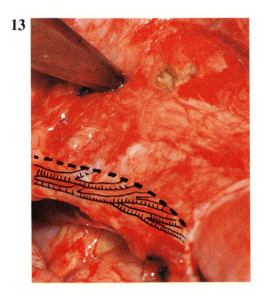

13

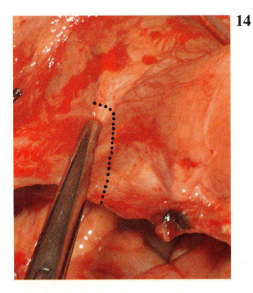

14

13 and 14

Figures 13 and **14** show some important points in surgical technique in a case where the uterine vessels were not traumatised. The prominent uterine vessels are outlined in **Figure 13** and the broken line indicates the lateral aspect of the cervix. The scissors are used as a retractor so that the bladder is clear of the operation area and will not be damaged when the uterus is cut across to be removed. **Figure 14** emphasises the point of placing the forceps at right angles to the uterus to prevent tearing downwards at the point of the forceps. A generous cuff of tissue is left beyond the forceps in detaching the pedicle across the dotted line and the muscle of the cervix is actually cut into beyond the broken line in the manner shown.

Stage IV: Removal of uterus

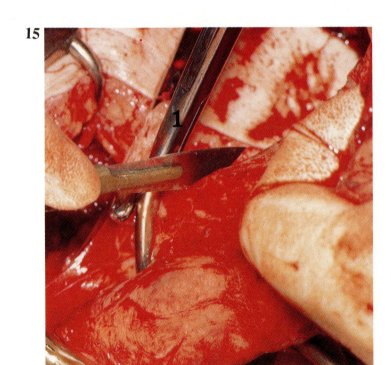

15

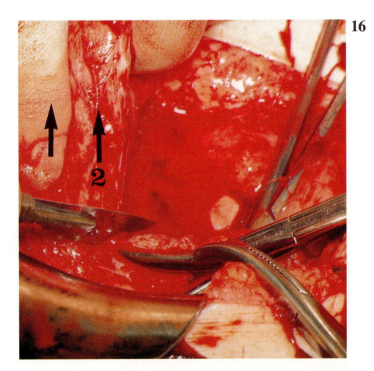

16

15 and 16

The curved forceps (1) clamps across the open cervix in **Figure 15**. It is often difficult to know the precise level because the cervix is torn into and is usually dilated, but it is a good rule to go straight across at a level where one can see the structures properly and be able to get good edges for subsequent closure. Any temptation to incise at a deeper level in the belief that a total hysterectomy will result should

be resisted. That is only possible when the vaginal angles have been properly defined and secured; without such preparation a full sized cervix is found at postoperative examination. The uterus is being detached with the scalpel at the level of the uterine isthmus on the right side. In **Figure 16** the uterus is held upwards (broad arrows) and removed as the left pedicle (2) is detached with the scalpel.

Stage V: Closure of cervical stump

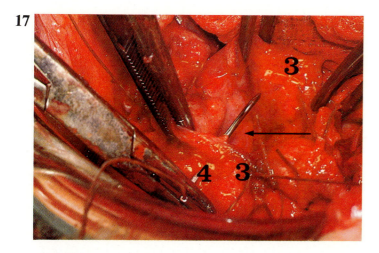

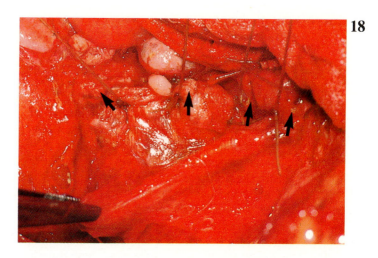

17 and 18
The thick wound edges (3) and (3) indicate that the tissue is cervical and this is closed by a series of interrupted stitches of PGA No. 1 suture (4). The case is a clean one and closure can be effected with safety. The first stitch is in place and the second being inserted (arrowed) in **Figure 17**. The cervical stump is closed in **Figure 18** and displayed on the uncut stitches.

Stage VI: Peritoneal closure

19
The round bodied needle (1) carrying a No. 000 PGA suture has closed the peritoneum medial to the right ovary (0) and indicated by the open arrow. The continuous stitch picks up posterior and anterior leaves of the peritoneum (black arrows) as it progresses across the upper surface of the cervical stump. It remains only to close the abdomen.

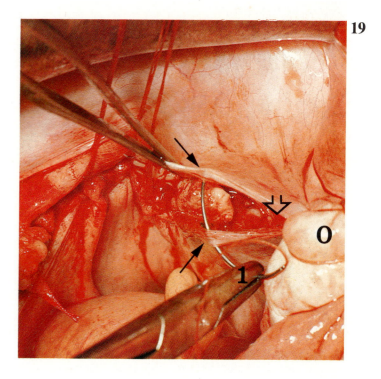

II: Total hysterectomy

The circumstances in which an experienced surgeon may remove both the uterus and the cervix when the clinical situation is not desperate have already been referred to. There are some occasions when total hysterectomy is positively indicated and the risks entailed have to be accepted. For example, there may be severe damage to the cervix from tears extending from the lower segment with bleeding from the cervix itself or the vaginal vault. There may also be indications that the uterus is infected following criminal or unskilled attempts at inducing abortion in the second trimester or as the result of clumsy or traumatic obstetrical interference to deliver the baby or control haemorrhage.

It is desirable to remove the damaged cervix and drain the pelvis in any of the circumstances mentioned. In abortion cases the uterus is less bulky than in the third trimester of pregnancy and the operation is correspondingly easier. The safety of the sub-total operation has been emphasised in this chapter, but readers should have little anxiety about the operation of total hysterectomy if they keep certain points in mind. The following are the more important safeguards to observe when doing a total hysterectomy in late pregnancy:

1. It is essential to obtain good separation of the bladder from the cervix by sharp dissection so that the bladder is well clear of the vaginal incision line when the uterus is ready for removal. This procedure also encourages the ureters to fall laterally and away from the site of operation.

2. As in the sub-total operation the uterine vessels should be carefully stripped of peritoneum so that they can be secured by the forceps close against the lateral wall of the upper cervix.

3. With the uterine vessels secured, the parametrium is clamped and cut close to the cervix taking bites of a size which will not slip from the forceps and can be easily ligated. It is important to keep close to the cervix, even to the extent of cutting into it rather than risk coming down on top of the ureteric tunnel with the ureter within it.

4. Once the parametrium has been detached and the utero-sacral ligaments divided the cervix and whole vaginal vault can be elevated and the vagina clamped across well below the level of the ureters and without damage to them.

5. Haemostasis should be meticulous since a dry wound makes for safety. If the pedicles are taken in controlled 'bites' with a protuding cuff of at least 0.5 cm and ligated as the operation proceeds, then blood loss should be under complete control. It is necessary to drain the pelvis if there is a risk of infection. This may be via a drain inserted through the vaginal vault as seen in **Figure 27**, or by the use of two Redivac suction drains inserted retroperitoneally.

In the case illustrated below only those steps particularly relative to total hysterectomy are shown.

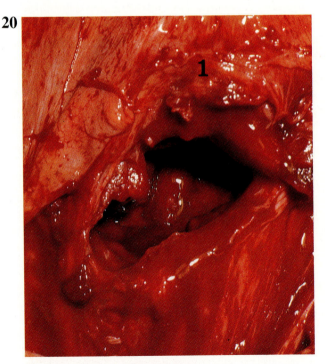

20 Appearances at laparotomy
A torn and lacerated anterior aspect of the lower uterine segment (1) following unskilled attempts at vaginal delivery. There was reason to believe that the patient might be infected.

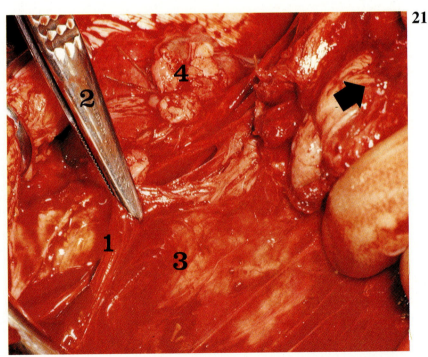

21 Deep reflection of bladder from cervix
The uterus is held upwards by the assistant in the direction of the broad arrow and the surgeon displaces the bladder (1) with the dissecting forceps (2) while dividing adhesions to ensure that the upper vagina (3) is reached and exposed. The uterine pedicle is numbered (4).

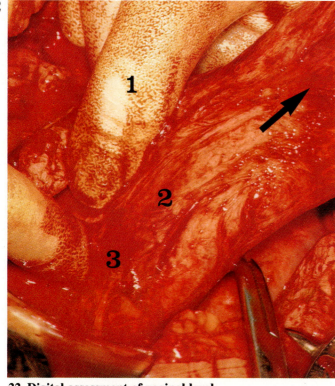

22 Digital assessment of vaginal level
With the uterus drawn up in the direction of the broad arrow the fingers in the posterior pouch and the thumb anteriorly (1) estimate the level of the cervix (2) and upper vagina (3). The manoeuvre is repeated from time to time during the operation.

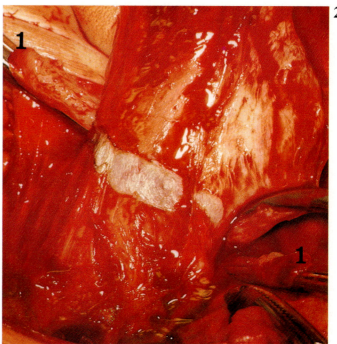

23 Securing uterine vessels
The straight clamping forceps (1) and (1) secure the parametrium on each side at right angles to the axis of the uterus and are detached with an 0.5 cm cuff of tissue which consists of cervical muscle in its medial part.

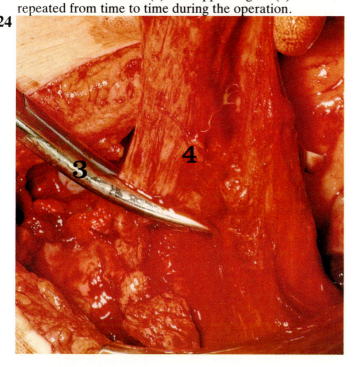

24 Securing vaginal vault
The curved forceps (3) secures the upper vagina at a level which will excise the traumatised and torn cervix (4). The parametrium has already been secured.

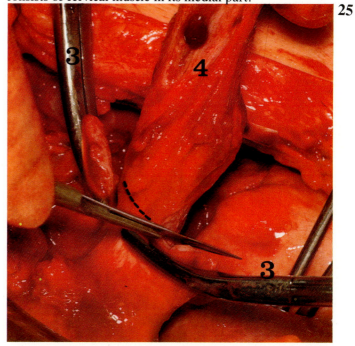

25 Removal of uterus
Note the considerable distance of the excision line (broken line) below the torn cervix (4). The pedicles secured during the operation have been ligated to get rid of the long heavy forceps which are an embarrassment in the wound during such an operation. The vaginal angle forceps are seen at (3).

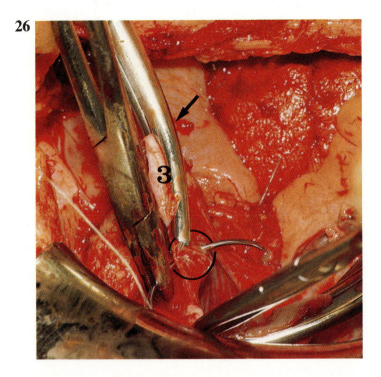

26

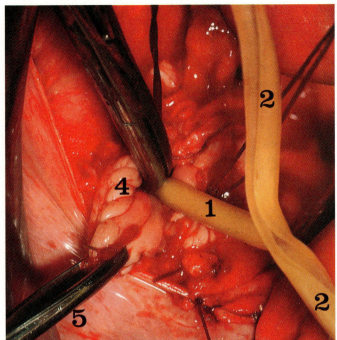

27

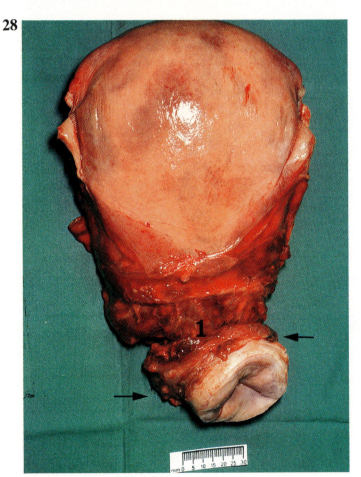

28

26 Securing vaginal angles
The right vaginal pedicle (3) is being transfixed prior to ligation and that is subsequently repeated on the other side. Note how the needle traverses the pedicle so that the first hitch of the ligature controls the paravaginal vessels as it comes under the point of the forceps in the area circled. The ligature is then tied under the heel of the forceps where arrowed.

27 Drainage of pelvis
A T-drain is inserted with the stem (1) being introduced into the vault of the vagina by forceps. Each arm (2) and (2) stretches towards the pelvic side wall under the closed peritoneum. The vaginal edge is numbered (4) and haemostasis has been obtained by an interlocking continuous suture. The Littlewoods forceps (5) support the vault during this manoeuvre.

28 Specimen
Although the operation suggested that detachment of the uterus took place well below the level of the cervix it will be seen that it has been removed with no great margin of tissue (arrowed). What appeared to be a complete cervical tear extending into the vagina was in fact localised to the upper cervix (1).

11: Uterine trauma from automobile accidents, assault, and other external sources

The adverse effects of moderate non-penetrating injuries such as falls, abdominal blows and less severe automobile accidents during pregnancy are surprisingly few. Miscarriage is less frequent than one might expect although in later pregnancy the membranes may rupture with early commencement of labour. Not infrequently there is an escape of liquor but the membranes seal off and the pregnancy continues.

There are sometimes cases of appallingly severe injury from blunt trauma. Some of these are the result of severe blows or kicks on the abdomen but the majority are the result of automobile accidents. In the present complex and dangerous world women at almost any stage of pregnancy have become accustomed to travel by car or plane and continue to participate fully in social and commercial life. Inevitably they have become more liable to serious accident and injury than formerly. Thus it is reported from Minnesota that in the decade up to 1960 trauma was the largest non-obstetric cause of death in pregnant women and half of these were due to automobile collisions[1]. Others found that 0.9 per cent of all maternal deaths in Oklahoma were caused by the automobile[2]. The possible obstetric and gynaecological implications are many and could only be covered in a specialist text such as that of Buchsbaum[3].

The authors are aware that gynaecologists are sometimes consulted by the traumatologist or casualty surgeon on the obstetric or gynaecological aspect of a multiple injury case and where there is doubt about the diagnosis of gynaecological involvement. It is therefore advisable to be aware of probable effects of such trauma and be able to draw on a sound knowledge of management even if that stems from the experience of others. In this section an attempt is made to provide some guidelines on this subject.

Pattern and type of automobile crash injuries

There are several general observations which should be kept in mind:
1. Obstetrical or uterine injury is invariably only a part of multiple body trauma which affects other vital structures to the extent of threatening the patient's life.

2. Head injury is the most frequent cause of death. Internal injuries may also be responsible by leading to exsanguination from rupture of major blood vessels such as aorta, pulmonary artery and renal artery. Rupture of the spleen, the liver and even the intestine is always more likely than uterine rupture; massive intra-peritoneal bleeding is the cause of death in such cases.

3. Quite apart from the effects of hypovolaemia pregnant women seem to have an increased susceptibility to neurogenic shock[4].

4. Nature provides a very efficient protective mechanism for the developing fetus. The uterus is protected within the bony pelvis in the first trimester of pregnancy and is unlikely to be injured. Thereafter, as an abdominal organ it becomes more vulnerable, but it is mobile and surrounded by soft cushioning organs such as bowel and bladder with the abdominal wall anteriorly and the whole bone and muscle structure of the back posteriorly. Within the uterus the fetus is surrounded by an insulating water jacket which gives a great deal of protection and dissipates traumatic forces. Thus automobile accidents of gross severity are reported with lower abdominal involvement and yet the fetus is not affected.

5. While the uterus and fetus are less likely to be damaged than almost any abdominal structure the fact remains that separation of the placenta and rupture of the uterus can occur, and in automobile accidents where there are pelvic fractures with bone displacement, rupture of the uterus, and separation of the placenta, are more liable to result. In a paper[5] on the incidence of such complications in a one-year series of 15 cases at the Baragwanath Hospital in Johannesburg, it is seen that pelvic fracture is not a necessary factor since in the series mentioned, 3 out of 4 assault cases without pelvic fracture had placental separation. Abruptio placentae is not necessarily associated with direct traumatic force and several authorities[3,6] believe that shock following trauma is the main cause of the actual placental separation.

6. When the uterus does rupture it is most likely to do so at the fundus and the clinical picture may not be dramatic or immediately apparent.

The use of seat belts

It is necessary to refer to seat belt restraint and its relationship to inflicted trauma before considering the pattern of injury that is to be expected in automobile accidents.

There is overwhelming evidence that the use of seat belts reduces maternal and fetal mortality and injury, and even if only by preventing ejection from the vehicle, they save many lives.

The surgeon considering the question of possible injury can expect no pattern to help him when a seat belt has *not* been worn. Any part of the body may be injured and it is usually quite impossible to work out the kinetics of the accident. Head injuries are frequent and are the most frequent cause of death in these circumstances. Multiple fractures are common and when these involve the pelvis and ribs they endanger the uterus and the fetus. Accidents in which the car has rolled over or somersaulted lead to complicated injuries as a result of the tumbling action of the occupant's body within the vehicle[7]. Ejection from the vehicle may occur and the effects of that are always serious.

It is estimated that the wearing of seat belts by pregnant patients reduces the death, injury and total mortality rate by at least half[4], and a major advantage is in preventing the serious effects of ejection from the car and roll-over within it.

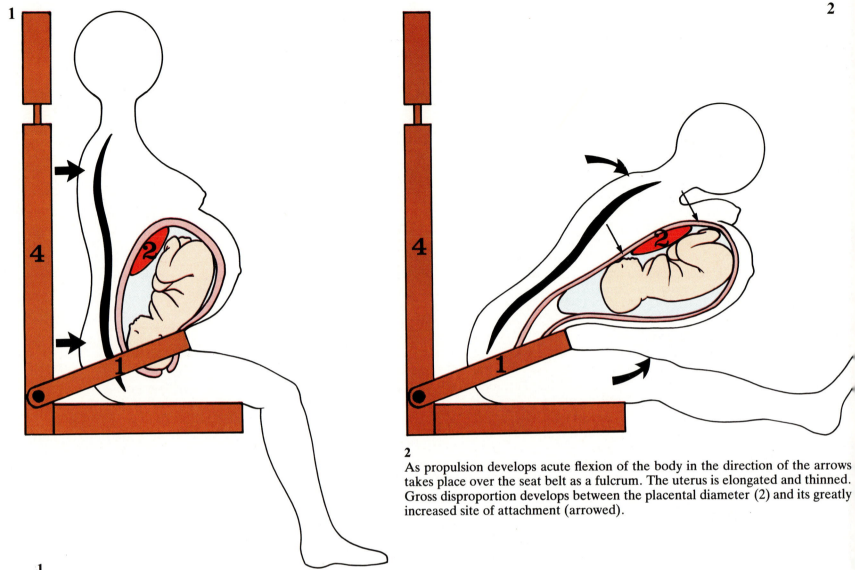

2

As propulsion develops acute flexion of the body in the direction of the arrows takes place over the seat belt as a fulcrum. The uterus is elongated and thinned. Gross disproportion develops between the placental diameter (2) and its greatly increased site of attachment (arrowed).

1

The initial stages of the forward propulsion of the body in a head-on crash. The seat belt (1) is fully extended and already the lower part of the body has moved forward in the direction of the arrow. The uterus is not yet distorted and the placenta (2) is unaffected.

Crash injury pattern in pregnant automobile victim wearing a seat belt

It is possible to study the pattern of injuries in head-on collisions where the woman in later pregnancy is wearing a seat belt. This is the most frequent type of accident and it is important to look at the forces involved and how they affect the body. For simplicity this is considered in relation to the lap belt only; there are some additional advantages in the chest or shoulder restraint systems, but they are not significant and the general principles are the same.

The lap belt applied across the upper thighs and around the pelvis fixes the pelvis to the seat of the car. On impact, the body attempts to continue its forward movement but is restrained and held stationary at pelvic level. The whole body jack-knives with the head, upper trunk and arms being thrown forwards and strongly flexed while the legs are extended to meet the trunk. Rebound follows completion of deceleration and when it occurs the upper body and head return through the same arc to an upright position and the legs return to a state of flexion. The very high tension on the seat belt during impact is now transferred to the supporting seat and the lower abdominal organs are compressed between the seat belt and the maternal spine. During the impact and rebound, pressure within the large pregnant uterus rises to levels 10 times that observed during labour. There is a concomitant rise in intra-peritoneal pressure but this is very much less than within the uterus.

The effect of these forces on the uterus in advanced pregnancy is shown on diagrams 1, 2 and 3. The mechanics of impact in pregnancy have been observed in the baboon[8] and the specific effects on the uterus

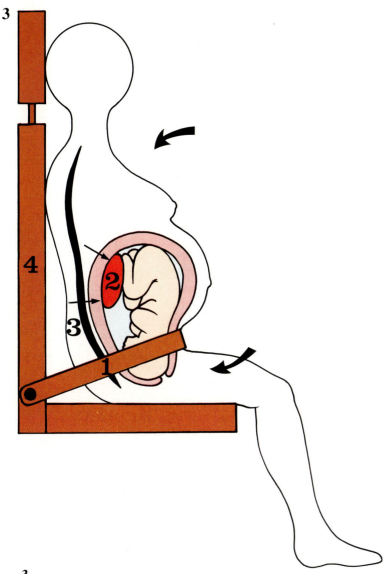

3
Following impact deflexion and recoil (in the direction of the arrows) takes place towards the back of the seat (4). The uterus is shortened, contracted and comes into collision with the vertebral column (3). Disproportion develops between the placental diameter and its reduced area of attachment.

studied from such information; with added clinical observation one can build up a reasonably accurate picture of what takes place.

(i) Risk of uterine rupture
During the collision the uterus follows the laws of inertia and continues in the direction the body is going until the body decelerates (**Figures 1** and **2**). The uterus is elongated and flattened against the anterior abdominal wall which is itself stretched forward as far as possible (**Figure 2**). The deformation of the uterus largely depends on the velocity of deceleration but also on the elasticity of the uterus. Abrupt deceleration can rupture the uterus directly but this is apparently quite unusual. With the recoil which follows and because of the elasticity of its wall the uterus shortens in the

opposite direction and is flattened against the posterior abdominal wall (**Figure 3**). The intra-uterine pressure at this stage is probably the highest achieved but the uterus is compacted rather than stretched and thus less liable to rupture. Even with very rapid deceleration the prospect of the uterus rupturing seems to be small; this is probably explained by the amount of elastic tissue in its wall.

(ii) Risk of placental separation
The forces involved are more likely to cause placental separation since that structure does not contain elastic tissue and cannot stretch or contract to adjust to increases or decreases in the area of its attachment to the uterine wall. The placenta is seldom torn or ruptured but frequently separated from the uterine wall. The anchoring villi are detached by the violent movements and the clinical condition resembles abruptio placentae. Retroplacental bleeding leads to further separation of placenta and membranes and the condition may be clinically concealed or revealed. This can be appreciated by studying figures 1, 2 and 3. In **1** the uterus has not yet been distorted and the placenta still occupies its normal area of the uterine wall. In **2** the uterine wall is stretched and thin, so that the area of placental attachment is greatly enlarged and the inelastic placenta is liable to be separated by shearing force. In **3** the uterus has contracted and been compressed to an abnormal degree with thickened walls and a greatly reduced area of placental attachment. The reverse type of shearing force to that seen in **2** is equally liable to cause separation. The elastic recoil of the uterine walls causes a powerful wave effect in the amniotic fluid at this stage and must also be disruptive at the placental site.

In one series of collisions which is reported[9], placental separation was only clinically apparent in 4 per cent of cases. In a certain number of cases the retroplacental haemorrhage remains limited; an area of the placenta becomes infarcted and the pregnancy continues to term. The larger haemorrhages are associated with premature labour with a high fetal mortality and in the severe cases there are immediate problems of maternal shock, severe blood loss and possibly hypofibrinogenemia.

Management

With multiple injuries the whole question of treatment must initially be in the hands of the traumatologist who will have to decide not only on what must be done but which injuries have priority. Where the gynaecologist is concerned in management decisions there are some basic considerations. Placental separation is always important, for apart from causing maternal death it is the most common cause of fetal death[9]. The pregnant victim should, therefore, be observed for abnormal uterine activity, tenderness and vaginal bleeding. If they are noted and if the patient is near term an immediate caesarean section may salvage the fetus. Otherwise bleeding may continue, the fetus dies unnecessarily and the mother's condition deteriorates with ensuing hypotension and shock. There is the additional danger of hypofibrinogenemia and the traumatologist would be advised of this possibility. It is also prudent to ensure that supplies of fibrinogen are available.

Penetrating wounds

Penetrating injuries of the abdomen by sharp metal objects, knives or bullets are much more infrequent and it is more difficult to assess the potential damage to the uterus and the fetus.

1. Gunshot wounds

Abdominal gunshot wounds are probably the most frequent and with the increasing violence and use of guns by criminals pregnant women are more exposed to such injury. Urban unrest and terrorist activity has also increased the incidence.

The pregnant uterus is sheltered by the pelvis in the first trimester but presents a considerable target thereafter, which because of its size and consistency, generally halts the flight of the bullet which may be found within it. The uterus and its contents, in fact, act as a shield which modifies the type of injury sustained and makes it less dangerous to the life of the mother. It does so because the normally vulnerable intestine is displaced from the line of fire by the enlarged uterus and also because the bulk of the uterus and its contents are sufficient to arrest the flight of the bullet. There is quite a low incidence of associated maternal injury[10].

Management
The modern view of treatment[10] is for early exploration to be performed in pregnant patients with gunshot wounds of the abdomen. Complete surgical exploration of the track or course of the bullet is essential and if access is obstructed by the presence of a large pregnant uterus, then caesarean section becomes necessary. There is some conflict of opinion on the details of how to treat these cases and clearly each must be judged on its merits.

2. Stab wounds

Stab wounds of the abdomen during pregnancy are infrequent and although the uterus is at great risk in late pregnancy there is not at present the same tendency to immediately explore the abdomen surgically. Previously all such cases had emergency operation but in 30 per cent of cases it was found that the peritoneum had not been penetrated and that in a further 15–20 per cent there was no injury that required repair. Treatment has therefore tended to become more conservative, at least initially, but maintaining very strict observational criteria. It must nonetheless be exceedingly difficult to maintain a policy of conservative management or inactivity in certain circumstances[11] and especially since the pregnant patient's abdominal wall may not respond to intra-peritoneal stimuli as quickly or to the same degree as in the non-pregnant state and thus masking signs of intraperitoneal leakage. A technique which may be of help is to employ a fistulogram[12] whereby the wound site is appropriately cleaned and a fine catheter passed into the track and fixed to the abdominal wall with a purse string suture.

A radio opaque substance is injected by syringe, the catheter is clamped and the patient's position changed so that antero-posterior and lateral abdominal x-rays can be taken. These are subsequently examined to determine if the contrast medium has entered the peritoneal cavity. If it has done so, it will be seen to have spilled widely and outline loops of bowel with pooling in the pelvis. Where the wound has not penetrated the peritoneum the contrast material is restricted to the abdominal wall and the case is recognised as a less serious one.

Management
This is again an individual matter and depends on the special circumstances. It may be taken as axiomatic that maintenance of the pregnancy should never compromise management of the maternal wound and, as in the case of gunshot wounds, if the gravid uterus limits exploration of the injury it should be emptied regardless of the stage of pregnancy.

The fetus has apparently a great capacity to survive such injuries and there is general agreement that the uterus also can often be conserved even if considerably traumatised. There are numerous reports of women having subsequent normal pregnancies.

12: Management of cervical neoplasia in pregnancy

1. Pre-malignant disease

The prevention of invasive cervical cancer is only possible if the pre-malignant lesions of dysplasia and carcinoma *in situ* (now referred to as CIN or cervical intraepithelial neoplasia) are detected and treated. Even though this can be done relatively easily the rate of this disease continues to remain high; only in selected countries where exfoliative cytological screening is efficient is the rate decreasing. This being so, and since women with cervical neoplasia are usually unwilling to come for cytological (detection) smear examination, an ideal situation exists for screening them when they come for ante-natal care in early pregnancy.

An abnormal smear in pregnancy probably indicates the presence of the premalignant CIN stage. Reference to Table I shows that in nearly 300 cases in which an abnormal smear was obtained in pregnancy, a histological diagnosis of CIN was found either during or after pregnancy in over 90 per cent. Less than 1 in 100 women had microinvasive or frankly invasive cancer and indeed no cases of frankly invasive cancer were missed. In only one case was a microinvasive cancer underdiagnosed initially as CIN 3. These excellent results were achieved because colposcopy was used in all cases. Although cytology remains the major screening method, colposcopy with its illuminated and magnified vision allows a *conservative* approach to be taken in the management of the abnormal pregnancy smear. This is principally because there is no evidence to suggest that the CIN lesion is more likely to progress to invasive cancer during pregnancy. Therefore this conservative approach can be accepted with safety.

Colposcopy in pregnancy

The physiological changes undergone by the cervix in pregnancy aid the detection of the premalignant (CIN) lesion. The atypical epithelium which harbours them usually appears white, or has a mosaic or punctated appearance when viewed colposcopically. In pregnancy these appearances are accentuated because they are seen against the darkish blue background of the extremely vascular and engorged cervix (**Figure 1**). With eversion of the endocervical epithelium which occurs from as early as the 10th week of pregnancy the upper extent of the atypical epithelium becomes easily visible (**Figure 1**), thus allowing the full extent of the potentially malignant area to be viewed and assessed.

Colposcopic examination

Two important observations must be made during the colposcopic examination; these are
- determination of the full extent of the atypical epithelium
- assessment of the epithelium as consistent with premalignancy or early malignancy.

The full extent of the atypical epithelium within the transformation zone must be seen before a satisfactory colposcopic opinion can be given. This means visualisation of the upper extent of the lesion; if it cannot be seen then the presence of early invasive cancer cannot be excluded. This is exemplified in the case shown in **Figures 3 to 5**. Whether the lesion is judged to be colposcopically consistent with a premalignant (CIN) stage will to some extent be determined by the experience of the examiner. Lesions not satisfactorily categorized must be submitted to biopsy. The cervix in **Figure 1** is consistent with CIN yet the cervix in **Figure 2** is not.

Biopsy under colposcopic control

If any doubt exists colposcopically on the presence of early *invasive* cancer (**Figure 2**), then a biopsy of the atypical epithelium must be taken for confirmation. This biopsy performed under colposcopic control and under anaesthesia is usually taken in the form of a wedge of tissue. It not only accurately removes the suspicious tissue, but also gives the pathologist an adequate amount of material on which to make a satisfactory diagnosis.

Cone biopsy, the traditional method for obtaining a cervical biopsy when colposcopy is not available should be avoided. The significant morbidity (approximately 30–40 per cent[1]) associated with its performance in pregnancy is too high for its routine use. In addition nearly 40 per cent of cone biopsies in pregnancy fail to remove the lesion.[2] Wedge biopsy offers an accurate and relatively atraumatic alternative (**Figures 10 to 15**).

Punch biopsy under colposcopic vision and *without* anaesthetic is used by many gynaecologists[3] to obtain histological confirmation of the CIN lesion. Others[4] dispense with it so long as they are satisfied that they have excluded the possibility of early invasive disease by colposcopy. Again, the capacity to do so will depend on the experience of the observer. Although the biopsy site after punch biopsy seems exceedingly vascular, haemostasis can be obtained by simple pressure with a tampon after the application of silver nitrate or Moncel's ferric subsulphate solution (**Figures 6 to 9**).

Colposcopic appearances of the cervix in pregnancy

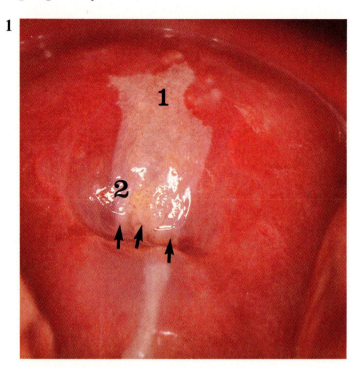

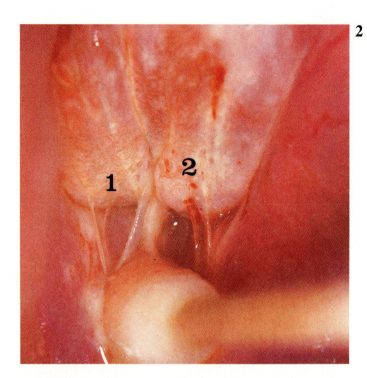

1 Premalignant lesion
A colpophotograph (X10) of a 22-year-old woman in her 10th week of pregnancy with an abnormal cytological smear (class 3) showing an area of atypical epithelium extending from the ectocervix (1) into the endocervical canal (2). The upper extent of the lesion is arrowed. Eversion of the endocervix has occurred, making it easy to visualise this upper extent. Biopsy revealed moderate to severe dysplasia (CIN 2–3).

2 Suspicion of early invasive lesion
A colpophotograph (X20) of a 38-year-old woman, para 4, with a class 4–5 smear at 18 weeks gestation. A small swab stick opens up the endocervical canal into which the atypical epithelium extends. The upper limit of this tissue cannot be seen. The epithelium at 1 and 2 was regarded as suspicious of early invasive cancer by the colposcopist and because of this and the non-visualisation of the upper extent, a wedge biopsy was undertaken. This showed the presence of carcinoma *in situ* (CIN 3) involving gland crypts but no early invasive cancer.

3 to 5 Early invasive (clinical) cancer in endocervical canal
Colpophotographs (X10) of a 34-year-old woman, para 4, presenting with a class 4–5 smear. The atypical epithelium (**Figure 3**) extends on to the ectocervix at (1) and into the endocervical canal at (2). A swab stick attempts to open the canal so as to visualise its upper extent. In **Figure 4** bleeding is produced as the swab stick passes into the endocervix and in **Figure 5** a pair of Desjardins forceps (used for viewing the endocervical canal) open the endocervix to show an early clinical invasive cancer at 3. The extent of the associated premalignant lesion is arrowed. This case shows the importance of proper visualisation of the upper extent of the atypical epithelium; if that is not seen, then the presence of early invasive cancer, as in this case, cannot be excluded.

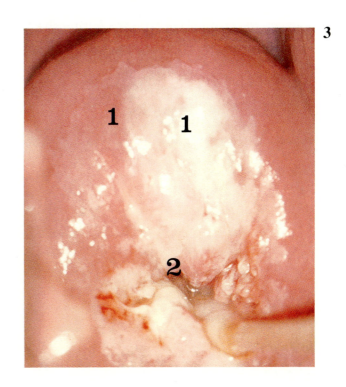

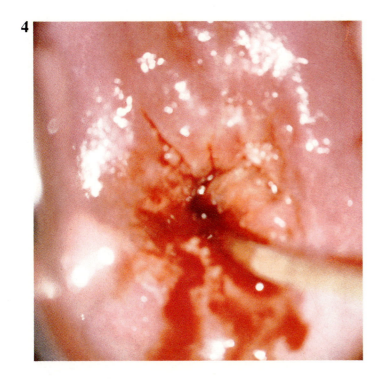

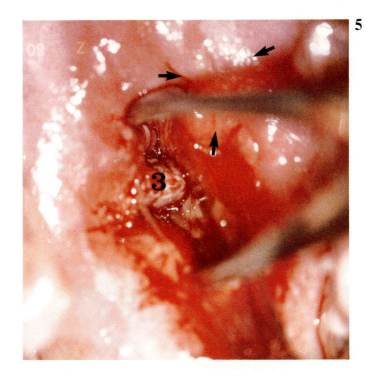

Punch biopsy of cervix

6 Premalignant lesion
Colpophotograph (X10) of a 24-year-old woman with a class 3 smear at 12 weeks of pregnancy. An area of atypical epithelium (white epithelium) exists

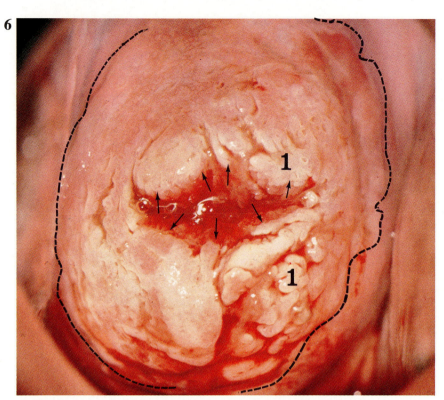

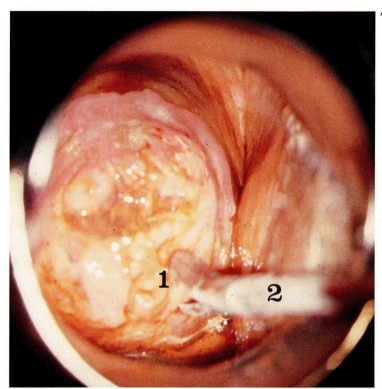

within the broken line and its upper extent is easily seen and is arrowed. No suspicion exists colposcopically of early invasive cancer. A punch biopsy will be taken from two areas (1) and (1) which show the most atypical change.

7 Biopsy procedure
A punch biopsy is about to be taken by the forceps (Patersons' colon forceps) (2) of one of the atypical areas (1). No anaesthesia is needed.

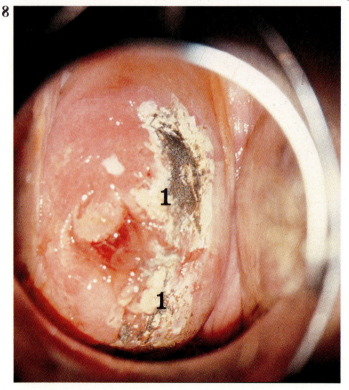

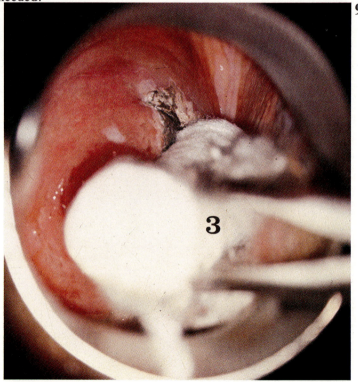

8 Post biopsy haemostasis
Biopsies have been taken at (1) and (1) and haemostasis has been achieved by the local application of silver nitrate.

9 Tampon insertion
Although haemostasis has been achieved a pressure tampon (3) is being inserted for 6 to 8 hours to achieve further protection. It is placed over the biopsy sites. In cases in which bleeding persists after silver nitrate application, it is suggested that a pressure tampon be applied for 4 to 5 minutes in the first instance; if this is successful a tampon can be inserted for 6 to 8 hours as in this case.

Wedge biopsy of cervix: to exclude early invasive cancer

10 and 11 Pre-clinical cervical lesion
Colposcopy of the cervix of this 32-year-old woman, para 2, with a class 4–5 smear in early pregnancy revealed atypical epithelium extending over the ecto and into the posterior region of the endocervix. This latter area was regarded by the

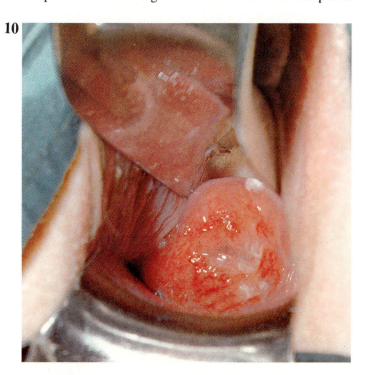

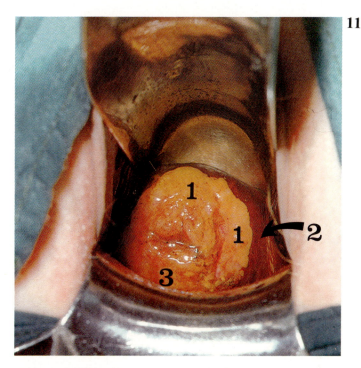

colposcopist as suspicious of early invasive cancer and so warranted a wedge biopsy. **Figure 10** shows the cervix with no apparent clinically abnormal features while in **Figure 11** the outline and extent of the atypical epithelium (1) after the application of Schiller's iodine solution becomes obvious. Normal, non-neoplastic tissue, should absorb the iodine solution and stain brown as seen at (2). The area containing the colposcopically suspicious lesion is at (3).

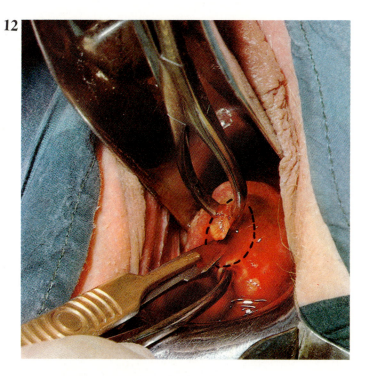

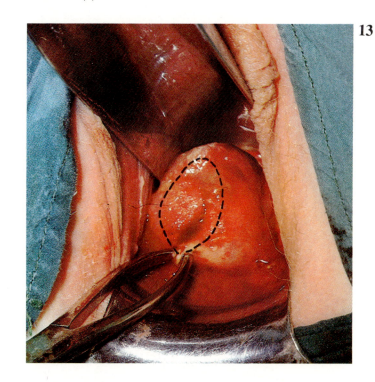

12 and 13 Excision of suspicious area
Two Littlewoods' forceps have been applied at the upper and lower extent of the suspicious area to be removed. Two ellipitical incisions (dotted lines) are made – one on the right (**Figure 12**) and one on the left side, so as to encompass the whole of the atypical area. The incision is carried 2 cm into the stroma so that the area of tissue removed is adequate for pathological assessment. Care must be taken so as not to abrade or damage the tissue during excision. **Figure 13** shows the area after the tissue has been removed.

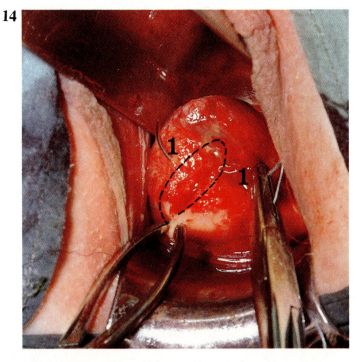

14

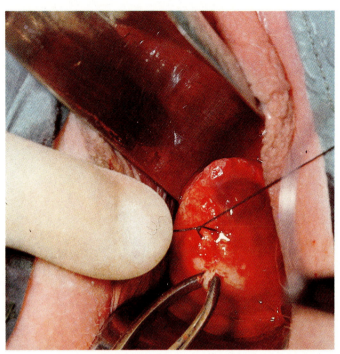

15

14 and 15 Resuture of biopsy site
The outline of the biopsy site can clearly be seen in **Figure 14** (dotted line). It is closed with interrupted sutures of 000 suture material. Occasionally, if bleeding is excessive, a figure of eight haemostatic suture has to be inserted instead of the simple interrupted suture. In **Figure 14** the first suture is inserted (1) and (1) and in **Figure 15** it is being tied. Only one other suture was necessary to produce complete closure and haemostasis.

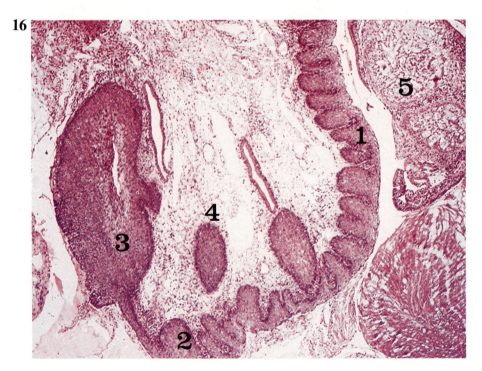

16

16 Biopsy specimen: CIN 3 (carcinoma *in situ*) with gland crypt involvement
The specimen shows the presence of severe dysplasia and carcinoma *in situ* (CIN 3) at (1) and (2) with extension into glandular crypts (3). The latter appearance is easily confused with that of early invasive disease, especially where a segment of CIN has been 'isolated' because of the plane of section of the specimen. It is purely an extension of CIN into a glandular crypt as seen at (4). However no breach of the basement membrane, which would suggest early invasive cancer, has occurred in any part of this section. Typical changes of pregnancy, i.e. micro-glandular hyperplasia are seen at (5).

TABLE 1

DIAGNOSIS OF THE ABNORMAL CERVICAL SMEAR IN PREGNANCY USING COLPOSCOPY

| Study | Patients Colposcoped | No Abnormality Detected *(Post Partum) | Histological Evidence of Disease (obtained by biopsy) | | | | | |
			CIN 1. (Mild Dysplasia)		CIN 2. (Mod. Dysplasia)	CIN 3. (Severe Dysplasia Ca. in situ)	Microinvasive Cancer	Invasive Cancer
Ortiz et al (1971)	47	4		6		37	—	—
Stafl et al (1973)	45	10	5		4	25	1	—
Abitbol et al (1973)	286		243			40(39)†	0(1)†	3
De Petrillo et al (1975)	159		130			24	2	3
Talebian et at (1976)	75	17	15		10	31	2	—
Benedet et al (1977)	123	10	8		8	95	2	—
Ostergard et al (1979)	161	37	53		33	37	—	1
Lurain et al (1979)	110	41	21		21	27	—	—
Singer et al (1980)								
McDonnel et al (1981)	170	70	27		20	52	1	
Total	1176	189	502	6	96	368	8	7

*Cytology and colposcopic biopsy negative in post partum period.
†Patient subsequently developed microinvasive cancer after initial CIN 3 diagnosis.

Summary: management of abnormal smear in pregnancy

The flow diagram (Table 2) represents a schema in which colposcopy plays an important role. Without colposcopy resort to cone biopsy becomes necessary in many cases.

TABLE 2

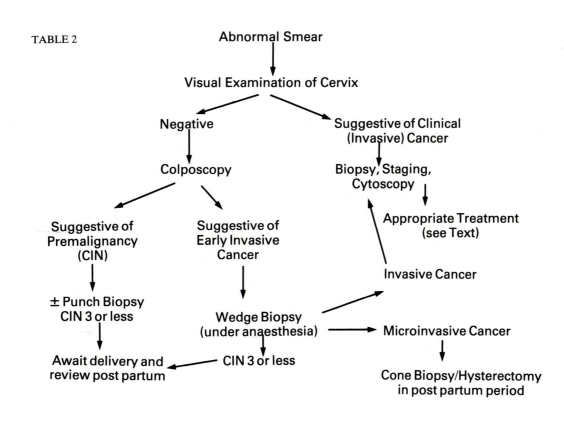

2. Malignant (invasive) disease

Malignant cervical disease usually presents in pregnancy without obvious clinical signs of disease. This produces problems in diagnosis as in the case illustrated by **Figure 17**. Even though this 33-year-old woman had a Class 3 smear during pregnancy, no treatment was instituted till nearly 4 months post-partum. In pregnancy no clinical signs of cervical cancer were obvious although it was reported that the cervix 'was eroded'. In the post-partum period an ulcerative and exophytic growth appeared in the posterior fornix and subsequent pelvic lymph node involvement was found during radical surgery. It is most likely that the 'eroded cervix' of pregnancy was indeed the early stage of this invasive cancer.

Because of bleeding or infection, the cervical smear may be reported as negative or even inflammatory despite the presence of invasive disease. The softness and hyperaemia of the cervix may also cause the examiner to underestimate the extent of the disease. In a recent study it was shown that 30 per cent of 113 patients with early clinical malignant disease had no symptoms when first seen.[5]

Treatment

The diagnosis will normally have been made by biopsy of an unsuspected preclinical or of an established clinical lesion. Certain factors in the management of these lesions must be taken into consideration:

—extent of disease (stage and histological type),
—duration of pregnancy,
—wishes of the mother concerning the pregnancy.

If the disease is histologically confirmed during pregnancy as a microinvasive carcinoma with stromal invasion limited to 3 mm beneath the surface and with no cancer invading the capillary lympathic space, it is probably reasonable to allow the pregnancy to continue, and, after delivery, treat the mother with either a cone biopsy or hysterectomy if sterilisation is required. If the disease is more advanced and a Stage I lesion is diagnosed then radical hysterectomy with pelvic lymphadenectomy after initial hysterotomy or caesarean section should be considered.

The exact mode of fetal delivery depends very much on the stage of the gestation. The wishes of the mother come foremost in deciding whether immediate treatment with sacrifice of the non viable fetus is chosen or whether a short delay is permissible to attain fetal viability. The latter alternative should not compromise the mother's chances of cure, and that ought to be assured as far as it is possible to do so.

In very early pregnancy the decision is relatively easy. Radical hysterectomy with lymphadenectomy (as in the case illustrated in **Figure 18**) can be done with the removal of the fetus in utero.

In later pregnancy the decision is much more difficult; usually fetal viability is awaited. With the expertise now available to perinatologists the necessary waiting time has decreased considerably over the last decade. Caesarean section is used to deliver the fetus and immediate radical hysterectomy with lymphadenectomy can be undertaken. If radiotherapy is to be used instead of surgery then it will commence as soon as the abdominal wound has healed. Whole pelvis irradiation precedes intracavity irradiation in such cases. In early pregnancy whole pelvis irradiation usually causes fetal abortion during treatment.

There is no evidence to suggest that pregnancy exerts a detrimental effect on cervical cancer. Several studies[5] now shown that stage for stage, the outcome in pregnant patients with cervical cancer is approximately the same as for non-pregnant patients.

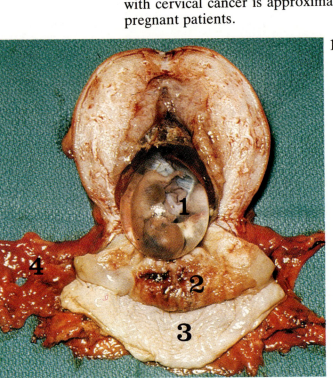

17

17
Invasive cervical cancer (1) diagnosed at 15 weeks post partum. It had already metastatised to the pelvic lymph nodes. It was considered to be a preclinical lesion during pregnancy (see text) yet presented with a Class 3 smear.

18
Radical surgery (Wertheims hysterectomy) specimen of an early pregnancy (1) in conjunction with a Stage 1 cervical cancer (2). A substantial amount of vagina (3) and parametrial tissue (4) has been removed.

13: Gestational trophoblastic disease

When dealing with the general subject of gestational trophoblastic disease in the Atlas, the authors have assumed that readers are familiar with the incidence and clinical features of the two principal divisions: the relatively benign but potentially dangerous hydatidiform (vesicular) mole and the malignant chorio-carcinoma or chorion epithelioma. Hydatid mole and chorio-carcinoma present very different clinical pictures and pose different problems of management; for that reason and also because it simplifies matters to do so, the two conditions are considered separately.

Hydatidiform mole

Relationship to chorio-carcinoma: essential follow-up

The woman who has hydatidiform mole is at considerable risk of developing subsequent chorio-carcinoma particularly in the succeeding two years. In the United Kingdom chorio-carcinoma is preceded by hydatidiform mole in about 50 per cent of cases, yet less than 5 per cent of patients who abort a hydatid mole later develop chorio-carcinoma and fewer than 10 per cent require treatment to eliminate persistent trophoblastic tissue[1]. Some 50 per cent of chorio-carcinoma cases follow normal pregnancy, abortion or labour without any evidence of hydatidiform mole at the time. Adequate screening of the hydatidiform mole group should, therefore, discover about half the total number of cases of chorio-carcinoma. Not only should patients with known hydatidiform mole be followed up carefully for at least two years, but the possibility of a trophoblastic tumour should be considered in every patient who has recurrent bleeding after delivery or abortion. Histological examination of curettings may give negative findings, sometimes because molar tissue is deeply embedded in the muscle wall of the uterus. Regular and routine estimation of gonadotrophins in the urine by radioimmunoassay is the best guide to early and certain diagnosis. (Report on confidential enquiries into maternal deaths in England and Wales 1973–75)[2]

To organise these important follow-up requirements a registration scheme was established in Great Britain by joint action of the Department of Health and Social Security and the Royal College of Obstetricians and Gynaecologists in January 1973 and the results have already more than justified this initiative. Referring to the project the Report emphasises that untreated chorio-carcinoma is nearly always fatal and that the chances of cure are diminished if the treatment is delayed. If treatment is begun within six months of evacuation of a mole the tumour can be eliminated in 95 per cent of cases. The ordinary pregnancy tests are not sufficiently sensitive to detect the relatively low levels of HCG present in early chorio-carcinoma and a reliable radioimmunoassay procedure is necessary.

Diagnosis

Prompt recognition of the condition depends on an acute awareness of the possibility where there is repeated bleeding in early pregnancy. Frank clinical evidence of the type illustrated in **Figure 1** is exceptional, and commendable reluctance to make a vaginal examination in an apparent case of threatened abortion excludes the evidence of a soft and over-bulky uterus and the ovarian enlargement due to theca-lutein cysts. An ultrasonic scan of the uterus presents a picture which is quite typical (see **Figure 2**) and is diagnostic so that the method deserves to be used more frequently as a primary diagnostic procedure than as a spectacular visual confirmation of the diagnosis.

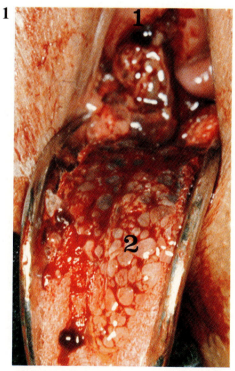

1 Clinical appearance
Unmistakable evidence of hydatidiform mole. With a Sims' speculum in the vagina the anterior lip of the cervix (1) is held in tissue forceps and a mass of vesicles (2) is being extruded into the vagina from the uterus.

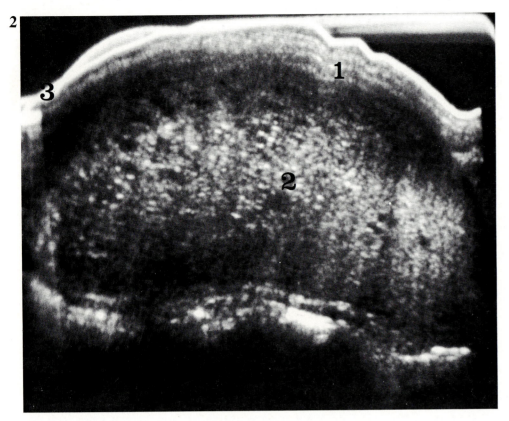

2 Ultrasonic scan
This longitudinal scan shows the typical 'snowstorm' appearance within the uterus. The various structures are designated as follows: uterine wall (1), hydatidiform mole (2), area of umbilicus (3).

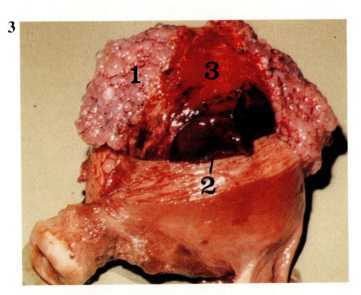

3 Hysterectomy specimen
The uterus is split open to show the pregnancy replaced by hydatidiform mole (1). In addition to the mass of vesicles the uterus contains old blood clot (2) and evidence of recent bleeding (3).

Treatment

The first requirement is to evacuate the uterus and as already seen the second is to keep the patient under observation for two years during which her HCG levels are monitored and with particular frequency in the first six months.

1. Prophylactic chemotherapy?

Such treatment at or soon after evacuation of the mole has been considered. It would be attractive if malignant cells could either be completely eliminated at this stage, or so reduced that subsequent treatment need only be minimal. Elston and Bagshawe[2] referring to several conflicting reports on the relationship between the degree of trophoblastic hyperplasia and subsequent development of chorio-carcinoma, studied 70 patients of their own with hydatidiform mole in 21 per cent of whom chorio-carcinoma developed. They found no relationship between the histological grade of hydatidiform mole and subsequent malignancy. There are various reports of prophylactic treatment being given. Results with Methotrexate were inconclusive although one group[3] reported on a series of 70 consecutive cases with more promising results. Comparing these results with those from the previous year's consecutive series there was a reduction in overall trophoblastic disease from 17.3 to 5.6 per cent. Goldstein[4] used Actinomycin D in 100 selected cases and observed 100 controls. In the treated group there were only 2 who subsequently showed evidence of trophoblastic neoplasm while there were 16 in the control group and 4 of these developed metastases. Unfortunately some of the treated group showed transient rises in serum transaminases, leucopenia, thrombocytopenia, stomatitis, skin eruptions and gastrointestinal symptoms and 32 of them suffered partial alopecia. He concluded that though prophylactic Actinomycin D reduced the incidence of neoplastic sequelae it did not avoid the need for systematic follow-up by sensitive gonadotrophin assay. Commenting on this study in a review article in the British Medical Journal[5] the writer concluded that where adequate follow-up facilities were available, the risk of prophylactic chemotherapy seemed greater than those of selective chemotherapy but where adequate gonadotrophin measurements could not be performed prophylactic chemotherapy in experienced hands might well reduce the risks. The present tendency is to discount the value of prophylactic treatment.

2. Surgical management

The fact that the uterus is soft, enlarged and vascular with molar invasion of the muscular wall means that it is extremely vulnerable to operative trauma with the risks of perforation, severe bleeding and subsequent sepsis. Dilatation of the cervix and even the most careful evacuation of the uterus with blunt curette and forceps was so often followed by complications such as a split cervix or a perforated uterus that at one time abdominal hysterotomy was accepted by many gynaecologists as the safest method of ensuring that the uterine cavity had been emptied; the method of course carries very obvious disadvantages. The advent of the suction apparatus for uterine evacuation as in therapeutic abortion has completely altered the picture, and the uterus can be safely and effectively emptied by this means (see pages 21–25). The equipment is seen in use in **Figure 4** and a kidney dish containing the uterine contents is shown as **Figure 5**.

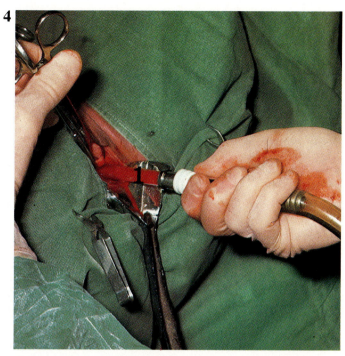

4 Evacuation of hydatidiform mole by suction curette
The equipment used for suction termination of pregnancy in the first trimester is ideal for this purpose. The procedure is seen in progress; the suction curette (1) is in the uterine cavity and the molar tissue is collected in the receiving bottle.

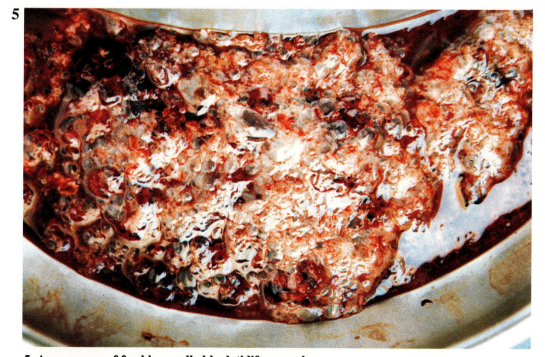

5 Appearance of freshly expelled hydatidiform mole
The patient was a 32-year-old gravida 2, para 0 with a uterine size of about 24 weeks. The cervix was softened by the application of prostaglandin before operation. The mass of vesicles in the kidney dish is only part of the molar tissue and blood clot removed from the uterus.

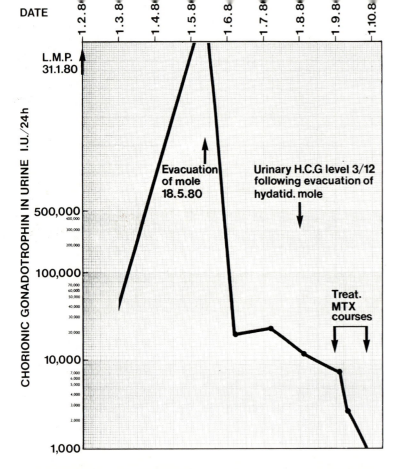

chorio-carcinoma and examine the results obtained before considering the surgical aspects of treatment. The Atlas is concerned with surgical treatment and the only absolute indication for its use is as an emergency measure to control massive haemorrhage. The relative indications for its use are still very much a matter of opinion and concern those patients who have not responded to chemotherapy. Only by a comprehensive study of routine management and its achievements can the practical surgeon assess the likely value of using surgical methods.

Diagnosis

The mandatory long term follow-up of hydatidiform mole by urinary HCG assays leads to the diagnosis in most of the cases of chorio-carcinoma. **Figure 6** typifies the progress of hydatidiform mole to chorio-carcinoma as indicated by the urinary HCG levels during follow-up and eventual successful treatment.

In the absence of a history of hydatidiform mole diagnosis of chorio-carcinoma depends very much on clinical awareness of the possibility. Cases are infrequent and the interval before malignancy manifests itself may be as long as five years, so that there is a tendency for them to be diagnosed later than one would wish. There should be no occasion for delayed diagnosis in a properly followed-up case of hydatidiform mole.

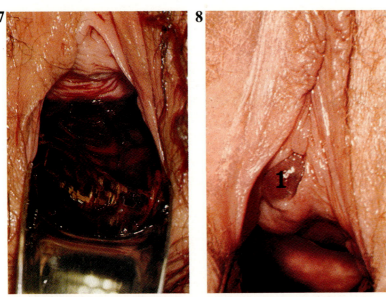

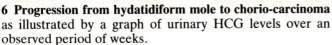

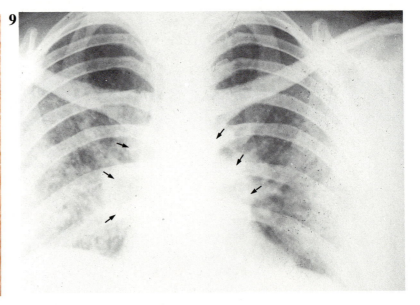

6 Progression from hydatidiform mole to chorio-carcinoma as illustrated by a graph of urinary HCG levels over an observed period of weeks.

7 and 8 Typical clinical representations of chorio-carcinoma
Figure 7 shows heavy vaginal bleeding in a post partum patient who had an enlarged uterus and raised urinary HCG levels. In **Figure 8** the bleeding has originated from an obvious periurethral metastasis (1).

9 Chest x-ray: chorio-carcinoma
Evidence of metastatic growth is seen throughout both lung fields. Sizeable nodules are particularly obvious in the hilar areas (arrowed).

The one symptom which should put the clinician on the alert and which usually presages the onset of malignancy is alarmingly heavy intermittent bleeding which is usually uterine (**Figure 7**) but may be from vaginal secondaries (**Figure 8**). There is often an associated blood-stained vaginal discharge. General symptoms and signs quickly follow. The patient looks and feels ill and often complains of dyspnoea and there may be haemoptysis or neural lesions. Pelvic examination may reveal vaginal secondaries while the uterus is usually enlarged and there may be cystic enlargement of the ovaries. A positive pregnancy test in the absence of pregnancy leads on to chest x-rays and HCG estimations which confirm the diagnosis.

Preliminary investigation and classification of chorio-carcinoma cases

The regime followed is that used at the Trophoblastic Screening Centre and Treatment Unit based at the Weston Park Hospital in Sheffield (Table 1). It is not thought that it differs in any essentials from what is done elsewhere. Initial tissue diagnosis is made at the referring centre or hospital and subsequently reviewed at the screening centre. Fresh tissue is obtained whenever surgical intervention is necessary otherwise structures are not disturbed more than is absolutely necessary (**Figures 10 and 11**). All patients have chest x-rays (**Figure 9**) and are evaluated with special reference to liver and renal function. A full metastatic search is routinely carried out but pelvic arteriography is only used in selected cases (**Figure 12**).

For comparison with other published results, patients are graded into 'Good' and 'Poor' prognosis categories using the criteria of Hammond et al.[11] 'Poor' prognosis patients are those with:

1. HCG values in excess of 100,000 IU per day.
2. Duration of symptoms in excess of four months.
3. Hepatic or intracranial metastases.

TABLE 1

TROPHOBLASTIC DISEASE INVESTIGATIONS

1. Routine
Full blood examination
Blood urea & electrolyte estimations
Liver function tests
Thyroid function tests
Chest x-ray
Creatinine clearance tests
H.C.G. assays

2. When indicated
Pelvic arteriography
Ultrasonic B-scan
Brain scanning (E.M.I.)
Whole lung topography

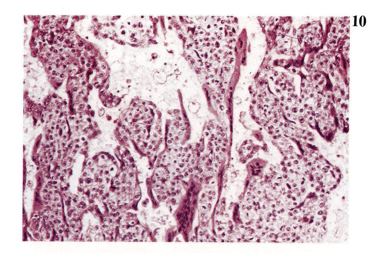

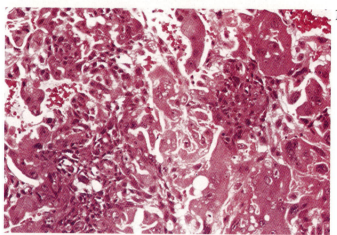

10 and 11 Histopathology of chorio-carcinoma
Figure 10 shows a well differentiated non metastatic chorio-carcinoma; **Figure 11** is of a less well differentiated and more clinically aggressive lesion.

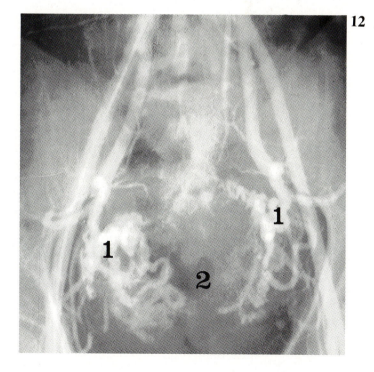

12 Pelvic arteriogram in a case of chorio-carcinoma
Increased pelvic vascularity with enlargement and varicosity of the uterine vessels (1) is seen. The relative avascularity at the centre of the intrauterine growth (2) is typical.

13

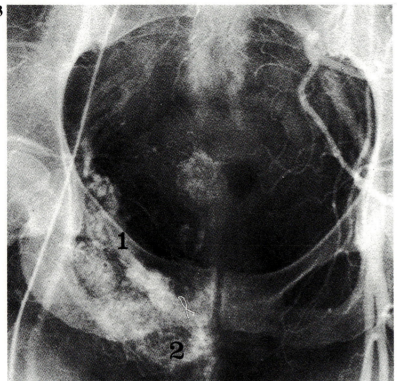

13 Pelvic arteriogram in case of extrauterine extension
The radiograph accurately delineates extension to the pelvic floor (1) and right paravaginal region (2).

14

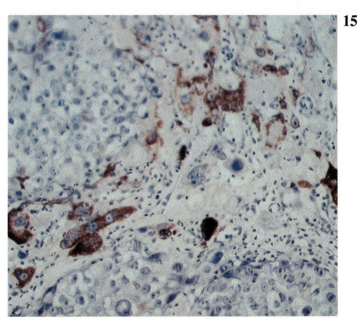

14
A haematoxylin and eosin preparation of a vulval deposit of choriocarcinoma. The tumour is haemorrhagic and appears undifferentiated. There was no history of a gestational carcinoma but the clear cell appearance of many cells and the deep eosinophilic staining of others, together with the haemorrhagic nature of the lesion were strongly suggestive of metastatic choriocarcinoma. (*H & E × 28*)

An interval of greater than two years following pregnancy or no history of antecedent pregnancy and with findings such as gross pulmonary infiltration, intracranial metastases or other metastases exceeding 5 cm in diameter all indicate a high risk category (**Figure 13**).

Because of the importance (and the difficulty) of definitively diagnosing the presence of secondary foci, increasingly sophisticated methods are used. Thus CAT scans have come to be used routinely if there is a suspicion of an occult secondary. Precise diagnosis in cases of possible clinical metastasis is also greatly aided by the use of the specific beta sub-unit of HCG in staining biopsy specimens. The method is explained in the legends for **Figures 14** and **15**.

15 Specific staining for metastatic choriocarcinoma
Shows the same lesion stained for the specific beta subunit of human chorionic gonadotrophin (HCG) using an indirect immunoperoxidase technique and affinity purified first and second antibodies. There are abundant bizarre, often multinucleate, HCG-positive giant cells in close apposition to the negative mononuclear clear cell areas. While the presence of beta HCG is not pathognomonic of choriocarcinoma, since extra gonadal tumours may secrete placental proteins, this appearance of the HCG positive giant cells, representing the malignant syncytiotrophoblast, in close opposition to the clear celled malignant cytotrophoblast, is typical. The immunoperoxidase stain confirmed the morphological suspicion that the lesion was metastatic choriocarcinoma (× *132*.)

Treatment: Chemotherapy

This is the primary method of treatment and is so overwhelmingly successful as to exclude almost the need for surgery in a therapeutic role. A summary of the principal chemotherapeutic operations and their administration is set out separately from this essentially surgical text in Appendix C, page 200. The results of treatment are also included.

The place of hysterectomy in the treatment of chorio-carcinoma

There are two situations in which hysterectomy may be required.
    (i) Initial uncontrollable haemorrhage
    (ii) Failed chemotherapy.

The first is when massive and life threatening haemorrhage occurs at the time of diagnosis and there is no possibility of satisfactorily controlling it before chemotherapy can be given. Some say that there is no place for hysterectomy in the treatment of choriocarcinoma but the authors cannot believe that the clinician has any choice in the circumstances described. Of the 58 cases of chorio-carcinoma in the first four years which were treated at the Sheffield Treatment Centre 4 needed immediate hysterectomy. Where it was necessary to perform hysterectomy for immediate

bleeding and so as not to prejudice subsequent treatment the policy was to give an initial double dose of methotrexate pre-operatively and continue the first course post-operatively so that the patient was 'covered' during a period when malignant trophoblastic cells would inevitably be released into the general circulation. There is no evidence that such treatment has any adverse effect on wound healing. Recognised authorities[23,3] generally agree the need for hysterectomy in the circumstances envisaged above (see **Figures 16** and **17**).

The second is when the response to chemotherapy in metastatic disease is unsatisfactory and the uterus is involved and enlarged by active tumour growth. Some surgeons are totally opposed to surgical intervention, maintaining that powerful forms and combinations of chemotherapy will bring such cases under control. Majority opinion is otherwise and Goldstein[24] believes that surgery is of help to the therapist in those cases with metastases where there is an enlarged uterus due to tumour growth. In many of these cases occult or impending perforation is encountered. In these circumstances hysterectomy should be performed, regardless of the patient's age, parity and plans for future childbearing. Chemotherapy has proved to be a poor substitute for surgery in such cases because of its

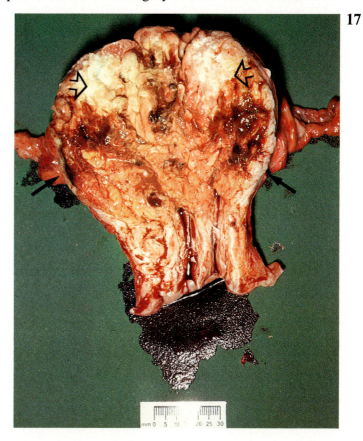

16

17

16 and 17 Specimen from a case of hysterectomy for uncontrolled bleeding
The uterus shows external evidence of growth on the anterior wall in the area indicated by arrows in **Figure 16**. In

Figure 17 the uterus has been split open to show involvement of practically the whole internal surface and with extension of the growth to the serosal surface anteriorly (arrowed) and across the whole of the fundus (open arrows).

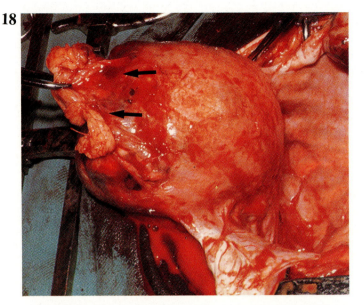

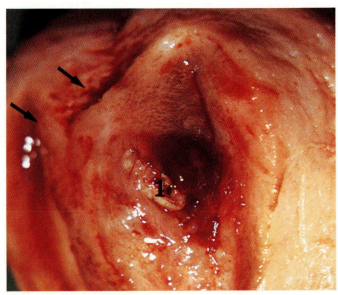

18 and 19 Hysterectomy and uterine specimens from a case of failed chemotherapy

The patient did not respond to massive multiple agent chemotherapy and laparoscopy showed a lesion extending through the fundus uteri. **Figure 18** shows the appearance at hysterectomy with the omentum adherent

at the site of the growth extension through the fundus (arrowed). **Figure 19** shows the interior of the uterus with the characteristic plum coloured chorio-carcinoma (1) which is largely buried in the uterine wall, but extends through to the serosal surface where arrowed.

difficulty in penetrating a large mass of rapidly proliferating tumour which is meantime providing a continuous threat of viable cells being widely disseminated from the uterus. Others[25,26] use hysterectomy in the type of case being described and there seems no doubt that it is now established procedure.

The last group[26] has in fact gone a stage further in using hysterectomy concurrently with chemotherapy which they still look on as the primary treatment modality. They were able to reduce significantly the duration of hospitalisation by the joint method and also the amount of chemotherapy used to achieve remission, regardless of whether or not metastases were present. They considered that surgical excision of chemotherapy-resistant foci of gestational trophoblastic disease was of benefit although less effective than initial operation. Any hesitation to embark on elective surgery during or immediately following a course of drug therapy because of the potential haz-

ards of infections and poor wound healing is dismissed by several authors[24,23,26]. Goldstein insists that surgery will always play an important part in the total management of the patient. In the initial 58 cases of the Sheffield series, hysterectomy was used in 8 cases where HCG levels remained high and intendive chemotherapy had not reduced the size of the uterus. In 3 of these laparoscopy had shown vesicular convolvement of the uterine peritoneal surface; 6 of the 8 had active residual disease confirmed histologically in the specimens (see **Figures 18** and **19**).

The place of surgery for secondary foci, where there is evidence that they are not responding to chemotherapy, is discussed in most articles on treatment. There is general agreement that lung secondaries frequently require thoracotomy and very occasionally a cerebral secondary may require neurosurgical excision. Unless they are bleeding heavily, vaginal secondaries are best treated non-surgically.

Hysterectomy for chorio-carcinoma resistant to chemotherapy–technique

Stage 1: Appearances at laparotomy

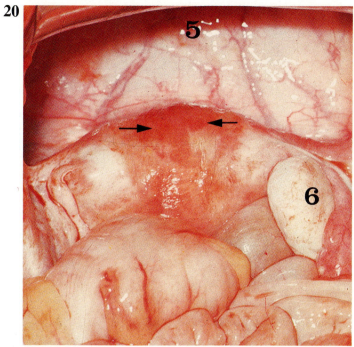

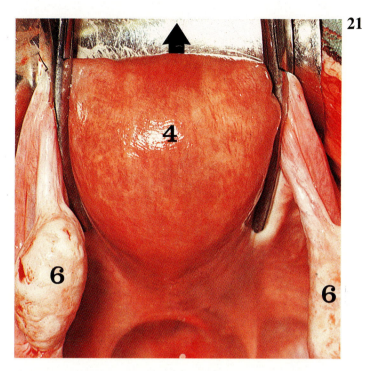

20 and 21

In **Figure 20** there is evidence of extension of the growth to the serosal surface on the anterior aspect of the fundus (arrowed); general discoloration of the fundus suggests that the spread is not entirely localised. In **Figure 21** the uterus is

lifted forwards in the direction of the broad arrow by the curved forceps on the broad ligaments and the posterior aspect of the uterus, the ovaries and the pouch of Douglas all appear normal.

Stage II: Securing upper uterine attachments

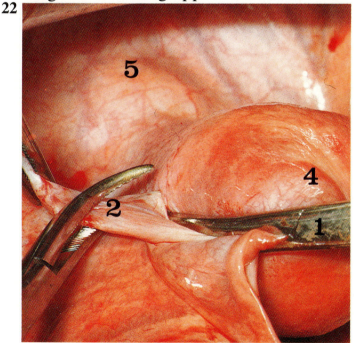

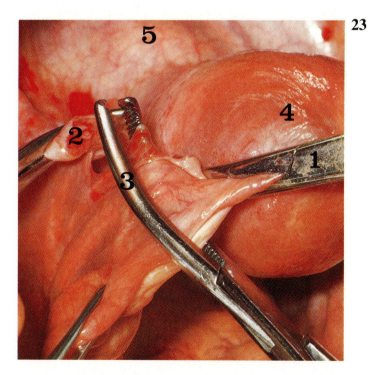

22 and 23

In **Figure 22** the heavy curved forceps (1) holds the left broad ligament while the Miles Phillips' forceps grasps the left round ligament prior to detaching it (2). In **Figure 23** heavy curved toothed forceps (3) enter the gap in the broad

ligament and grasp the remainder of that structure. The uterus is numbered (4), the bladder (5) and the ovary (6) when visible in the photographs.

163

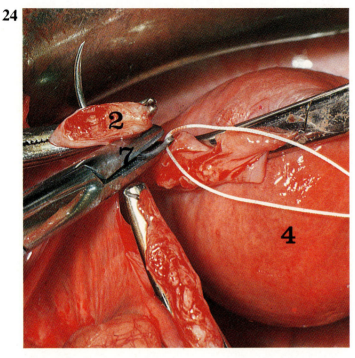

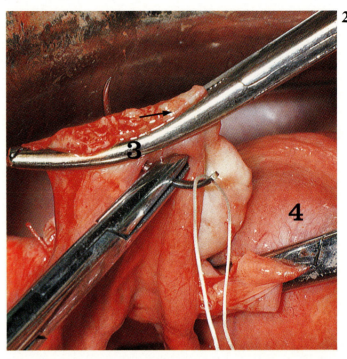

24 and 25
In **Figure 24** the round ligament pedicle is transfixed with a needle carrying a No. 0 PGA suture (7) prior to ligation. In

Figure 25 the same procedure is seen in progress on the broad ligament pedicle. The fallopian tube is included in the pedicle and its lumen is arrowed.

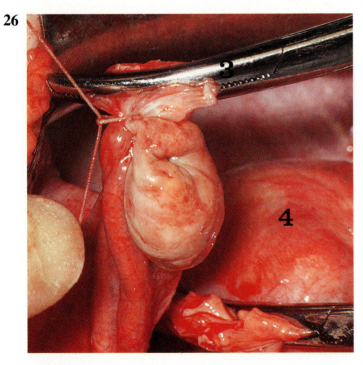

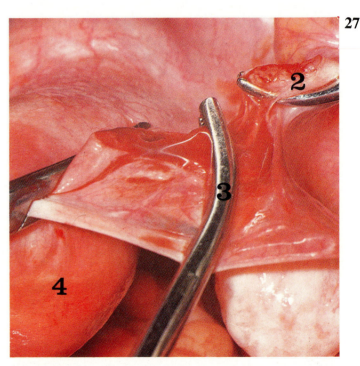

26 and 27
In **Figure 26** the broad ligament pedicle has been ligated under the point of the forceps and the ligature has now come

round under the heel of the forceps to complete the ligature which is being tied. **Figure 27** shows a similar procedure on the opposite side; the same numbers apply.

28

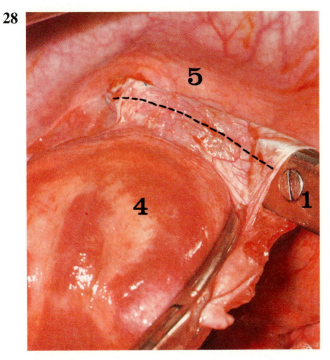

29

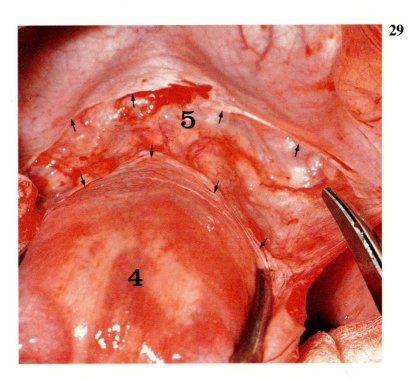

28 and 29
Figure 28 shows the scissors (1) elevating the peritoneum between the uterus (4) and bladder (5) prior to dividing it along the broken line. In **Figure 29** the division of the peritoneum has been completed and the cut edges are denoted by fine arrows. The bladder is now bare of peritoneum where numbered (5).

30

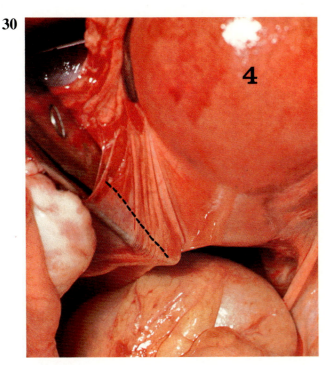

31

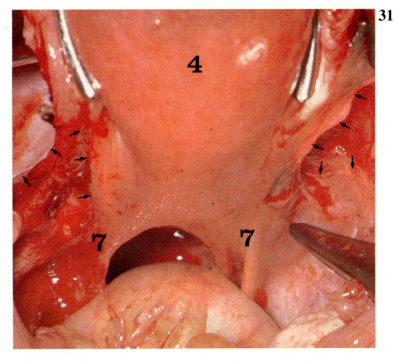

30 and 31
In **Figure 30** the scissors define and elevate the posterior layer of the broad ligament on the left side prior to cutting it along the broken line to expose the uterine vessels and the utero-sacral ligaments. In **Figure 31** the same procedure has been completed on the right side. The cut peritoneal edges are denoted by fine arrows and the uterine vessels lie in the angle between them. The utero-sacral ligaments are prominent (7) and (7).

Stage IV: Reflection of bladder from uterus; definition of uterine vessels

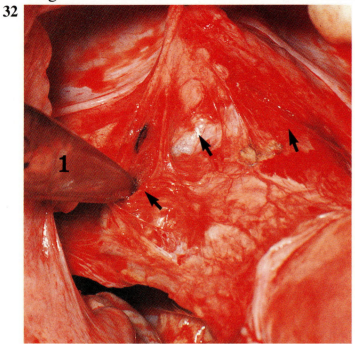

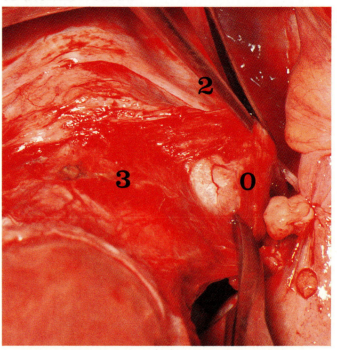

32 and 33

In **Figure 32** the scissors (1) are used partly to cut and partly as a blunt dissector in detaching and reflecting the bladder off the anterior aspect of the cervix and lower uterus. The line of separation is arrowed. **Figure 33** shows a further stage

of the same manoeuvre with the fine dissecting forceps (2) separating loose connective tissue to define the uterine vessels in that area (0). The cervix is denoted (3) in these and succeeding photographs.

Stage V: Securing uterine vessels

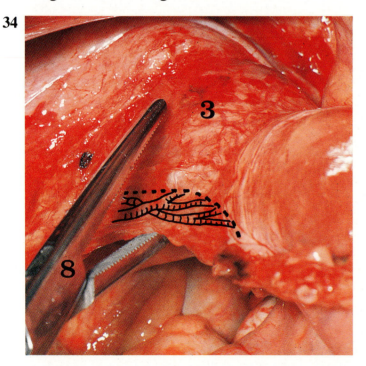

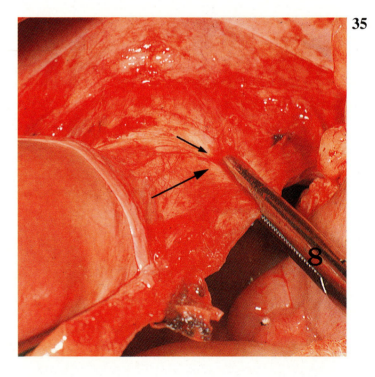

34 and 35

The uterine vessels are outlined and the edge of the cervix is designated by a broken line in **Figure 34**. The heavy straight Kocher forceps (8) clamps the leash of uterine vessels at right angles to the axis off the uterus and is firmly placed up against the lateral aspect of the cervix. In **Figure 35** the same

procedure is carried out on the opposite side. Note how the toothed upper point of the forceps pulls the tissue laterally (where arrowed) in making sure that the forceps is firmly against the cervix.

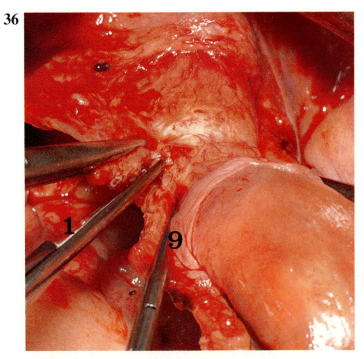

36

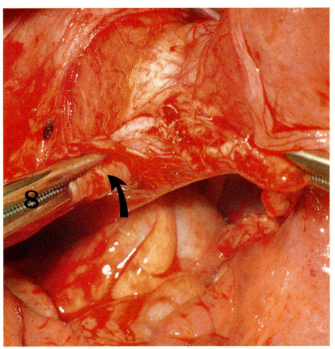

37

36 and 37
The uterine vessels have been secured distally on the uterine edge to prevent blood back flow (9) and the scissors (1) cut between the forceps in **Figure 36**. In **Figure 37** note how the detached uterine pedicle is stripped off the lateral aspect of

the cervix by rotating it with the attached forceps acting as a lever in the direction of the arrow and pushing it distally at the same time. This is a useful procedure for liberating the cervix and giving access to the vaginal vault without causing bleeding by cutting with the knife or scissors.

Stage VI: Securing utero-sacral ligaments

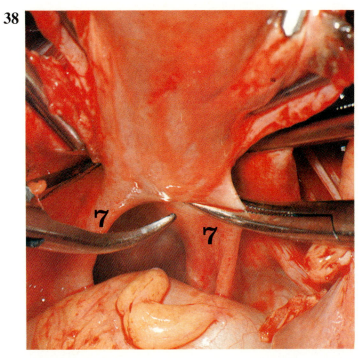

38

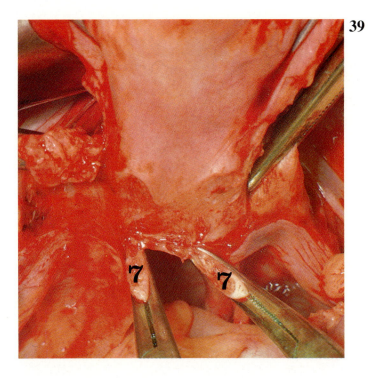

39

38 and 39
The right utero-sacral ligament (7) has already been clamped by curved forceps on the right side and the procedure is being repeated on the left. Note that the clamps

are still on the uterine vessel pedicles. Both utero-sacral ligaments have been detached from the uterus in **Figure 39** and are held in forceps.

Stage VII: Removal of uterus at vaginal angles

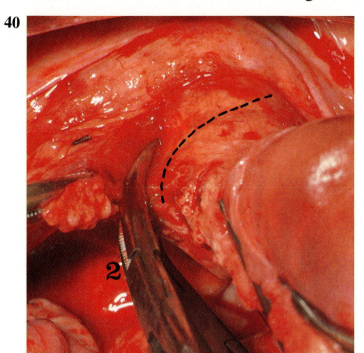

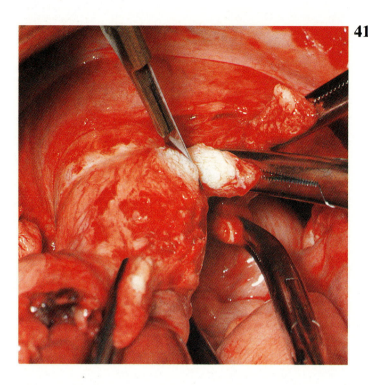

40 and 41
With the forceps on the uterine artery pedicle pushed distally, the surgeon should check that it is possible to approximate the anterior and posterior vaginal walls between finger and thumb beyond the cervix. If so there is adequate access and the vagina can be opened and cut across at the level of

the broken line. A heavy curved forceps (2) is applied to the left vaginal angle just distal to that line. In **Figure 41** the procedure is repeated on the right side and the scalpel is seen cutting into the vagina to leave at least an 0.5 cm cuff of tissue distal to the forceps.

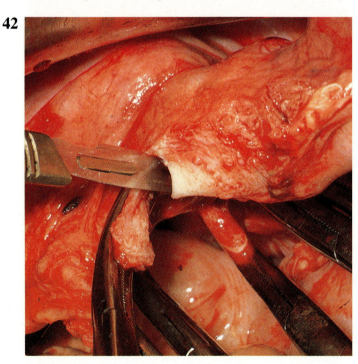

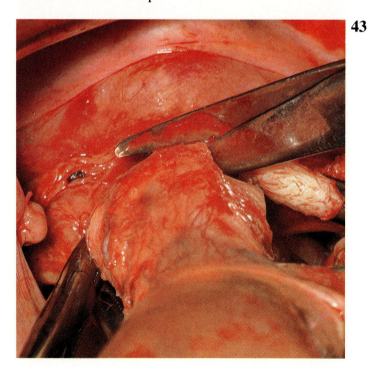

42 and 43
The uterus is seen being detached with the scalpel at the vaginal angle on the left side in **Figure 42** and in **Figure 43**

the scissors complete the division of the anterior vaginal wall to remove the uterus.

Stage VIII: Securing vaginal angle pedicles

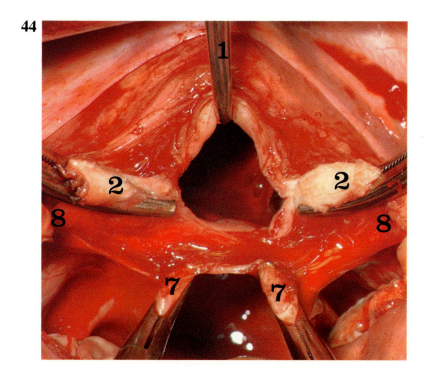

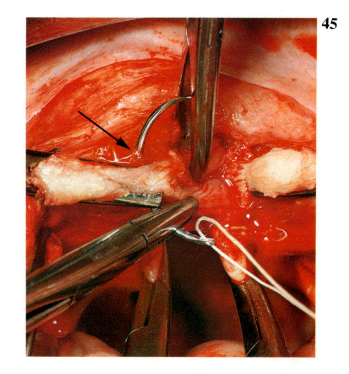

44 to 46

The vaginal angles are secured by forceps (2) and (2) in
Figure 44 and the utero-sacral ligaments are numbered (7)
and (7). A tissue forceps (1) holds the anterior vaginal edge.
The uterine pedicles (8) and (8) are just visible at the edges
of the photograph. In **Figure 45** the left vaginal angle pedicle
is transfixed by a needle carrying a No. 1 PGA suture
(arrowed) preparatory to ligature. The same is being done
on the right side in **Figure 46** and the left pedicle (2) has
already been tied off.

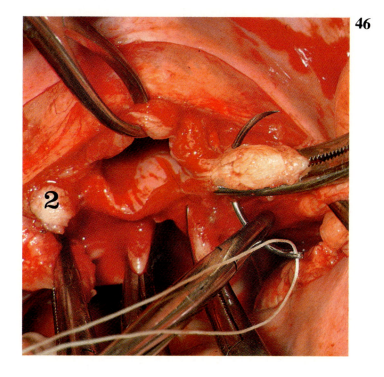

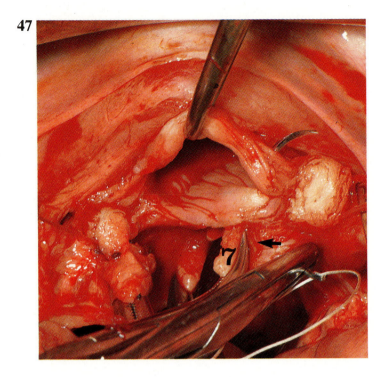

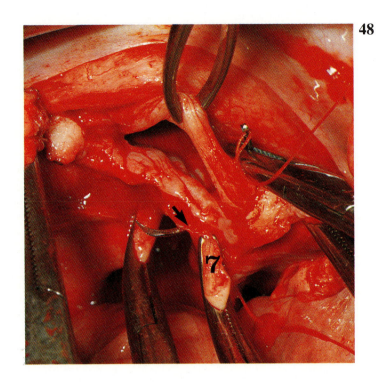

47 to 49

The vaginal vault is closed by two mattress sutures which include in their grasp the utero-sacral pedicles. This both ensures haemostasis and supports the vault on the utero-sacral pedicles. In **Figure 47** as the needle enters the posterior vaginal edge it takes a bite of the lateral aspect of the utero-sacral pedicle (7) where arrowed; the point of the needle then emerges through the anterior vaginal edge. In **Figure 48** the needle returns by a similar route to complete the mattress stitch and picks up the medial edge of the utero-sacral pedicle (arrowed). In **Figure 49** the mattress stitch is being tied off (arrowed) and includes the utero-sacral ligament within it at a level just proximal to the holding forceps which is removed as the pedicle is ligated. The procedure is repeated on the other side.

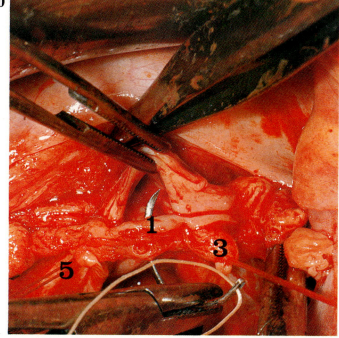

50
In this photograph the mattress stitches (3) and (3) have been completed and the central point of the vault is closed by a single through and through stitch (1).

Stage X: Ligation of uterine pedicles

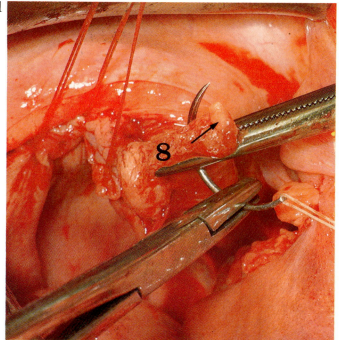

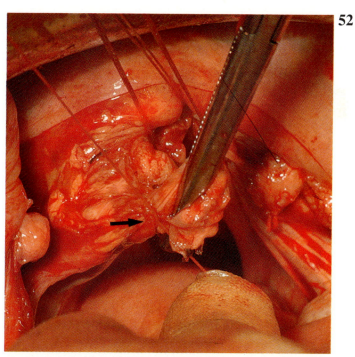

51 and 52
In routine hysterectomy it is generally preferable to secure the uterine vessels as the operation proceeds (see description in Vol. 2 of the Atlas, pages 57 and 58). This leaves the pelvis clear of instruments and gives somewhat better access. The uterine pedicle forceps have been retained in place here because all the tissues are soft and far more vascular than normal, so that it is easy for a ligature to be pulled or torn off. If that were to happen, if is difficult to recapture the pedicle without danger to the ureter. In **Figure 51** the right uterine pedicle (8) containing the uterine artery (arrowed) is transfixed with a needle carrying a No. 1 PGA suture prior to ligation behind the considerable cuff of tissue which lies beyond the forceps. In **Figure 52** the left pedicle is being tied off (arrowed) under the forceps which is about to be removed.

53

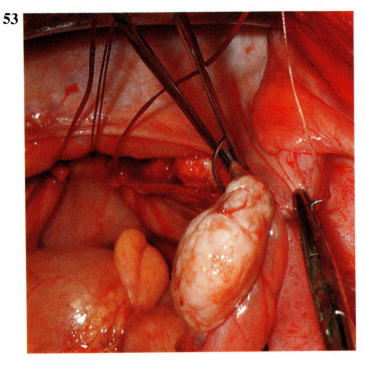

54

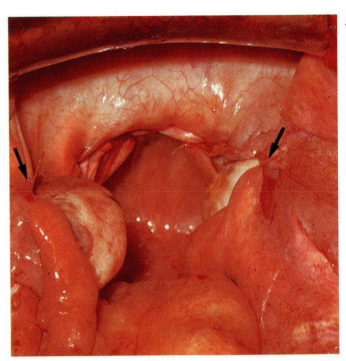

53 and 54

In **Figure 53** the needle carrying a 000 PGA continuous suture closes the right side of the peritoneal opening medial to the right ovary. It unites the edges close across the medial aspect of the ovarian pedicle. The stitch is tied off as an anchor (arrowed), and then proceeds across the pelvis to be completed (also arrowed) medial to the left ovary in **Figure 54**. The wound is neatly closed and the pelvis dry.

55

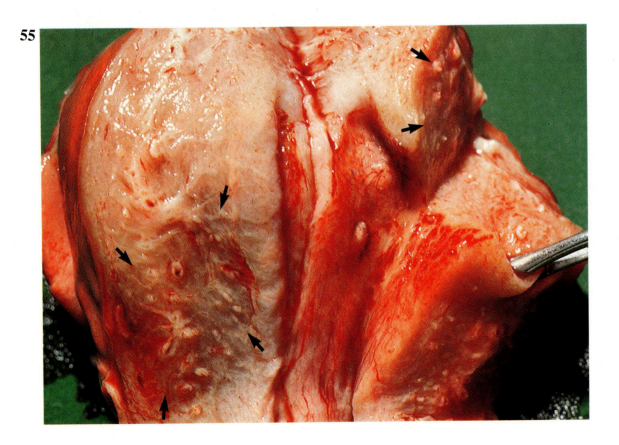

55 Specimen

A plum coloured chorio-carcinomatous nodule (arrowed) which is largely buried in the uterine wall is typical in its position and appearance. The uterus has been cut open to show the extension of the growth towards the anterior serosal surface where it was seen clinically.

14: Amniocentesis

In recent years there has been a dramatic increase in the employment of amniocentesis in both early and late pregnancy. This is mainly because of the development of techniques for more accurate diagnosis of congenital abnormalities and for the evaluation of fetal maturity. Once considered a hazardous procedure it is now regarded as relatively safe especially if employed with ultrasonic guidance; the risk of entering the placenta or damaging vital fetal tissues has been significantly reduced.

In this chapter the indications for amniocentesis will be briefly discussed. The use of ultrasonography with the procedure and the actual technique itself will be explained and illustrated.

1. Indications for amniocentesis

These are conveniently divided into those applying in early or late pregnancy.

(a) Early pregnancy indications

Most amniocenteses done between 15–18 gestational weeks are for a genetic indication. The cells of the amniotic fluid are cultured and biochemical and chromosomal studies performed. Indications are:
— maternal age – over 35 years of age
— elevated alpha-fetoprotein (serum)
— previous offspring with chromosomal abnormality
— previous infant with a neural tube defect
— parent with chromosome abnormality
— metabolic disorder carrier state.

(b) Late pregnancy indications

The indications are less in the late stage of pregnancy and consist of:
— assessment of Rhesus disease or other blood group immunisations (excluding ABO incompatability).
— determination of fetal maturity by estimation of sphingomyelin/lecithin (L/S) ratio.
— determination of fetal 'well being' as judged by evidence of meconium staining of the liquor; white blood cells or bacteria are looked for by some clinicians in cases of premature rupture of membranes.

2. Timing of early pregnancy amniocentesis

The ideal seems to be between 15–18 weeks as prior to this time the amount of amniotic fluid is limited (i.e. 50 ml at 12 weeks, 100 ml at 14 weeks, 175 ml at 16 weeks and between 250–325 ml at 18–20 weeks). The placenta occupies a relatively large area of uterine surface as compared to later in pregnancy. This is seen diagramatically in **Figures 13** and **14.**

3. The use of ultrasound in amniocentesis

Before the development of ultrasound, amniocentesis was performed without visual control. Since its introduction the position of fetus and placenta can be easily determined with resultant minimal risk of inflicting damage on them and of creating haemorrhage during puncture. By employing specially constructed ultrasonic aspiration transducers it is possible under visual control to position and maintain the needle in the amniotic fluid, placing it in a position away from fetus and placenta. This technique is described on page 178.

Diagnostic ultrasound imaging should be used as a preliminary procedure to amniocentesis. By employing B-Scan ultrasound, preferably with a gray scale display, valuable information regarding the position of the placenta and fetus as well as the distribution of amniotic fluid can be obtained. The initial screening technique involves the obtaining of an image by longitudinally moving the transducer from the pubis towards the umbilicus. Ultrasonograms are recorded first from the midline (as in **Figure 1**) and then at uniform distances (usually 2 cm) on either side (**Figure 2**). When the complete uterus has been examined longitudinally, transverse sections are obtained starting from the level of the pubis and moving towards the umbilicus at 2 cm intervals (**Figure 3**). In analysing the ultrasonograms four features are determined i.e. (1) placental localisation, (2) fetal position and structures, (3) urinary bladder and (4) amniotic fluid distribution.

The placenta must be accurately localised including its outer borders so that the area for needle placement will avoid any contact with placenta or fetal parts. Doppler ultrasonic techniques for placental localisation are not as useful as B-mode images, especially those obtained with a visible type of display; gray scale, either static or real time is an even better mode of display. The technology in this field is developing so rapidly that the authors recommend the reader to recent texts on the subject.[1,2]

The primary purpose of ultrasonic scanning is to determine the most desirable site for needle puncture. The scanner looks for collections of amniotic fluid that are free from fetal parts (**Figures 2** and **3**).

The presence of an anterior placenta makes the obtaining of a blood-free specimen difficult. In **Figures 4** to **6** two such placentae are seen; in one of them (**Figure 4**) the placenta extends into the lower segment and so needle placement would need to be in the fundal area while in the other (**Figure 6**) the placenta covers the whole anterior surface and puncture through the placenta may be unavoidable. Sometimes in later pregnancy where there is an anterior placenta in the upper half of the uterus, it will be necessary to puncture in the lower segment and so it is necessary to shield the fetal pole (either breech or head) from possible contact with the inserted needle (**Figure 15**).

Occasionally the operator may need to hand elevate the fetal pole out of the pelvis; this is a procedure which requires some skill. When the placenta is implanted over the entire anterior uterine wall as in **Figure 6** amniocentesis may be made safer by using ultrasound to decide where to traverse the placenta.

The operator in this situation should keep his needle away from the chorionic plate, the area where the umbilical cord is inserted and an area congested with blood vessels. The cord can usually be demonstrated on ultrasound as seen in **Figures 2** and **3.**

Ultrasonography in amniocentesis

1 to 3 Ultrasonograms of a 20 weeks fetus

Grey scale B-Scan ultrasonograms showing placental and fetal structures. In **Figure 1** a midline longitudinal scan shows the placenta (1) extending along the posterior superior border; the fetus with its head (2) and trunk (3) is clearly seen. The fetal heart is at (4). In **Figure 2** taken 2 cm lateral to **Figure 1** a clear area indicating a collection of amniotic fluid is visible at (5). It is situated at 4.9 cm distance (as indicated by the horizontal line) from the skin surface. The umbilical cord is easily seen (6) as is the maternal bladder (7) in both **Figure 1** and **2. Figure 3** is a transverse scan taken to show the posterior placenta (1).

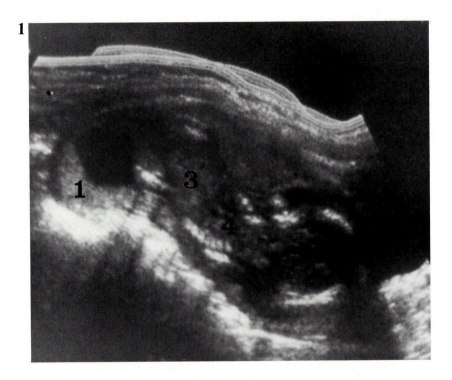

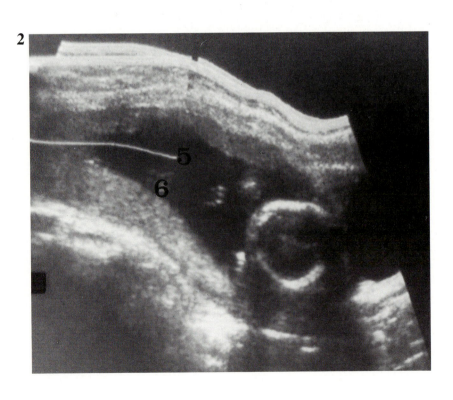

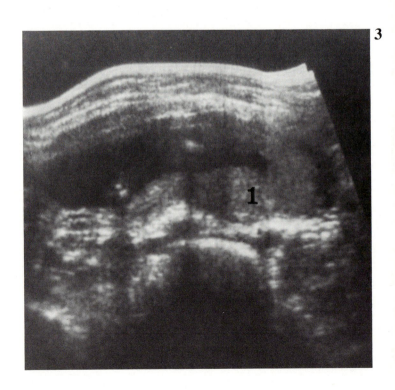

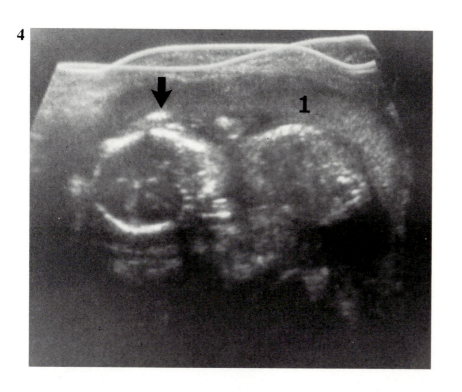

4

4 to 6 Anterior placentae
Ultrasonograms show examples of anterior situated placentae (1). In **Figure 4** its lower border extends into the lower segment (thin arrow) and its upper border (thick arrow) lying as it does below the fundus allows a clear area in which to insert the needle into the amniotic fluid. This area was confirmed and outlined by a further scan (**Figure 5**) taken laterally to that in **Figure 4**. **Figure 6** shows that there is a clear area (2) for aspiration; the fetal head (3) trunk (4) and umbilical cord (5) are all clearly seen. The placenta (1) covers the whole anterior uterine wall and needle puncture still needs to be through the placenta; obviously the cord (at 5) has to be avoided. The clear area of fluid is at (2).

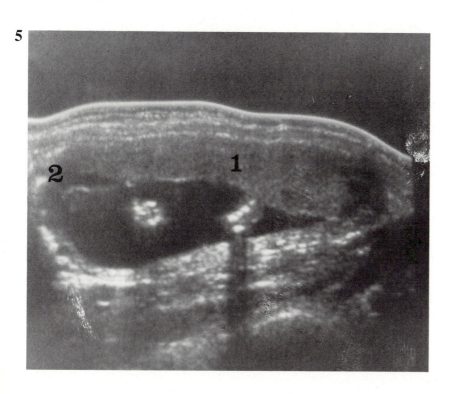

5

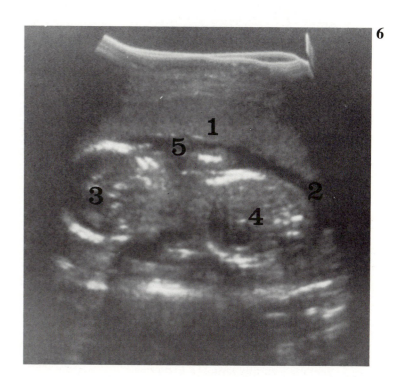

6

Technique of amniocentesis

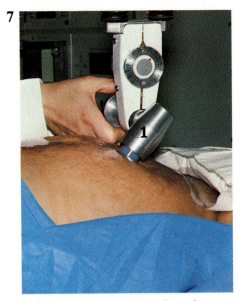

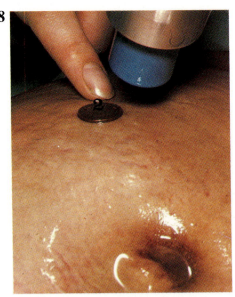

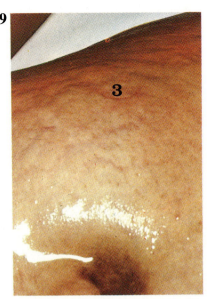

7 to 9 Determination of aspiration site in early second trimester
The determination of the site for aspiration by ultrasound has been discussed above. in **Figure 7** the

B-Scan transducer (1) has located a suitable pocket of fluid and in **Figures 8** and **9** a 'pressure' mark on the skin is being made by a coin (2) placed directly over this

collection of fluid. At this site (3) the local anaesthetic (if used) will be injected and the aspiration needle subsequently inserted. The umbilicus is at (4).

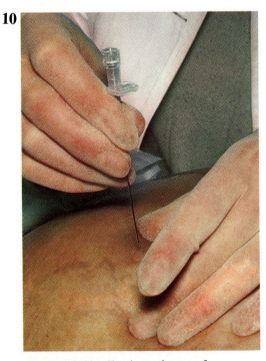

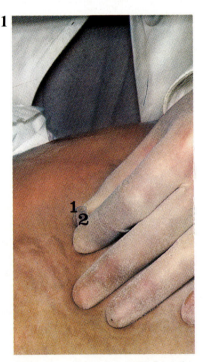

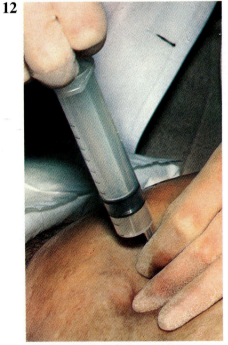

10 to 12 Needle insertion and aspiration
The abdomen has been suitably prepared with an antiseptic agent and sterile drapes applied. Some clinicians infiltrate the abdominal wall with local anaesthetic but the authors do not use it on the grounds that it only increases the number of needle insertions and the procedure can be performed painlessly in any case. In **Figure**

10 the operator is steadying the injection site with one hand while with the other is inserting a 9 cm (3½ inch) 20 gauge spinal needle with stylet into the skin and abdominal wall. A brisk and rapid needle insertion is recommended because a slow movement results in the uterine wall being pushed away without actual puncture of the amniotic sac. Once the needle is in position as in **Figure 11,** the

stylet is removed and a drop of amniotic fluid (1) is looked for as it emerges from the needle (2). If none appears the needle is rotated 90° and if still unsuccessful, then the needle is briskly advanced still further. Once the drop has appeared a syringe is attached as in **Figure 12** and liquor is aspirated. Once the required volume is obtained, the needle is quickly withdrawn.

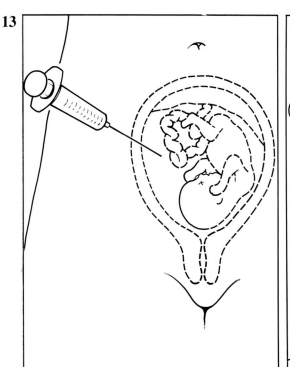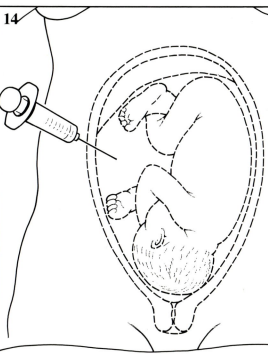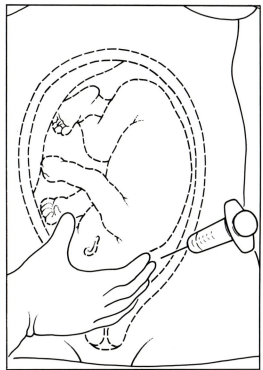

13 to 15 Site of amniocentesis: diagrammatic representation
The site of the needle insertion varies according to the stage of pregnancy and the fetal position. Ultrasound will obviously locate the most suitable collection of amniotic fluid for aspiration during early pregnancy as shown diagramatically in **Figure 13.** The placenta is relatively large compared with the uterus, fetus and amniotic fluid volume. Because there may be a placenta along two thirds of the uterine cavity surface it can be difficult to obtain fluid without passing through the placenta.

In later pregnancy the uterus grows and the placenta although larger in size, occupies a relatively smaller area of the uterine cavity. This being so, the needle is inserted so as to avoid the placenta and the large bulk of the fetal body. It is aimed at that region where the small fetal parts are present as shown in **Figure 14.** Occasionally as when the fetal back lies in an anterior position, it may be found necessary to position the site of needle entry to lie in an area behind the fetal neck as seen in **Figure 15.** The operator's hand, in such circumstances, shields the fetal head.

4. Problems encountered with amniocentesis

Various conditions of the mother or her pregnancy may impair the satisfactory performance of this procedure. Maternal conditions include obesity, abdominal scars or rotation of the uterus. The placenta which is hydropic, or large as with multiple pregnancy or anterior presents a problem. A reduction in amniotic fluid as found with growth retardation, certain congenital abnormalities or post maturity also adds to the difficulty of amniocentesis.

(a) Maternal conditions
Obesity
In such cases the needle needs to traverse the thick abdominal as well as the uterine wall. This may mean inserting the needle so deeply that the hub indents the abdominal wall.
Abdominal scars
These suggest the presence of intra-abdominal adhesions but do not contraindicate the procedure. Care must be taken especially if peritonitis followed a ruptured appendix or pyosalpinx.
Uterine rotation
When rotation is marked the uterine vessels are rotated into an anterior rather than a lateral position and become liable to damage during amniocentesis. This is particularly so if a suprapubic approach is used.

(b) Placental conditions
Hydropic placenta
Difficulty is encountered because the needle tip becomes lodged in the substance of the oedematous placenta and neither fluid or blood can be aspirated. In such cases it is essential to use ultrasound to locate small areas of fluid.
Multiple gestations
Both sacs must be aspirated so that the tests are specific for each and ultrasound again must be used. Methylene blue instilled into the first sac will allow the operator to differentiate it from the second.
Oligohydramnios
Even small pockets of fluid can usually be detected by ultrasound and can be aspirated. If it is meconium stained it indicates fetal distress.

(c) Other problems
Blood stained liquor
It is only when the needle is within the myometrium with its large venous sinuses or in the placental substance that blood will be obtained. Careful note should be made as to whether the blood appeared on insertion or withdrawal or if it was present in the fluid itself. Blood usually appears as the operator readjusts the needle after entry into the sac and if this occurs then a

change of syringe is advised. Any blood that has contaminated the specimen should be removed by immediate centrifugation of the specimen.

Maternal isoimmunisation may occur from the passage of as little as 0.3 ml of fetal blood. This may be critical in those cases where the mother has low levels of Rhesus immunisation; such a small transplacental haemorrhage may induce an anamnestic response and result in a high level of immunisation.

Many clinicians routinely administer 50 ug of Rh. immune globulin to cover the risk of Rh. immunisation in the Rhesus negative patient. This is obviously unnecessary if the father is Rh. negative.

Urine contamination
Urine obtained by inadvertent entry into the bladder is similar to amniotic fluid in appearance and it may need spectrophotometric scanning to differentiate it from liquor.

Amniocentesis (fetoscopy) under ultrasonic guidance

Techniques and apparatus have been developed whereby a continuous ultrasonic image is obtained of the intrauterine contents during amniocentesis. Various transducers (1 in **Figure 16**) have been adapted for use with an aspiration needle. The simplest type as shown diagrammatically in **Figure 16** has a central lumen for the passage of the needle (2) which on entering the amniotic space (3) produces an echo recordable on an A-mode type of display (4). The distance from transducer at the skin surface to the needle tip can be measured.

Aspiration – transducers connected to B-Scan displays (real time) have now been developed allowing changes in the size and position of the liquor pool to be continuously monitored. Two such devices are seen in **Figures 17** and **18. Figure 17** is of a real time imaging machine with multiple crystal transducers which has a central lumen for needle placement (1). This machine has the advantage of real time B-Scan imaging with the ability to detect the needle pathway from any desired position. In **Figure 18** a central slot has been made into

the transducer (1) through which a needle (2) can be inserted. The transducer can be removed once the needle is in place and has the advantage that an endoscopic needle can be directed into the amniotic space. The endoscope contains fibreoptics so that the fetus and placenta can be visualised. This endoscopic technique of fetoscopy allows fetal blood sampling to be obtained from the chorionic plate or more recently from the umbilical cord, and is of particular value in the mid trimester diagnosis of haemoglobinopathy, B-thalassaemia. The incidence of immediate fetal death following fetoscopy is low (<2 per cent) but the risks of spontaneous abortion (4 per cent) and prematurity (15 per cent) are significant and often associated with amniotic fluid leakage.

The authors have not attempted to present photographs of fetoscopy. At its present state of development it is an extremely difficulty and highly specialised technique, which needs to be available in a few referral centres only. The technique is well described elsewhere and the reader is referred to these reports.

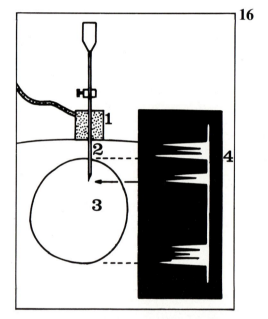

16

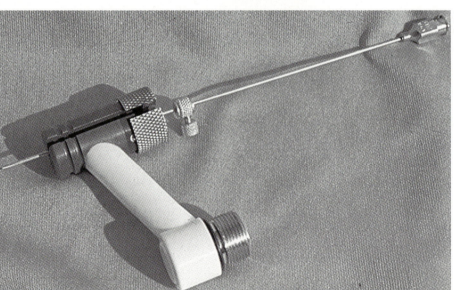

18

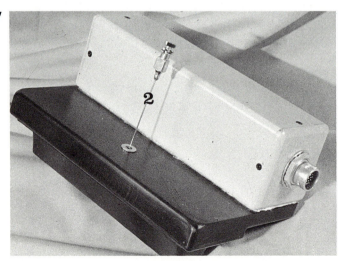

17

15: Anaesthetic and resuscitative aspects of obstetric surgery

by Dr A G D Nicholas, Consultant Anaesthetist, Jessop Hospital for Women, Sheffield

This chapter deals with obstetrical problems and decisions which concern both the anaesthetist and the obstetric surgeon. The safety (and sometimes the life) of the pregnant patient is at risk, and in most cases the welfare of the fetus is also involved; it is therefore important that the clinicians jointly make the correct decisions in initiating treatment.

The anaesthetist, in his or her own field, has the responsibility of selecting the most suitable form of anaesthesia for the individual case, and the principal considerations influencing that decision are discussed in a short review of the available methods on pages 179–181. Local infiltration analgesia is only briefly considered since its major use during pregnancy is for first trimester termination. Spinal and epidural analgesia are covered in some detail because they may be used in elective caesarean section; the former technique is less commonly employed although still favoured in some centres. General anaesthesia is still regarded as the normal method in use for caesarean section and is the type of surgery dealt with in this volume. Complications of the method in relation to gastric reflux, intubation failure and postural hypotension are discussed in detail.

In obstetric surgery, anaesthetic as well as purely surgical considerations are frequently complicated and influenced by accompanying haemorrhage. This is often severe before treatment begins and usually persists during the subsequent operation. The surgeon is likely to be fully occupied in delivering the fetus and arresting the haemorrhage so that the anaesthetist is effectively in sole charge of blood transfusion and maintenance of the patient's circulation. It is essential in such circumstances to have immediately available a safe and familiar regime which is at the same time flexible; such a programme is outlined in a brief review of the management of severe haemorrhage and hypovolaemic shock.

An additional short section deals with the prophylaxis and early management of venous thrombotic disease in obstetric surgery.

A. Anaesthesia and analgesia in obstetric surgery

I. Local infiltration analgesia

The method may occasionally be indicated for abdominal delivery when an anaesthetist is not available. Severe airway problems may sometimes contra-indicate general anaesthesia where alternative regional block methods are considered to be unsuitable. Local infiltration is safe if the total dose of the solution is within safety limits. Each layer of tissue must be injected separately but even then the analgesia may vary in effectiveness.

Routine precautions
(i) Patients should breathe an oxygen enriched atmosphere to maintain fetal oxygenation and prevent maternal toxic cerebral effects.
(ii) An anticonvulsant drug such as diazepam 10 mg should be available for intravenous use if toxic effects are noted.
(iii) Care should be taken to avoid intravenous injection of the drug.
(iv) A safe total dose should not be exceeded.

Suitable drugs
(i) 0.5 per cent Lignocaine with 1 : 400,000 adrenalin – maximum dose for the average patient is 400–500 mgms.
(ii) 0.25 per cent Bupivicaine plain or with 1 : 400,000 adrenalin – maximum dose for the average patient is 150–200 mgms.

II. Spinal analgesia

The administration and the risks of spinal analgesia are relative to the extent of the block required. In the description here, lower segment caesarean section is envisaged, but many of the procedures where it is used (e.g. forceps delivery, retained placenta etc) require a much less extensive analgesia. A dose of 0.6–1.0 ml of heavy nupercaine would be adequate for the latter. The method has recognised advantages in obstetrical surgery but it has equally definite disadvantages.

Advantages
1. It is a quick and essentially simple procedure.
2. The small amount of drug required has no toxic effect on the mother or fetus.
3. Good analgesia is obtainable in 10–15 minutes by a standard technique.

Disadvantages
1. It is a 'one shot' method so that an inadequate block cannot be 'topped up'.
2. A too high block may result in the quick onset of hypotension and respiratory inadequacy which both demand rapid correction.
3. Despite the use of a fine 25 gauge needle, 10–15 per cent of patients develop 'spinal' headaches. This is not a serious disadvantage in a resting post-operative patient.

Routine procedure when using a spinal technique for lower segment caesarean section

1. The patient is starved of food for 12 hours.
2. Antacids are given in 2 doses: 30 minutes and 5 minutes before surgery – 15 ml sodium citrate.
3. An intravenous infusion is established before surgery begins and 1 litre of Hartmann's solution is infused over 15–20 minutes.
4. One ampoule of ephedrine (30 mg) or of methyl-amphetamine (30 mg) is drawn up in a 2 ml syringe.
5. Under aseptic conditions a lumbar puncture is done in the lateral position at L.3/4 interspace and 1.4–1.8 ml heavy nupercaine or amethocaine is injected over 5–10 seconds.
6. The patient is kept on her back with the shoulders elevated by pillows for 1–2 minutes to increase the thoracic curve and prevent the spread of the block above T6–T7.
7. The patient's legs are raised and the thighs flexed to reduce lumbar lordosis and facilitate even spread of the drug.
8. After 2 minutes the patient is turned on to her other side in a lateral tilt position and in a 10–15° head down inclination until the block is established.
9. The patient breathes an oxygen enriched atmosphere and 10–15 mg of the vasopressor drug is injected intramuscularly. The remaining drug is kept in reserve and given in small intravenous doses if required to maintain the blood pressure.
10. The anaesthetist stays at the patient's head to reassure her, check the blood pressure and administer oxygen and anti-emetic drugs if required.
11. It is vitally important to ensure that patients having spinal analgesia are not left in positions which would induce the inferior vena caval syndrome.

High standards of drug preparation, modern aseptic techniques and the use of fine gauge needles (SWG 22–25) and bacterial filters all contribute to a virtual absence of infective or neurological complications. If hypotension is avoided and the mother is adequately oxygenated the fetus is born in excellent condition and drug depression does not occur.

III. Epidural (lumbar) analgesia

Epidural block analgesia has become part of the routine management of labour in selected cases. In these and in its extended use for caesarean section it has these *advantages*:

1. The slow onset of block provides a gradual and recognisable onset of hypotension and respiratory inadequacy if these develop.
2. The epidural catheter allows topping up an inadequate block or prolonging analgesia postoperatively.
3. When used for pain relief in labour the block can be extended for forceps delivery or caesarean section. It is simple to top up the block with a dose that will provide analgesia from T6–7 to S5.
4. The epidural space is very resistant to infection.
5. Spinal headache does not occur unless the subarachnoid space has been accidentally 'tapped'.
6. The risk of gastric inhalation is very small (as it is with spinal analgesia).

The method also has *disadvantages*:

1. It takes some time to initiate a block (e.g. 30–40 minutes) for caesarean section, so that it might be inappropriate as a standard procedure in a busy unit.
2. Block onset is slow (15–35 minutes) and somewhat unpredictable in spread.
3. A moderately large dose of analgesic is required and will have some depressant effect on the neonate.

There are some distinct contraindications to the use of epidural block

1. Cases of ante-partum haemorrhage.
2. Patients with haemorrhagic diseases.
3. Patients on anticoagulant drugs.
4. In the presence of local or general infection (principally urinary tract infection and infected liquor)[1].
5. In active neurological disease.
6. Spinal skeletal deformities may make the method difficult or dangerous.
7. In the presence of fetal distress.

Precautions in use

These are as for spinal analgesia. The means of resuscitation and the drugs to facilitate endo-tracheal intubation must always be at hand whenever this technique is used.

IV. General anaesthesia

(in particular relation to caesarean delivery)

Despite improvements in ante-natal care in many centres throughout the world and despite better anaesthetic techniques there is a continuing maternal mortality and morbidity associated with caesarean section due principally to 3 main conditions. These are:

1. Regurgitation of solid or liquid gastric contents into the oesophagus with subsequent aspiration into the lungs. Vomiting frequently causes similar effects.
2. Failure to perform endotracheal intubation and to maintain an adequate airway. This leads to hypoxia sometimes complicated by gastric regurgitation which further accentuates the severity of the condition.
3. Obstruction of the inferior vena cava and the aorta during the period of anaesthesia resulting in maternal and fetal hypoxia.

It might therefore appear that general anesthesia should be avoided in caesarean section although there are many definite indications for its use. Clearly the highest standard of practice must be established and maintained or it will be replaced by local techniques which may prove to have corresponding disadvantages. A hastily embarked-on local technique may encounter difficulties and complications which render it more dangerous than general anaesthesia would have been.

General anaesthesia is the method of choice in cases of urgency such as prolapsed cord, bleeding from the placental site and severe fetal distress. It is predominantly in this group that disasters are liable to occur.

Technique of general anaesthesia

(i) Preparation for general anaesthesia in operative delivery

1. Premedication is best avoided in operations which include delivery of the fetus.
2. Anticholinergic drugs should not be used prior to endotracheal intubation as they lower the tone of the gastro-oesophageal sphincter.
3. An intravenous infusion is started before anaesthesia commences as on occasion blood loss may be rapid and reach a total of 2–2½ litres.
4. The patient should be blood grouped and cross matched and at least 1 litre of compatible blood be available in the operating room.
5. Pre-oxygenation with 100 per cent oxygen at a flow of 8–10 litres per minute for 3–5 minutes is an essential precaution. The pregnant patient has an increased oxygen consumption and when lying down she also has an increased closing volume and less efficient ventilation/perfusion ratios which may lead to reduced arterial oxygen levels[2]. The importance of preoxygenation, if one subsequently encounters problems with endotracheal intubation, is obvious.

(ii) Essential operating room equipment
1. A tilting operating table
2. Efficient suction apparatus
3. Endotracheal tubes of all sizes and including micro-laryngeal tubes
4. Stilettes and bougies (over which an endotracheal tube can be passed)
5. A cardiac monitor
6. Blood warming equipment
7. Pressure infusion bags
8. A mechanical respiratory ventilator.

(iii) Anaesthetic induction agents
Intravenous induction agents must not be used where difficulties with endotracheal intubation are anticipated. Thiopentone, 200–250 mg intravenously retains its place as the drug of choice. Suxamethonium, 100 mg intravenously is then given as a muscle relaxant. When relaxation occurs intubation is carried out without prior inflation of the lungs. Cricoid pressure is applied during the procedure.

(iv) Maintenance of anaesthesia
Certain problems are to some extent inseparable from the administration of general anaesthesia:
1. 'Awareness' developing during a combination of light anaesthesia with high inspired oxygen levels
2. Drug depression of the fetus
3. Inadequate fetal oxygenation
4. Inadequate placental blood flow.

These 4 items may respectively be countered by the following 4 measures:
1. The use of 0.5 per cent halothane with a 50/50 mixture of N_2O and O_2: other similar techniques are suggested[3,4].
2. Use of the drugs mentioned in 1, plus 4 mg pancuronium bromide intravenously to allow intermittent positive pressure respiration during the operation. This should be done while the suxamethonium is still acting; to prevent awareness developing.
3. Inspiration of an increased concentration of oxygen by the mother improves fetal welfare[5]. An anaesthetic mixture containing at least 50–60 per cent of O_2 is now recommended. Overventilation of the patient may be a factor in reducing fetal oxygenation and should be avoided.
4. Falls in cardiac output due to inferior vena caval occlusion should be avoided. The use of 0.5 per cent halothane may prevent reflex vascular changes due to the effects of surgery, and so avoid placental vaso-constriction.

The post-delivery phase
The following factors have a bearing on management:
1. Uterine retraction will return approximately 500 ml of blood to the general circulation, compensating for a blood loss at delivery that is, on average, 750–1000 ml.
2. The rise in the central venous pressure (CVP) following delivery of the placenta and fetus is mainly due to the 0.5 mg ergometrine still widely given at delivery.
3. Ergometrine presents dangers from its alpha effect which increases peripheral resistance, venous return and therefore cardiac work, besides affecting the calibre of the coronary vessels. This may last for 1–2 hours and the myocardial stress may be dangerous in cardiac or toxaemic patients. By causing vomiting at a time when laryngeal reflexes have not returned or in the presence of already established lung soiling it could be fatal. Syntocinon is the preferred alternative to ergometrine. Given as 20 units in 500 ml of Hartmann's solution at operation it does not affect venous return, produces a vaso-dilatation and is non-emetic. A second 500 ml of Hartmann's solution containing 20 units of syntocinon is given over 4 hours postoperatively to prevent uterine relaxation.

V. Possible hazards from general anaesthesia at delivery

Obstetrical operations where the fetus is delivered under anaesthesia present 3 problems of particular concern to the anaesthetist:

1. Delayed gastric emptying and the full stomach

Aetiology
1. Delayed gastric emptying is common in pregnant women after the 34th week and is worse in those with heartburn. The delay is accentuated by painful labour and narcotic analgesic drugs.
2. Pregnant women secrete a highly acid gastric juice in the third trimester and in labour.
3. Gastro-oesophageal reflux with heartburn occurs in 45–75 per cent of pregnant women and is due to an incompetent gastro-oesophageal sphincter.
4. Injudicious feeding of the patient in labour or the unexpected and rapid onset of labour after a meal.

Clinical effects
1. Regurgitated or vomited gastric contents may be inhaled into the lungs.
2. Solid food may cause airway obstruction with immediate asphyxia and lung collapse or later lung abscess formation.
3. Acid liquid contents will cause inflammatory changes in the lungs (Mendelson's syndrome) with the possible development of pulmonary oedema, right heart failure and even death.

(i) Passing a stomach tube
(ii) Giving a dilute solution of apomorphine (3mg in 10ml normal saline) until nausea starts. Intravenous atropine will terminate the effects after the patient has vomited once or twice.
Neither method is pleasant and may not ensure a completely empty stomach. They are only used if local analgesia is contraindicated and the stomach is known to be full.

4. Increase gastric peristalsis and emptying by giving Metoclopramide 10mg intravenously at least 30 minutes before the operation. It is not given if labour is established or narcotic agents have been given.
5. Increase the tone of the gastro-oesophageal spincter by the same medication[6]. Avoid using atropine, glycopyrrolate and pethidine as all these drugs reduce spincter tone[3].
6. Neutralise the acid gastric juice by antacid mixtures.
   (i) Mist. Magnesium Trisilicate 15–20ml. Taken orally 30 minutes and 5 minutes before induction of anaesthesia; it will give a gastric pH of above 2.5. The aluminium salts are considered more irritant to the lungs.

2 Cricoid pressure
Clinical demonstration of the method of applying cricoid pressure to prevent gastric regurgitation.

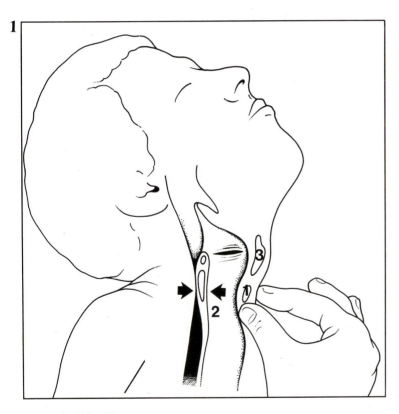

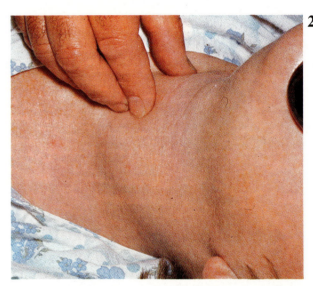

   (ii) Sodium Citrate in 0.3 molar solution is used in the same dosage and manner. It has the advantage of being a clear solution which if inhaled is less likely to damage the lungs.
7. Depress hydrochloric acid secretion. Cimetidine, an H_2 receptor blocker acts in this way. 200mg given intravenously 60–80 minutes before anaesthesia gives a significant drop in acidity. If there is time for the drug to be given it is probably the safest method. It must be combined with a single dose of sodium citrate or magnesium trisilicate to neutralise any remaining acid gastric juice.
8. Cricoid pressure
   When anaesthesia is induced cricoid pressure must be used to prevent regurgitation of gastric contents. As described by Sellick[7] it depends on the ability of the ring shaped cartilage when pressed posteriorly to compress the oesophagus against the bodies of the cervical vertebrae, thus occluding the oesophageal lumen. The chin should be extended and in the midline. (**Figures 1** and **2.**)

1 Cricoid pressure
Diagram to show mechanism of occluding the oesphagus by posterior pressure on the ring-shaped cricoid cartilage (1). The arrows indicate the area of obstruction of the oesophagus. The trachea is numbered (2) and the thyroid cartilage (3).

Management
1. Patients should be starved for 12 hours before elective caesarean section.
2. Patients in labour should receive no food and only occasional ice cubes to suck.
3. A full or partially full stomach may be emptied prior to giving an urgently required anaesthetic – by one of the following methods:

2. Respiratory problems arising from failed endotracheal intubation

The sequelae of such a failure in an obstetrical case can be both rapid and tragic. The surgeon working in areas where skilled anaesthesia is not available should therefore ensure that he or she has the capacity to intubate (and do a tracheotomy) if required. Those concerned will doubtless seek instruction in intubation which appears a simple enough procedure but requires practice to be done with any facility – or at all, in difficult cases. The first essential is to use the laryngoscope correctly and this is shown diagrammatically in **Figures 3** and **4.** The next step is to introduce the tube into the trachea and the endotracheal tube and malleable director which aids its introduction are seen in **Figure 5.** The essential steps of the procedure are illustrated (**Figures 6** to **10**).

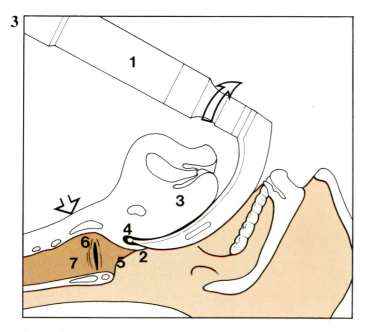

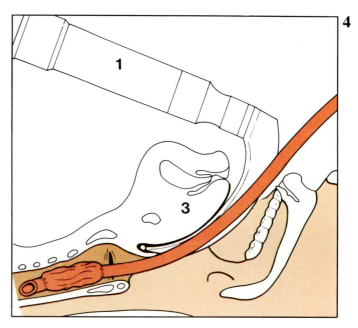

3 and 4 Diagrammatic representation of laryngostomy
The first step is to position correctly the patient's head by flexing the neck on a small but firm pillow placed beneath the occiput and extending the head at the atlanto-occipital joint. The mouth is then opened and the Macintosh laryngoscope (1) introduced on the right side to visualise the epiglottis (2). The tongue (3) is meantime kept depressed and to the left. Once the epiglottis has been seen, the tip of the laryngoscope is passed into the vallecula (4). The next step is very important and entails gently lifting the laryngoscope upwards and distally by its handle in the direction of the broad arrow. There must be no deviation or angulation from this line, otherwise the tip of the laryngoscope will lift the larynx (5) and obscure it from view. Teeth, gums and lips can all be damaged by such angulation.

If there is difficulty in visualisation of the larynx at this stage, pressure is exerted externally on the neck at the level of the open arrow to bring it back into view. Once the larynx is visible the endotracheal tube is passed along the right side of the mouth so that its tip comes to lie between the vocal cords (6). The tube is then centralised and advanced into the trachea (7) until the proximal end of the cuff lies just below the vocal cords.

The tube should always be allowed to maintain its original curve in the first instance as its shape is appropriate to most cases. If the tube does not follow the required line of approach to the larynx, then the malleable introducer shown in **Figure 5** is used to alter the curvature as required.

Correct placement is ensured by inflating the cuff with air to eliminate leakage around the tube and by ausculation of the lungs during positive pressure ventilation.

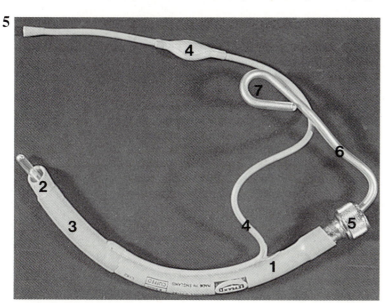

5 Endotracheal tube
The tube (1) is semi-rigid with an obliquely cut tip (2) and an encircling cuff (3) which can be inflated with a syringe via the narrow tube (4). The Nosworthy metal connector (5) fits the endotracheal connection to link up with the anaesthetic circuit. In the lumen of the tube is a malleable plastic coated metal director (6) which is of sufficient length to control the tip of the tube when it is manipulated by the proximal 'handle' (7). The tip of this director should not protrude beyond the tube as shown in the photograph as it could create a false passage. The size of tube for an average female patient has an external diameter of 7.5 or 8mm.

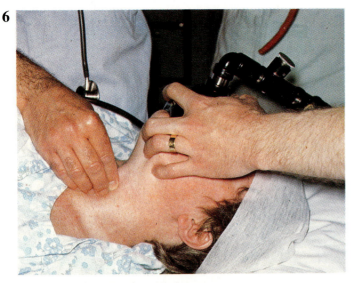

6 Endotracheal intubation – technique
Anaesthesia has been induced and oxygen is being administered preparatory to passing the laryngoscope. Note that the chin is extended and supported by the fingers of the left hand while cricoid pressure is applied by an assistant.

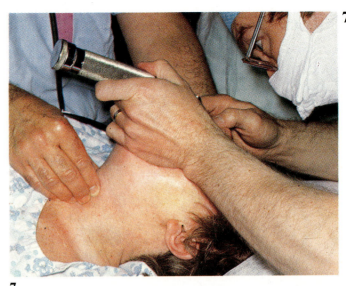

7
The mouth is kept open and the head extended with the assistant's right hand while the laryngoscope is introduced with the left hand. The edge of the left hand rests on and supports the patient's chin as the tip of the instrument is introduced under vision. Cricoid pressure is maintained.

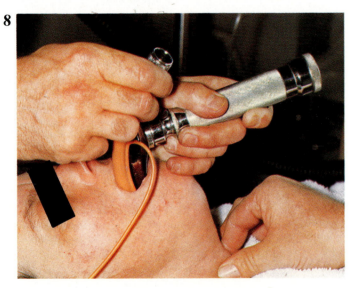

8
From the other side, the endotracheal tube is seen being introduced into the trachea under vision. The director is not in use at this stage. Cricoid pressure is maintained.

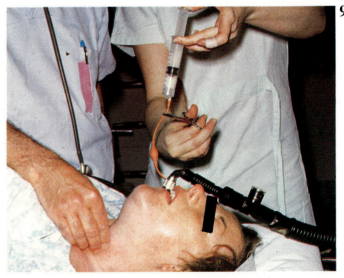

9
The tube is in place; this is checked by pressure on the chest and noting expulsion of air through the tube. The connection to the anaesthetic circuit has been made and the cuff within the trachea is inflated via the narrow tube with a syringe before clamping off the inflation tube with a fine forceps.

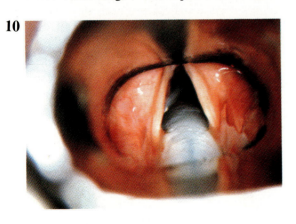

10
Endotracheal photograph of vocal cords as seen during intubation.

Failed intubation procedure

1. When attempted endotracheal intubation has failed, adequate oxygenation becomes the first requirement. Cricoid pressure is maintained to prevent regurgitation of gastric contents, and the patient's lungs are inflated with oxygen until spontaneous respiration returns.
2. If the operation is not considered urgent, the patient is allowed to wake up and the situation is reassessed. Local spinal or epidural block analgesia may be suitable alternatives.

3. If the operation must proceed, inhalation anaesthesia is used with the patient in the lateral and head down position. Oxygen and halothane is the most suitable mixture and as anaesthesia deepens ether is added (after giving intravenous atropine). When an ether content of 15 per cent is reached, the halothane is discontinued. The operation can be performed under ether with spontaneous ventilation.

4. Before proceeding further it is always worth performing laryngoscopy to reassess the situation, once anaesthesia is deep enough and the jaw is relaxed. Under these conditions one is not under pressure; there is plenty of time because the patient is breathing spontaneously. It may be possible to pass a smaller endotracheal tube or a microlargyngeal tube. The passage of an endotracheal tube may be aided by first passing a Toronto catheter (14 or 16 size) or the smallest size oesophageal bougie, and threading the endotracheal tube over either of those. If this is successful, the relaxant technique of anaesthesia described may then be used. Otherwise it is a case of continuing with spontaneous ventilation.

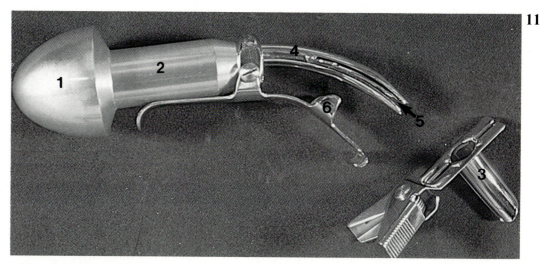

11 Penlon tracheotome
The various parts of the instrument are numbered thus: 1. handle, 2. shank, 3. expanding cannula, 4. introducer (trochar), 5. scalpel blade, 6. swing stop bar.

Tracheotomy

Where there is a problem with intubation it may become difficult to maintain the airway. Cases of laryngeal oedema due to severe toxaemia or fluid overloading present similar problems. In such cases tracheotomy is used to establish an airway through the crico-thyroid membrane.

Methods of tracheotomy
The Penlon Tracheotome (manufactured by Penlon Ltd., Abingdon, Berks) is shown in **Figure 11** and is inserted as demonstrated in the consecutive-step **Figure 14.** The instrument gives a good airway through the crico-thyroid membrane and is easily connected up to the breathing circuit. The tracheostomy tube and necessary equipment for the procedure are shown on **Figure 12.**

The compact and efficient Cawthorne Emergency Laryngostomy Tube (Down Bros Ltd.) shown in **Figure 13** provides a narrow airway which might make it difficult to maintain anaesthesia. Nonetheless it is easy to use in difficult situations and might on occasion be life-saving.

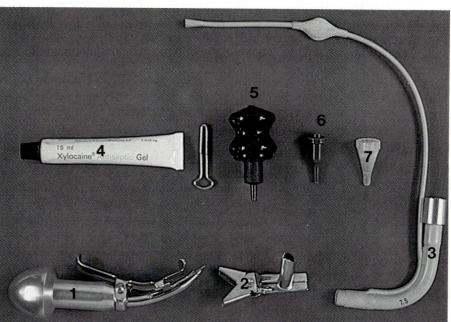

12 Tracheotomy instruments
The various items are numbered thus: 1. Penlon tracheotome, 2. expanding (split) cannula, 3. endotracheal tube, 4. analgesic ointment, 5. inflating bellows for endotracheal tube, 6. non-return valve for pilot tube, 7. nozzle for tube of analgesic ointment.

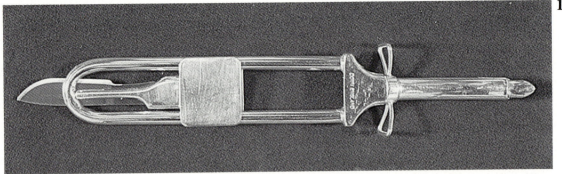

13 Cawthorne emergency laryngostomy tube
The scalpel blade is retractable within the frame of the instrument. The small laryngostomy tube
fits over the trochar, but with the tip of the trochar projecting beyond it. The tube is left *in situ*
when the trochar is withdrawn. It has metal loops to take attaching tapes for fixation.

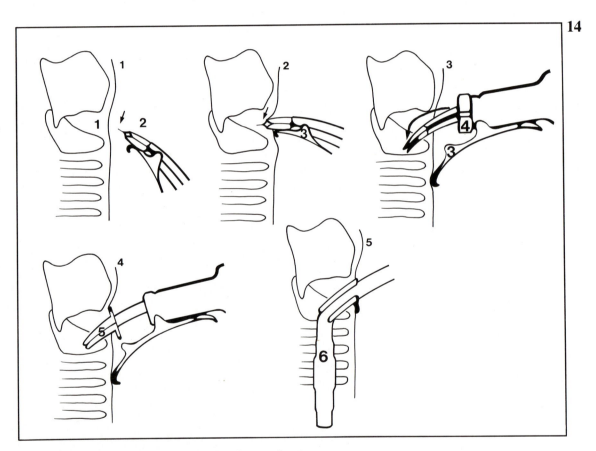

14 Technique of tracheotomy using Penlon tracheotome
1. The crico-thyroid space is located at (1) and the tracheotome (2) is ready for use. The
   scalpel blade is arrowed.
2. The blade is thrust into the crico-thyroid membrane where arrowed. Deep penetration is
   prevented by the swing-stop bar (3).
3. The swing-stop is now released. The trochar is fully advanced forwards and downwards in
   an arc indicated by the curved arrow. The thrust is arrested by the fixed guard (4). Note
   that when the swing-stop is released, the scalpel blade retracts into the introducer.
4. The metal cannula (5) is now advanced along the trochar to a fully inserted position with
   its flange on the skin surface.
5. The cuffed tracheostomy tube (6) is inserted through the split cannula which can be
   levered open to accommodate it.

3. Maternal and fetal hypoxia relating to inferior vena caval and aortic compression

This well recognised clinical syndrome has already been referred to in Chapters 1 and 9. Pressure on the inferior vena cava leads to a reduction in maternal cardiac output and placental blood flow. The degree of resultant hypotension depends very much on the collateral venous drainage and **Figure 15** shows the usual anatomy of the paravertebral venous plexus which is the main collateral route. The total collateral circulation is normally inadequate for effective blood return in pregnancy. Those women apparently immune to the syndrome have in some cases been shown to have more and larger collateral veins than is normal. That the condition does not solely concern the inferior vena cava is clear from **Figures 16** and **17** where the aorta and the common iliac arterial flow is distorted

and impeded by the heavy uterus so that placental supply must be further affected.

Development of the syndrome is avoided by attention to the position of the patient. Other benefits accruing when the mother is maintained in an efficient lateral tilt on the labour or operating table (**Figure 18**) include an improvement in the biochemical state of the fetus at delivery with a reduction in the need for resuscitation at that time. It should be remembered that the fall in cardiac output as a result of vena cava block may also be aggravated by the effects of regional analgesia or general anaesthesia. Further protection of the fetal state can be ensured by avoiding the supine position in the labour ward and during transport to the operating room[9].

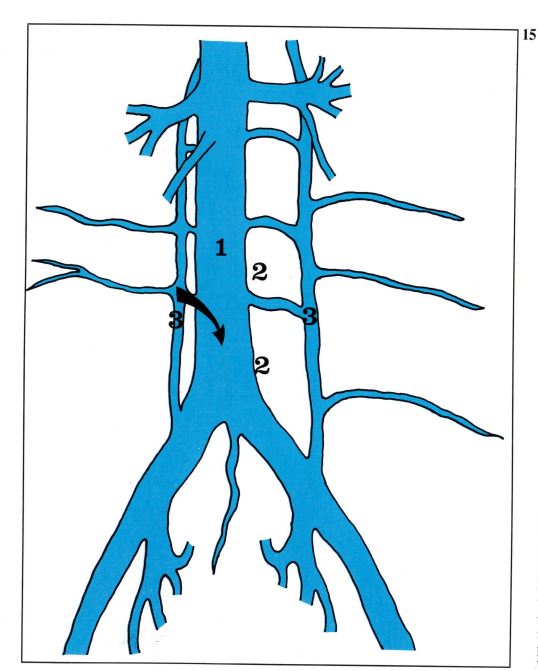

15

15 Tracing of a radiograph to show the inferior vena cava and its collateral (paravertebral) circulation

When the inferior vena cava (1) is compressed against the vertebral bodies (2) at the level arrowed, venous return can only be via the paravertebral (3) and epidural veins. The latter are very small and are not shown. The tracing shows that the paravertebral capacity is quite inadequate to replace that of the inferior vena cava.

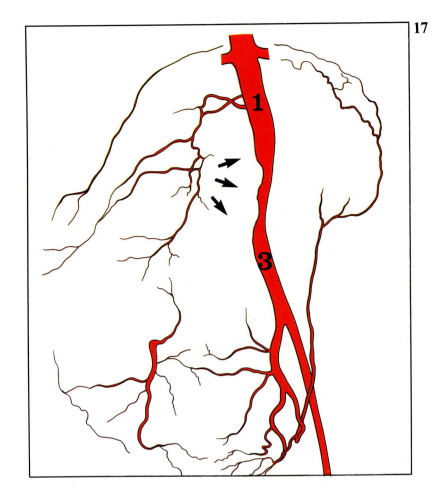

16 and 17 Extent to which aorta and common iliac arteries may be compressed by late pregnancy uterus
Bieniarz et al[8] in a series of arteriographic studies showed that the relaxed late pregnancy uterus may compress and displace the abdominal aorta especially at L4-5 level. They also showed that the contracting uterus could greatly narrow the aorta and even occlude the right common iliac artery. Our diagrams based on the original arteriograms illustrate such effects and the principal areas of compression by the relaxed and contracting uterus are arrowed in **Figures 16** and **17** respectively. The aorta is numbered (1), the right common iliac artery (2) and the left common artery (3).

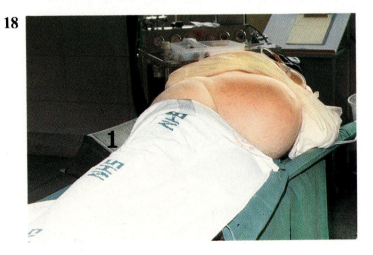

18 Left lateral tilt for caesarean section
The waterproofed sorbo rubber wedge (1) under the patient's right buttock maintains her in a 30° lateral tilt.

B. The management of haemorrhage and its sequelae

Primary replacement of simple blood loss from various obstetrical causes may at any time have to take account of possible dangerous escalations of the haemorrhagic state. Thus a deficiency of certain blood clotting factors may develop during massive blood replacement. The dangerous condition of disseminated intravascular coagulation is a further possible development which is particularly associated with bleeding in severe accidental haemorrhage, amniotic fluid embolism or intrauterine fetal death.

The increase in blood volume during pregnancy has been referred to (Chapter 1) and allows the patient, for example, to withstand blood losses of 1–1.5 litres at caesarean section without detriment.

Treatment of haemorrhage

This is directed towards:
1. Early establishment of one or two safe intravenous transfusion lines.
2. Maintenance of body temperature.
3. Adequate oxygenation of the tissues.
4. Maintenance or restoration of adequate circulatory fluid volume and cardiac output.
5. Maintenance of peripheral tissue perfusion.
6. Maintenance of adequate haemoglobin level.
7. Arrest of the haemorrhage.

Vasco-constriction may make intravenous infusion difficult to establish. If a vein on the arm or hand can be entered with a 20 gauge needle on a 20 ml syringe and a tourniquet is kept on the upper arm it is possible to distend the venous system with 20 ml volumes of normal saline until there is a large vein capable of taking a 16 or 18 gauge catheter. Once a vein has been cannulated a pressure infusion bag (Fenwal, **Figure 19**) may be used to accelerate transfusion.

Body temperature is maintained to safeguard liver metabolism, myocardial function and prevent peripheral vaso-constriction. The survival blanket (**Figure 20**) is used and if possible the transfused stored (cold) blood is passed through warming equipment (**Figure 22**).

Oxygen is given to increase oxygen carrying power in the plasma and compensate for the loss of haemoglobin carrying capacity. It will also help to combat the effects of the decreased pulmonary blood flow which impairs the ventilation/perfusion ratios. If air hunger is present intermittent positive pressure respiration may be needed until blood loss is controlled.

An adequate circulatory volume and peripheral perfusion enables calcium ions to be mobilised from the body stores so that parenteral calcium gluconate is less often needed unless there is electrocardiographic evidence of hypokalaemia or there is a continuing poor response to the rapid infusion of large amounts of blood. To restore adequate oxygen carriage the haemoglobin must of course be replaced.

In many cases of acute obstetric haemorrhage surgical intervention is required to stop the bleeding while the patient is still in poor general condition. Resuscitation and transfusion must go hand in hand so that there is minimal delay in commencing surgery. Delay means further blood loss with loss of clotting factors and the possibility of a bleeding diathesis developing while resuscitation is still taking place.

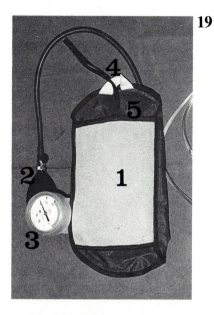

19 Pressure infusion bag
The Fenwal pressure infusion bag (1) is an inflatable jacket with a bulb pump (2) and a pressure gauge (3). It has a tape (4) to suspend it from a drip stand and it accommodates within it the compressible plastic blood or IV fluid container (5). It is seen in use in **Figure 22**. (Fenwal Laboratories, Branch of Travenol Laboratories Inc, Illinois, USA.)

Maintenance/restoration of circulating fluid volume
The first problem is to assess the amount of fluid required and this is done by continuous assessment of the clinical condition. Pulse rate, blood pressure, electrocardiograph, the state of the peripheral circulation, the jugular venous pressure and if necessary the central venous pressure are continually monitored as fluid replacement takes place. Where the circulatory volume is low a head-down tilt is maintained to encourage venous return and aid cardiac filling. Pressure infusion bags will permit the rapid replacement of fluid (**Figure 19**).

20

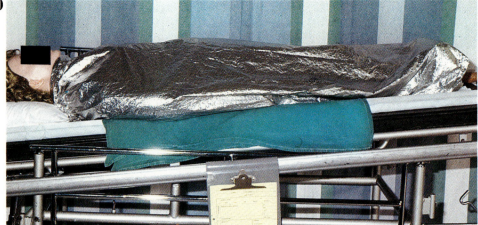

20 Survival blanket
The blanket is tucked in firmly to insulate the body; only the patient's head is uncovered. Note the 15° head-down tilt for a shocked patient.

Replacement of blood volume

The continuing assessment of the patient's clinical condition by the methods already in use will indicate the amount and type of blood which is appropriate.

Stored blood – is usually CPD blood, i.e. 63 ml of citrate phosphate dextrose in 420 ml of whole blood. It is the standard replacement blood for severe haemorrhage.

Fresh blood – is indicated when large amounts of blood (in excess of 2½–5 litres) are required. This is in order to maintain adequate levels of the clotting factors.

Autologous blood transfusion – may be vital if fresh blood is not available, or when a clotting screen cannot be carried out or the concentrates of the necessary clotting factors are not available.

The various blood preparations available for transfusion and their characteristics are presented as a table in Appendix D (page 201). The principal blood extracts are seen ready for use in **Figure 21**.

The following fluids are used as required in the individual case:

1. *Hartmann's solution* (Ringer-lactate)
One litre may be given while blood is being cross matched. If haemorrhage is profuse a further 500–1000 ml may be given after every 1.5–2.0 litres of blood. Improved tissue perfusion is obtained as a result of the decrease in blood viscosity. Renal function is likewise protected by the induced diuresis.

2. *Dextran*
Dextran has a molecular weight of 70,000 (Dextran 70 in 0.9 per cent saline or 5 per cent dextrose) and has an estimated half life of 6 hours. It is a suitable alternative to Ringer-lactate in amounts of up to 1000 ml.

3. *Gelatin solution* (prepared by hydrolysis of animal collagens) may interfere with cross matching by causing red cell rouleaux formation. It is currently marketed as Haemaccel (Hoechst) which is a 3 per cent solution with a colloid osmotic pressure equivalent to plasma and capable of being used until blood becomes available.

4. *Human plasma protein factor*
This solution is said to be free of the risk of hepatitis and may be used as a volume expander.

21

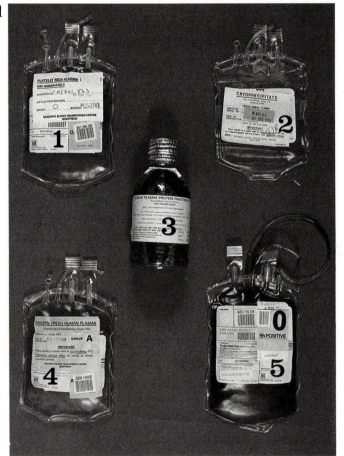

21 Blood extracts
The various extracts are numbered thus: 1. platelet rich plasma, 2. cryoprecipitate, 3. human plasma protein fraction, 4. frozen fresh human plasma, 5. concentrated red cells.

C. Hypovolaemic shock due to haemorrhage

This is the commonest type of shock encountered in obstetrics and care is essential to ensure that any contribution of a cardiogenic or endotoxic nature to the overall clinical state, is recognised.

Clinical signs

The patient is pale, sweating and anxious or may have some clouding of consciousness. Peripheral cyanosis is present and there is vasoconstriction, tachycardia and hypotension (although young pregnant women may maintain a blood pressure of near normal till large amounts of blood have been lost). Air hunger is obvious and there is oliguria.

Management

This would include the following requirements:
1. Administration of 100 per cent oxygen at a rate of 8 litres per minute.
2. Patient in 15° head-down tilt.
3. Patient covered with survival blanket.
4. Pulse, blood pressure and ECG being continually recorded.
5. Temperature of the rectum and of the big toe being recorded to estimate core-peripheral temperature gradient (thus assessing improving or failing peripheral perfusion).
6. Two intravenous transfusion lines in place with blood warming equipment (**Figure 22**) to prevent body cooling. Pressure infusion bags (i.e. Fenwal type) (**Figures 19** and **22**) enable rapid transfusion to be given and blood filters (**Figure 23**) remove any particulate matter from stored blood.
7. Patient is catheterised and urine output recorded.
8. Initiation of central venous pressure (CVP) monitoring. This can give rise to complications if the internal jugular or subclavian vein is used in the acutely ill patient. A simpler or safer alternative is to use the external jugular vein as illustrated and described on pages 192–193. This gives all the required information in assessing replacement needs.
9. Insertion of an arterial line into the radial or dorsalis pedis artery so that acid-based estimations and the need for bicarbonate therapy can be assessed (**Figures 24** and **25**).

10. Assessment of blood volume
(i) If CVP, core-peripheral temperature gradient and urine output are restored to normal, blood volume and peripheral perfusion should be satisfactory. CVP should be 8–10cm of H_2O. Core-peripheral temperature gradient should be 4°C and urine output 40–50ml per hour.
(ii) Pulse, blood pressure and acid-base balance should rapidly return to normal and if the bleeding has been arrested the patient will quickly regain a satisfactory general condition.

Management of the deteriorating situation

If a shocked lung syndrome has developed with superimposed cardiogenic or endotoxic shock, or in the presence of disseminated intravascular coagulation, the patient should be transferred to an intensive care unit.

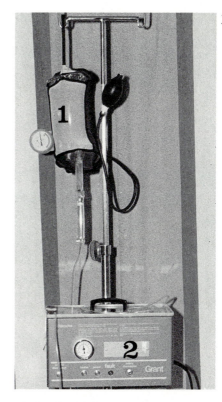

22 Blood transfusion in shock
Rapid replacement is aided by the Fenwal pressure bag (1) and body heat is conserved by passing the infusion through the blood warming equipment (2). (Fenwal Laboratories, Branch of Travenol Laboratories Inc, Illinois, USA.)

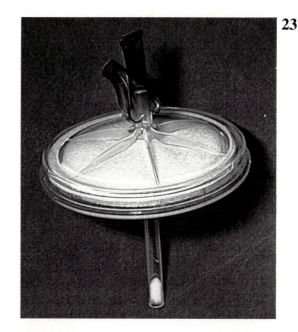

23 Blood filter
20 Micron High Capacity Transfusion Filter for removal of microaggregates from whole blood or red blood cells. (Fenwal Laboratories, Branch of Travenol Laboratories Inc, Illinois, USA.)

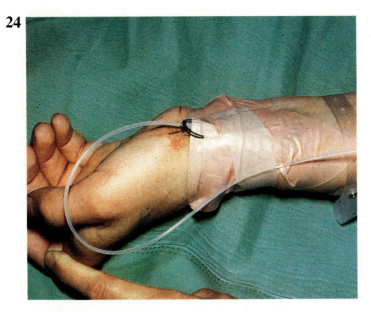

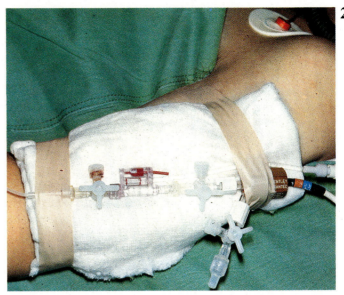

24 and 25 Arterial Line
Figure 24 shows the monitoring catheter in the right radial artery. The automatic flushing system for the arterial line and the transducer are seen in **Figure 25.**

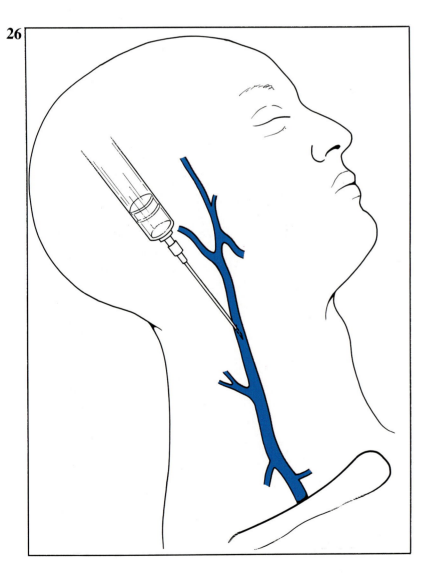

26 to 28 Diagrammatic illustration of the steps in catheterisation of the external jugular vein
1. puncture of the external jugular vein (**Figure 26**);
2. passage of the introducer through the needle into the vein (**Figure 27**); 3. after withdrawal of the needle, passage of the catheter over the introducer into the vein (**Figure 28**).

Estimation of CVP by catheterisation of external jugular vein

The safest methods of measuring central venous pressure are to use either the cephalic vein in the arm or the external jugular vein but in both cases there may be difficulty in passing the catheter into the superior vena cava or right atrium.

A simple safer alternative is to place a large bore intravenous cannula in the external jugular vein and insert through it a flexible tipped introducer of the type shown in **Figure 29**. With assistance and a little patience it is then possible to manipulate a large bore intravenous catheter over the introducer into the right atrium of the heart or the superior vena cava. The patient's head may need to be altered in position to enable the introducer to pass through the valves at the lower end of the external jugular vein. **Figures 26** to **28** summarise the intravenous insertion technique in diagrammatic form; the necessary equipment is seen in **Figure 29** and a monitor system is shown established in **Figure 30**. **Figures 31** to **36** illustrate the successive stages of the procedure.

27

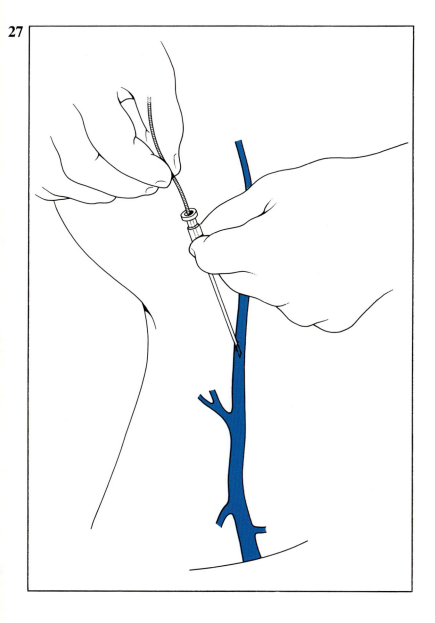

28

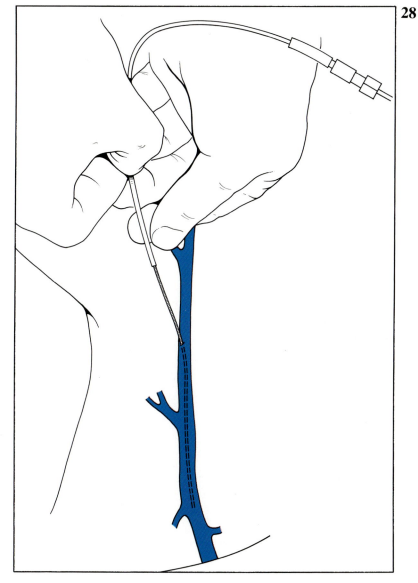

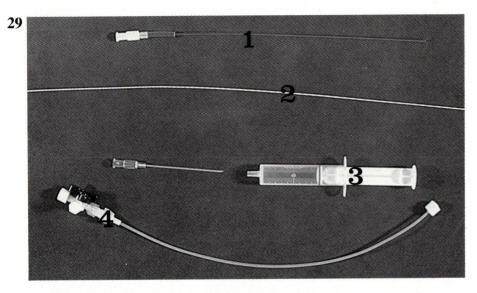

29 Equipment for intravenous installation of central venous, pressure line
1. Central venous catheter, 2. introducer with flexible tip, 3. syringe and intravenous cannula, 4. connecting tubing and 3-way tap.

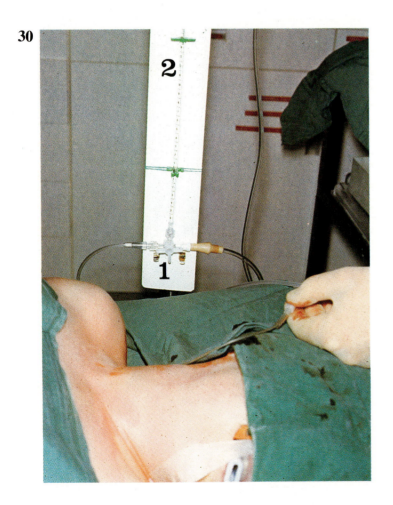

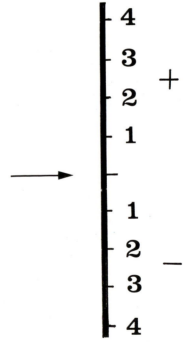

30 CVP line and monitoring scale in place
1. 3-way tap, 2. Scale showing zero, with plus and minus readings (in cm of water). The arrow indicates zero on a simplified diagram in CM scale.

The zero line is kept level with the patient's mid-axillary point and should be checked by using a spirit level. This essential point is not demonstrable on this photograph.

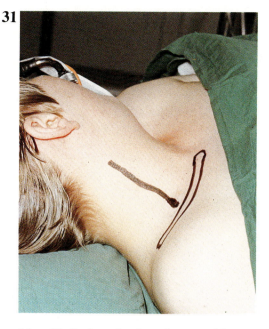

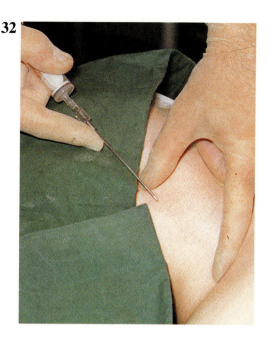

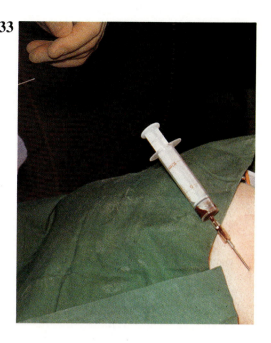

31 to 36 Catheterisation of external jugular vein

In **Figure 31** the patient is supine with the head turned to the opposite side. The vein is surface-marked and the clavicle outlined. If the vein is not easily visible

pressure with a finger tip just above the mid-clavicular point will distend it (**Figure 32**). That the vein has been

entered in **Figure 33,** is shown by the blood withdrawn into the barrel of the syringe. In **Figure 34,** the flexible tip of

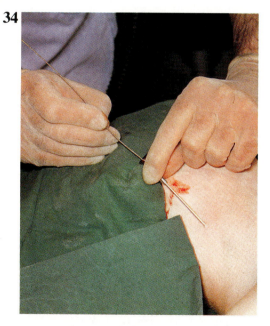

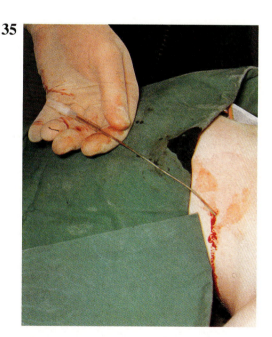

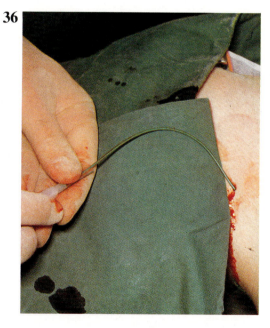

the introducer is fed into the vein through the needle which is subsequently withdrawn over it. The position of the patient's head is centralised as the introducer is advanced towards the superior vena cava and some manipulation is necessary to negotiate the valves of the lower end of the external jugular vein. In

Figures 35 and **36** the central venous catheter is threaded over the introducer and the introducer withdrawn. The catheter is connected to the 3-way tap as shown.

The intravenous infusion is commenced to clear the catheter before a reading is taken and the respiratory swing checked. The presence of respiratory swing confirms that the catheter is correctly placed.

D. Disseminated intravascular coagulation (DIC)

This complication and its management has been referred to in Chapter 8. The incidence, possible anticipation and treatment of the condition are of immediate concern to the anaesthetist. Conditions associated with the development of DIC are:

1. Endotoxic shock
2. Prolonged shock of any aetiology
3. Placental abruption (severe accidental haemorrhage
4. Amniotic fluid embolus
5. Pre-eclamptic toxaemia (severe/fulminating type and eclampsia)
6. Intra-uterine fetal death
7. Hydatidiform mole
8. Massive haemorrhage
9. Massive pulmonary embolus.

In any of these situations screening for coagulation defects should be carried out early to allow the haematologist time to obtain fresh blood for transfusions. In patients where screening has not been carried out spontaneous haemorrhages may occur. Absent or poor clot formation may be noticed during surgery and bleeding may commence from recent venepuncture sites. Where coagulation screening can be carried out at intervals, the lack of certain factors can be correctly assessed and replacement therapy given. In massive transfusion (5 litres or more) the deficiencies of clotting factors may vary substantially from patient to patient.

The following preparations should be available to combat haemorrhage and associated DIC especially when fresh blood is difficult to obtain.

Fresh frozen plasma
Cryoprecipitate: Factor VIII Deficiency
                 Fibrinogen Deficiency
Platelet Rich plasma   Thrombocytopenia
Platelet concentrate
Factor IX concentrate.

The amounts to be given will depend on the results of the coagulation screening tests and the close co-operation of a haematologist is required to ensure efficient therapy.

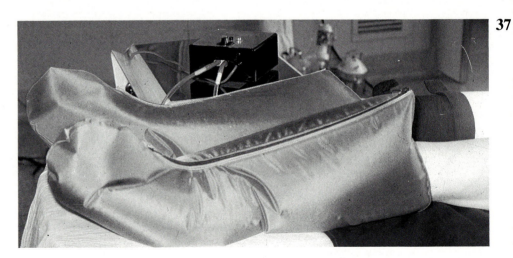

37 Inflatable boots worn by patient during operation in high risk thrombo-embolic cases.

E. Prevention of pulmonary embolism

Reference to the condition has been made in Chapter 9 (page 112); the relative figures of its incidence are seen in the Report on Confidential Enquiries into Maternal Deaths in England and Wales 1973–1975[10]. Many patients die immediately or within 2 hours of a pulmonary embolism, so that treatment is generally of little avail. The important requirements are:
1. Identification of patients at risk and the institution of prophylactic treatment.
2. Early diagnosis of thrombo-embolism at a stage when effective treatment can be given.

Risk factors

The following factors appear to be important[10]:

1. Obesity
For example, 12 of the 38 women who died and were reported in the Confidential Enquiry were overweight (76 Kg +); Another 3 were described as obese.

2. Restricted activity
Bed rest may have been a contributory factor in 7 cases in the above enquiry report.

3. Suppression of lactation by oestrogens
Four patients (19 per cent) in the report were known to have had lactation suppressed by this means.

It is emphasised that increasing age and parity and operative procedures all increase the risk of thrombo-embolism. Bed rest followed by caesarean section produces a high risk of the complication.

Diagnosis

This is generally based on the following:

1. Clinical evidence
Calf tenderness, oedema of the leg and increased warmth are all suspicious findings. The lower limbs are measured at the same level on thigh and calf and differences of 2 cm in circumference are significant.

2. Ultrasound scanning
The Doppler method is easy to carry out in obstetric units. The probe is placed first on the popliteal and then femoral vein. The normal 'swoosh' ('a' wave or augmentation wave) heard with increase in blood flow following calf compression is absent where there is blockage. The method is considered 85–95 per cent accurate for major vein thrombosis[11].

3. Isotope venography and lung scanning
99 m Te (technetium) is used[12] with an injection into the dorsal vein of each foot. The calf veins, the ilio-femoral segment and the lung fields can all be examined. The method is very accurate for the diagnosis of ilio-femoral thrombosis and even more so for demonstrating lung emboli.

Prevention is directed at the high risk group; treatment is instituted when the diagnosis is established or confirmed by techniques such as isotope venography.

Prevention

The following measures are of value:
1. Patients suffering from varicose veins should wear supportive elastic stockings during pregnancy.
2. In late pregnancy the possibility of inferior vena caval compression should be explained to patients. They are advised to avoid lying on their backs at night or when resting, e.g. because of pre-eclamptic toxaemia. Patients in labour are nursed in the sitting or lateral position and lateral tilting of the table is used at caesarean section.
3. Inflatable leggings which are alternately inflated and deflated by an electric pump may be fitted during operative procedures to prevent venous stasis. (**Figure 37**).
4. Dextran 70 solutions given during and after anaesthesia and operations to a total volume of 1 litre have been shown to reduce the incidence of venous thrombosis following pelvic surgery[13].
5. Patients with a history of deep vein thrombosis or pulmonary embolus should have long term subcutaneous heparin therapy during pregnancy and the puerperium. Sodium heparin 5000 units in 0.2 ml is the preparation of choice[14]. Some obstetricians advise that self-administration be taught and the lateral abdominal wall used as the site of injection. 5000 to 7000 IU 12 hourly is usually adequate but may need to be increased to 10,000 IU 12 hourly in late pregnancy. With increased dosage it is advisable to measure heparin blood levels. A plasma level of 0.05–0.3 IU/ml is effective and safe.

Appendix A: Acute defibrination syndrome (Disseminated Intravascular Coagulation (DIC))

Basic principles in management
by Pierre Cotteel

There are certain established facts in relation to the condition and in practice the following should be taken into account:

General considerations

1. Primary fibrinolysis is rare.
2. Disseminated Intravascular Coagulation precedes severe haemorrhage and diminished blood coagulation.
3. The initial causative factor is a severe local lesion which leads to an upset of the clotting mechanism (e.g. gross obstetric injury, difficult delivery or prolonged caesarean delivery, intra-uterine death – in general those conditions which cause abnormally heavy or prolonged bleeding and including uterine atony and severe vaginal and perineal tears).
4. The clotting mechanism is a dynamic process and normally retains a balance between production and destruction especially in regard to fibrinogen.

Development of the condition

1. The local lesions cause a micro-coagulation which at first is in the form of localised micro-emboli but these are later disseminated throughout the body.
2. There is diminished fibrinogen because of its conversion to fibrin.
3. The fibrin blocks the small blood vessels and causes diffuse intravascular coagulation. This is the first stage of the condition.
4. The drop in the fibrinogen is followed by reduced blood coagulating power and bleeding. This is the beginning of disordered blood coagulation.
5. A vicious circle ensues – there is an increase in fibrinolytic activity to enable the blood to permeate the vessels and clear up the areas of micro-embolism. This secondary fibrinolysis is often in excess of what is required and leads to a worse and less easily reversed state than existed in the first place. The blood is unable to clot and is in fact haemolysed.

Treatment

(1) Management should be active and urgent and is aimed at treating the cause before a vicious circle develops.
(2) Treatment may be directed towards rapidly re-establishing a normal clotting mechanism without laboratory aid and without risk:

   Replace the patient's blood loss by whole blood or preferably by packed cells and above all give fresh frozen plasma which is rich in coagulation factors.
   Each estimated litre of blood lost would be replaced by 3 units or *culots* (each approximately 200 ml) of packed cells and **adequate** amount of fresh, frozen plasma; transfused under pressure (see Blood Preparations, Appendix D).

(3) Treatment may be indicated by laboratory guidance when that is available. It is important to have a full and urgent report for two reasons: (i) to judge the gravity of the situation (most of the parameters are upset whatever the exact diagnosis) and (ii) to know if it is indeed a case of DIC or one of fibrinolysis. The most helpful tests and which are specific for DIC are these:

   (i) increase in coagulation time
   (ii) a real drop in platelets (thrombopenia)
   (iii) a normal Von Kaula test (upset in fibrinolysis).

I. If it is a case of DIC (the more likely diagnosis):
HEPARIN is given to dissolve the micro-clots. Fibrinogen is then no longer broken down and increases in amount.
— recommended dosage: 5 mg/Kg/24 hours.
— in practice: 50 mg intravenously immediately and repeat up to a total of 200 to 300 mg depending on the laboratory reports.

II. If it is a case of fibrinolysis:
FIBRINOLYTICS are given
— aminocaproic acid (Haemocaprol) 20 ml intravenously, then 20 ml in an intravenous drip over 2 to 3 hours.
— aprotinine (Iniprol) 1–4 million units intravenously, and then depending on laboratory results.

Dangers of giving the wrong treatment

1. If heparin is given in a case of fibrinolysis:
there are no clots to dissolve so that the treatment aggravates the haemorrhage by further lessening coagulation and depressing fibrinogen.

2. If fibrinolytics are given in a case of DIC
there is an aggravation of the condition by diminution of fibrinogen and an increase of fibrin. Haemorrhage increases.

These dangers are relatively greater because one is dealing with a dynamic condition which is changing all the time and more quickly than the laboratory can keep pace with. The results are not always relevant at the time they are received since they report on a situation which has already passed. It is therefore preferable to use frozen plasma and fibrinogen (2–4 grams); the latter is very useful in either of the two conditions as it is nearly always deficient. If other methods fail heparin may be given but should be used cautiously because it carries some risk. Nonetheless it sometimes offers the only possibility of improving the situation.

Appendix B: Essential prerequisites in caesarean section

This list of important considerations and requirements is incomplete but includes items which the authors consider essential and even elementary.

1. A fully trained surgical team

The fact that the lives of two individuals are at stake makes the operation a uniquely important one. The condition of pregnancy itself brings additional problems to both the surgeon and anaesthetist and the possibility of severe unexpected haemorrhage is always present. The surgeon performing the operation should be fully trained and have adequate experience of operative delivery. Junior surgical staff should be meticulously trained and do the operation under supervision until they are judged to be competent. The same standard of competence applies in the specialty of anaesthesia.

2. Satisfactory condition of the patient

Patients in shock or in need of immediate resuscitation should not be operated on until blood volume has been re-established and the state of the clotting mechanism is known.

In non-emergency circumstances conditions such as anaemia, ketosis and oedema should be corrected or stabilised pre-operatively.

3. Anaesthetic safeguards

The specialist anaesthetists have brought the standard and safety of anaesthesia to a very high degree and most surgeons tend to leave the choice of method to their colleagues. This has happened in the United Kingdom where the general wellbeing of both the mother and the fetus during delivery has primarily become the clinical concern of the anaesthetist (see Chapter 15, page 179). Such ideal conditions are far from universal and many surgeons must take the decision regarding the type of anaesthesia to be given and carry the major responsibility for subsequent events. Some surgeons rely very much on epidural block but it is not always available nor necessarily appropriate to the case. Where general anaesthesia is employed or indicated the patient should be in the operating room prepared and ready for the operation before induction of the anaesthetic and a cuffed endotracheal tube should always be inserted. The Confidential Report[2] clearly indicates that the surgeon who does not always have an experienced anaesthetic colleague must keep himself informed on anaesthetic matters since it is rightly implied that he bears a major responsibility regarding the provision of the anaesthesia.

4. Anticipation of haemorrhage, sepsis and pulmonary embolus

These 3 conditions together constitute the major cause of death in caesarean section and should as far as possible be anticipated by sound and careful surgery. A caesarean section should never be commenced unless at least 1 litre of cross matched blood has been provided and is immediately available. The methods of minimising blood loss are discussed on page 114.

Sepsis and pulmonary embolus can both be reduced by adopting surgical measures which allow the uterus and the abdominal wall to heal neatly and strongly without interference from uterine contraction and normal abdominal movement. This entails the routine use of a lower abdominal transverse incision, a transverse opening of the lower uterine segment and early ambulation.

Reference to the Confidential Report[2] reveals that of the 38 deaths due to pulmonary embolism studied in the years 1973–75 6 followed caesarean section and a further 2 were known about but not reported on. In 4 of the 6 cases the clinical history of findings might have indicated an increased risk of pulmonary embolism and 4 had been resting antenatally for hypertensive diseases of pregnancy. Operative delivery or surgical intervention during pregnancy increases the risk of embolism and it is therefore important to anticipate the condition in two ways. One is to identify the patients at risk and treat them prophylactically, the other is by making an early diagnosis of thrombotic precursors and commencing treatment without delay.

5. Presence of specialist paediatrician at delivery

Circumstances which dictate the need for caesarean section ideally require the presence of a paediatric colleague to assume the immediate neonatal care of the child. The unhappy scene where both surgeon and anaesthetist are deflected from their own urgent affairs by joining the midwives in a worrying wrangle as to how the unresponding baby should be dealt with should be avoided.

6. Avoidance of unnecessary accompanying surgical procedures

There has usually been prior discussion and agreement where sterilisation is required but in emergency conditions this may not be known about and enquiries should be made regarding that and the opportunity given to the couple to submit any particular request about the operation. It is not necessary to discuss sterilisation here; suffice to say that if it is considered necessary this is a very suitable opportunity to do it.

Other additional surgical procedures at the time of caesarean section are frequently requested or asked about; the most frequent of these are routine appendicectomy, myomectomy and removal of an ovarian cyst. The authors consider it quite wrong to do appendicectomy at this time. Unnecessarily opening the bowel in the presence of blood in the peritoneal cavity is a recipe for peritoneal infection and it has been pointed out[5] that additional trauma to the bowel and peritoneal cavity in conjunction with a large uterus contributes to postoperative ileus and morbidity.

There are many good reasons for not doing myomectomy at the time of caesarean section. Only if a fibroid is in the line of the incision or on a narrow pedicle which can safely be ligated should it be considered.

Ovarian cystectomy is rather different since the ovary is not enlarged and vascular to the same extent. If the cyst is obviously benign and of follicular or dermoid type, it should be removed. The operation must be done with the utmost attention to haemostasis and reconstruction of the ovary, as there is always the risk of slow blood loss and collection to form a haematocele in the pouch of Douglas.

Appendix C: Chemotherapy in chorio carcinoma

Following the pioneer work of Li and his co-workers[6], chemotherapy has remained the primary treatment in gestational trophoblastic tumours. There is a wealth of published work dealing with treatment of this disease[7,8,9,10,11]. Techniques for the radioimmunoassay of chorionic gonadotrophin (HCG) and the beta sub-unit of HCG have been greatly refined[12,13,14,15]. The long term consequences of the use of cytotoxic agents in women of childbearing age has been a matter of some concern and the long term follow-up reports have helped to allay these fears[16,17,18,19]. With regard to actual clinical management and treatment protocols, these differ in different centres but are in essence the same. The methods described here are orthodox and are those employed in Sheffield.

Treatment methods

The minimum requirement for treatment is elevation of HCG values 6 weeks after evacuation of a mole. Initial treatment irrespective of risk category is by 'single agent'. The cytotoxic agent used is methotrexate (MTX) with citrovorum factor (CF) rescue. The 'standard' regime as advocated by Bagshawe[7] was initially used in all patients and has been the basis of all treatment protocol since. The standard MTX-CF regime consists of methotrexate 50 mg i.m. starting on Day 1 and repeated at 48 hour intervals for 4 doses (total 200 mgm). Each dose of methotrexate is followed at 30 hours by citrovorum factor (6 mg i.m.). This constitutes one 'course' of treatment. It was customary initially to give patients in the 'low' risk category only 4 courses with rest periods of 7–10 days between but experience showed that a higher remission rate was obtainable by giving the full 6 courses in all cases. 'Medium' and 'High' risk patients always received 6 courses of treatment. Table I summarises the standard regime.

The chemotherapy regime is remarkable in the almost total absence of detectable toxicity. There is no evidence of myelosuppression or renal or liver function impairment; all three parameters are monitored before treatment, between courses and when therapy is complete. Minor discomfort is experienced by a few patients in the form of mild conjunctivitis, small gingival ulcers and pleurodynia. All patients are ambulant throughout treatment (unless confined to bed by the gravity of their illness), no barrier nursing is necessary and patients are discharged home after the last dose of CF. The type of response to therapy as indicated by the urinary HCG levels varies in individual patients (**Figure 1**).

Patients resistant to the initial MTX-CF regime are treated by 'triple agent' regimes using combinations of the following agents, actinomycin D, cyclophosphamide, vincristine, vinblastine, adriamycin and bleomycin (Table II). Patients are deemed to be in remission after 4 normal HCG assays of urine at weekly intervals. Further follow-up is bi-weekly and monthly urinary HCG assays for the first year and 3 monthly for the second year.

Table 1

GESTATIONAL TROPHOBLASTIC DISEASE

STANDARD CHEMOTHERAPY REGIME

METHOTREXATE (MTX) 50 mgm IM per dose
CITROVORUM (FOL) 6 mgm IM per dose

DAY 1	1 MTX	3 MTX	5 MTX	7 MTX	
					ONE COURSE
	2 FOL	4 FOL	6 FOL	8 FOL	

REST 7 – 10 days

REPEAT 4 courses – local disease
6 courses – metastatic or extensive disease

IF NO SIGNIFICANT FALL IN HCG LEVELS AFTER 3rd COURSE,
CONSIDER COMBINED CHEMOTHERAPY

Table 2

GESTATIONAL TROPHOBLASTIC DISEASE

SPECIALISED TREATMENTS

COMBINATION CHEMOTHERAPY
    CYCLOPHOSPHAMIDE
    VINCRISTINE   (VARYING
    ADRIAMYCIN   COMBINATIONS)
    BLEOMYCIN

RADIOTHERAPY
    WHOLE CRANIUM + INTRATHECAL MTX.
    WHOLE PELVIS + CONED BOOSTER DOSAGE
        TO VULVO-VAGINAL SECS.
    LOCALISED LUNG LESIONS –
        MEGAVOLT. NARROW FIELD

SURGERY
    HYSTERECTOMY
    LOBECTOMY

Figure 1

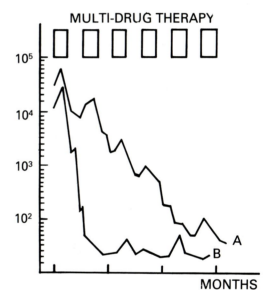

Values of human chorionic gonadotrophin in the urine during six courses of cytotoxic chemotherapy for choriocarcinoma showing step-wise reduction and different rates of response in two patients.

Results

Published results confirm the enormously successful use of chemical agents in the curative treatment of neoplastic disease[20,21,22]. The Sheffield results are equally good: thus in the first 4 years 58 patients were treated as the remission rate in the non-metastatic trophoblastic disease group (45 patients) was 100 per cent. In the metastatic trophoblastic disease group (13 patients) the disease-free remission rate was 92.3 per cent. The overall remission rate was 98.3 per cent.

There has been no evidence that initial treatment with a single agent MTX, using relatively high doses, prejudices subsequent response to combination therapy if resistance is recognised early.

The success in the treatment of gestational trophoblastic disease has brought in its wake an understandable concern about the long-term consequences of known mutagenic and oncogenic agents in young women of childbearing age and their offspring. Pregnancy in women successfully treated has been the subject of several papers[16,17,19]. It is reassuring that in over 200 recorded pregnancies there has been no increase in congenital abnormalities. It will, however, be a long time before sufficient data is available on incidence of recessive mutations and their consequences in second and third generation offspring of treated patients.

APPENDIX D

TABLE OF BLOOD PREPARATIONS AVAILABLE FOR TRANSFUSION AND THEIR MAIN CHARACTERISTICS

Type	Volume	Storage	Shelf Life	Indications
Whole blood	420 ml of blood in 63 ml Citrate-phosphate dextrose (CPD)	At 4°C ± 2°	21 days (but up to 28 days)	Massive haemorrhage
Concentrated red cells (packed cells, plasma reduced blood)	Approx 200 ml of citrated plasma removed from whole blood. Haematocrit 60–70%	At 4°C ± 2°	21 days (but up to 28 days)	(1) After moderate haemorrhage (2) Anaemia – when response to haematinics too slow or when no response to haematinics
Frozen fresh plasma (FFP)	Approx 200 ml	–22°C	6 months	To replace clotting factors after massive blood replacement. (approx 500 ml FFP per 10 units whole blood)
Platelet rich plasma (PRP)	Approx 200 ml	4°C with gentle agitation	48 hours (approx)	Bleeding due to thrombocytopenia
Platelet concentrate	Approx 20 ml	As PRP	As PRP	As PRP
Human plasma protein fraction	400 ml containing 18 grams of protein	2°–25°C – in dark	3 years	Plasma volume expander – burns, massive haemorrhage
Cytoprecipitate	10–20 ml	–22°C	6 months	Factor VIII deficiency. Fibrinogen deficiency.
Dextran sedimented blood	Approx 500 ml	4°C ± 2°	< 12 hours	Patients with WBC or platelet antibodies

Others: Factor VIII concentrate
Factor IX concentrate
Salt poor albumin
Human immunoglobulins
Frozen red cells

References

1: Surgical anatomy

1. Walters, W. A. W., Macgregor, W. G. and Hills, M. (1966). Cardiac output at rest during pregnancy and the puerperium. *Clinical Science* **30**, 1.
2. Hytten, F. E. and Lind, T. (1973). *Diagnostic Indices in Pregnancy*. Ciba Geigy Ltd., Basle.
3. Green, G. E. (1974). *Surgical Disease in Pregnancy* (pp. 33–44). Eds. H. K. Barber and E. A. Graber. W. B. Saunders Co., Philadelphia.
4. MacGillivray, I., Rose, G. A. and Rowe, B. (1969). Blood pressure survey in pregnancy. *Clinical Science* **37**, 395.
5. Colditz, R. B. and Josey, W. E. (1970). Central venous pressure in supine position during normal pregnancy. *Obstetrics and Gynecology* **36**, 769.
6. Assali, N. S. (1972). *Pathophysiology of Gestation* (Vol. I). Academic Press, New York.
7. Lees, M. M., Scott, D. B., Slawson, K. B. and Ken, M. G. (1968). Haemodynamic change during caesarean section. *J. Obstet. Gynecol. Brit. Comm.* **75**, 546.
8. Barber, H. K. and Graber, E. A. (1974). The acute abdomen in pregnancy – editorial comment. *Surgical Disease in Pregnancy* (pp. 110–111). Eds. H. K. Barber and E. A. Graber. W. B. Saunders Co., Philadelphia.
9. Pritchard, J. A. (1965). Changes in the blood volume during pregnancy and delivery. *Anaesthesiology* **26**, 393.
10. Cruikshank, D. P. (1979). Anatomic and physiologic alterations of pregnancy. *Trauma in Pregnancy* (pp. 26 & 27). Ed. H. J. Buchsbaum. W. B. Saunders Co., Philadelphia.
11. Brinkman, C. R. and Woods, J. R. (1979). Effects of hypovolaemia and hypoxia upon the conceptus. *Trauma in Pregnancy* (pp. 52–79). Ed. H. J. Buchsbaum. W. B. Saunders Co., Philadelphia.
12. Dilts, P. V., Brinkman, C. R., Kirschbaum, T. H. and Assali, N. S. (1969). Uterine and systemic hemodynamic interrelationships and their response to hypoxia. *Am. J. Obstet. Gynecol.* **103**, 138.
13. Greiss, F., Anderson, S. G. and King, L. C. (1972). Uterine vascular bed: effects of acute hypoxia. *Am. J. Obstet. Gynecol.* **113**, 1057.
14. Makowski, E. L., Hertz, R. H. and Beschia, G. (1973). Effects of acute maternal hypoxia and hyperoxia on the blood flow to the pregnant uterus. *Am. J. Obstet. Gynecol.* **115**, 624.
15. Brinkman, C. R., Weston, P., Kirschbaum, T. H. and Assali, N. S. (1970). Effects of maternal hypoxia on fetal cardiovascular hemodynamics. *Am. J. Obstet. Gynecol.* **108**, 288.
16. Greiss, F. (1967). A clinical concept of uterine blood flow during pregnancy. *Am. J. Obstet. Gynecol.* **30**, 595.
17. Pitkin, R. M. (1978). Morphologic changes in pregnancy. *Gynecologic and Obstetric Urology* (pp. 375–381). Eds. H. J. Buchsbaum and J. D. Schmidt. W. B. Saunders Co., Philadelphia.
18. Schulman, A. and Herlinger, H. (1975). Urinary tract dilatation in pregnancy. *British Journal of Radiology* **48**, 638–645.
19. Bieniarz, J. and Crottogini, J. J. *et al.* (1968). Aorta-caval compression by the uterus in late human pregnancy. *Am. J. Obstet. Gynecol.* **100**, 203..

2: Therapeutic (induced) abortion

1. Cates, W., Grimes, D. and Smith, J. C. (1977). The risk of dying from legal abortion in the United States, 1972–75. *Int. J. Gynaecol. Obstet.* **15**, 172–76.
2. Late consequences of abortion. *British Medical Journal* (1981). **282**, 1564–5.
3. Burnhill, M. S. (1979). Reducing complications of first trimester abortion. *Contemp. Ob. Gyn.* **13**, 145–166.
4. MacKenzie, I. Z. and Fry, A. (1981). Prostaglandin E_2 pessaries to facilitate first trimester aspiration termination. *Brit. J. Obstet. Gynecol.* **88**, 10, 1033–1037.
5. Grimes, D. A. and Cates, W. (1979). Complications from legally induced abortion: a review. *Obstet. Gynecol. Survey* **34**, 177–191.
6. Daling, J. R., Spadoni, L. R. and Emanuel, I. (1981). Role of induced abortion in secondary infertility. *Obstet. Gynecol.* **57**, 59–61.
7. Haslap, S., Shiono, P., Ramcharan, S. *et al.* (1979). A prospective study of spontaneous fetal losses after induced abortions. *N. Engl. J. Med.* **301**, 677–81.
8. World Health Organisation Task Force on sequelae of abortion. Gestation, birth weight and spontaneous abortion in pregnancy after induced abortion. *Lancet* (1979). **1**, 142–5.
9. Obel, E. B. (1979). Risk of spontaneous abortion following legally induced abortion. *Acta. Obstet. Gynecol. Scand.* **58**, 485–90.
10. Grimes, D. A. and Cates, W. (1979). The comparative efficacy and safety of intraamniotic prostaglandin $F_2\propto$ and hypertonic saline for second trimester abortion: a review and critique. *J. Reprod. Med.* **22**, 248.
11. Duenhoelter, J. H. and Grant, N. (1976). Concurrent use of prostaglandin $F_2\propto$ and laminaria tents for induction of mid-trimester abortion. *Obstet. Gynecol.* **47**, 469.
12. Midwinter, A., Sheperd, A. and Bowen, M. (1973). Continuous extra-amniotic prostaglandin E_2 for therapeutic termination, effectiveness of various infusion rates and dosages. *J. Obstet. Gynecol. Brit. Comm.* **80**, 371–3.
13. Smith, D., Twiggs, H. and Craft, I. (1981). Prostaglandins in gel for mid-trimester abortion. *Brit. Med. J.* **282**, 2012.
14. Abramovici, H., Rofe, A. and Atad, J. (1981). Termination of mid-trimester missed abortion by extraovular instillation of normal saline. *Brit. J. Obstet. Gynecol.* **88**, 9, 931–3.
15. Eaton, C. J., Cohn, F. and Bollinger, C. C. (1972). Laminaria tent as a cervical dilator prior to aspiration type therapeutic abortion. *Obstet. Gynecol.* **39**, 533–7.
16. Golditch, C. M. and Glasser, M. B. (1974). Use of laminaria tents for cervical dilatation prior to vacuum aspiration abortion. *Am. J. Obstet. Gynecol.* **119**, 481–5.
17. Lischke, J. H. and Goodlin, R. C. (1973). Use of laminaria tents with hypertonic saline amnioinfusion. *Am. J. Obstet. Gynecol.* **116**, 586–7.
18. Garrioch, D. B., Gilbert, J. K. and Plantevin, O. M. (1981). Choice of ecbolic and the morbidity of day care termination of pregnancy. *Brit. J. Obstet. Gynecol.* **88**, 1029–32.
19. Grimes, D. A., Schultz, K. F. and Cates, W. (1977). Mid-trimester abortion of dilatation and evacuation. *N. Engl. J. Med.* **296**, 1141–5.
20. Hodari, A., Perlata, J. and Quiroga, P. (1974). Dilatation and curettage for second trimester abortion. *Am. J. Obstet. Gynecol.* **127**, 850–854.
21. Speroff, L., Cates, W. and Barr, M. (1979). Is there a best way to do mid-trimester abortions? *Contemp. Ob. Gyn.* **13**, 106–141.
22. Russell, K. P. and Ballard, C. A. (1974). Surgical aspects of abortion. *Surgical Disease in Pregnancy* (pp. 470–483). W. B. Saunders & Co., Philadelphia.

23. Barber, H. R. K. and Graber, E. A. (1974). Surgical aspects of abortion – editorial comment. *Surgical Disease in Pregnancy* (p. 483). W. B. Saunders Co., Philadelphia.

3: Spontaneous abortion

1. Report on Confidential Enquiries into Maternal Deaths in England and Wales, 1973–1975. (1979). (p. 9). H.M.S.O., London.
2. Rees, E. (1980). The treatment of pelvic inflammatory disease. *Am. J. Obstet. Gynecol.* 138. No. 7 (ii) (pp. 1042–1047).
3. Embrey, M. P. (1981). Prostaglandins in human reproduction. *British Medical Journal* **283**, 1563.
4. Embrey, M. P., Graham, N. B. and McNeill, M. E. (1980). Induction of labour with a sustained-release prostaglandin E$_2$ vaginal pessary. *British Medical Journal* **281**, 901.
5. Southern, E. M., Gutknecht, G. D., Mohberg, N. R. and Edelman, D. A. (1978). Vaginal prostaglandin E$_2$ in the management of fetal intrauterine death. *Brit. J. Obstet. Gynecol.* **85**, 437–441.
6. Bartlett, J. G. (1979). Anaerobic infections of the pelvis. *Clin. Obstet. & Gynecol.* **22**, 351–360.
7. Borden, G. W. and Hall, W. H. (1951). Fatal transfusion reactions from massive bacterial contamination of blood. *New England Journal of Medicine* **245**, 760.
8. Braude, A. I., Siemienski, J., Williams, D. and Sanford, J. (1953). Overwhelming bacteremic shock produced by gram-negative bacilli. A report of four cases with one recovery. *Univ. Mich. Med. Bull.* **19**, 23.

4: Surgical treatment of recurrent abortion

1. Shirodkar, V. N. (1968). Long-term results with the operative treatment of habitual abortion. *Obstet. Gynecol. Survey* **23**, 553.
2. McDonald, I. A. (1980). Cervical cerclage. *Clinics in Obstet. Gynecol.* (Vol. 7:3). Operative Obstetrics (pp. 46–47). Ed. I. MacGillivray. W. B. Saunders Co., London.
3. Shirodkar, V. N. (1955). A new method of operative treatment for habitual abortion. *Antiseptic* **52**, 229–235.
4. Shirodkar, V. N. (1960). Habitual abortion in the second trimester. *Contributions to Obstetrics and Gynaecology* (p. 1). Livingstone, London.
5. McDonald, I. A. (1978). Incompetence of the cervix. *Australian and New Zealand Journal of Obstetrics and Gynaecology* **18**, 34–37.
6. Barter, R. H. and Parks, J. (1958). Myoma utery associated with pregnancy. *Clinical Obstetrics and Gynecology* **1**, 519.
7. Babaknia, A., Rock, J. A. and Jones, H. W. (1978). Pregnancy success following abdominal myomectomy for infertility. *Fertility and Sterility* **30**, 644.
8. Jones, H. W. and Wheeless, C. R. (1969). Salvage of the reproductive potential of women with anomalous development of the mullerian ducts 1868 – 1968 – 2068. *Am. J. Obstet. Gynecol.* **104**, 348.
9. MacNaughton, M. C. (1981). Chairman of Joint Medical Research Council/Royal College of Obstetricians and Gynaecologists Project: 'Evaluation of Cervical Cerclage by Randomised Trial'. Commenced 1981.

5: Ectopic pregnancy

1. Garcia, C. R., Bronson, R. A., Ledger, W. J. and Marshall, J. R. (1980). The atypical ectopic: Early detection, effective treatment. (Symposium.) *Contemp. Ob. Gyn.* **16**, 92–103.
2. Westrom, L. (1980). Incidence, prevalence and trends of acute pelvic inflammatory disease and its consequences in industrialized countries. *Am. J. Obstet. Gynecol.* 138. No. 7 (ii) (pp. 880–890).
3. Kleiner, G. J. and Roberts, T. W. (1967). Current factors in causation of tubal pregnancy: a prospective clinico-pathologic study. *Am. J. Obstet. Gynecol.* **99**, 21.

4. Report on Confidential Enquiries into Maternal Deaths in England and Wales, 1973–1975. (1979). (pp. 98–102). H.M.S.O., London.
5. Shoen, J. A. and Nowak, R. J. (1975). Repeat ectopic pregnancy: a 16-year clinical survey. *Obstet. Gynecol.* **45**, 542.
6. Hallatt, J. G. (1975). Repeat ectopic pregnancy: a study of 123 consecutive cases. *Am. J. Obstet. Gynecol.* **122**, 520.
7. Boronow, R. A., McElin, T. W., West, R. H. and Buckingham, J. C. (1965). Ovarian pregnancy: a report of 4 cases and a 13-year survey of the English literature. *Am. J. Obstet. Gynecol.* **91**, 1095.
8. Campbell, J. S., *et al.* (1974). Acute hemoperitoneum, IUD, and occult ovarian pregnancy. *Obstet. Gynecol.* **43**, 438.
9. Pratt-Thomas, H. R., White, L. and Messer, H. H. (1974). Primary ovarian pregnancy: presentation of ten cases, including one full-term pregnancy. *South Med. J.* **67**, 920.
10. Beacham, W. D., Hernquist, W. C., Beacham, D. W. and Webster, H. D. (1962). Abdominal pregnancy at Charity Hospital in New Orleans. *Am. J. Obstet. Gynecol.* **84**, 1257, 1962.

6: The acute abdomen in pregnancy

1. Brant, H. A. (1967). Acute appendicitis in pregnancy. *Obstet. Gynecol.* **29**, 130.
2. Babaknia, A. and Parsa, H. (1977). Appendicitis during pregnancy. *Obstet. Gynecol.* **50**, 40.
3. Mattingly, R. F. (1977). The vermiform appendix in relation to pregnancy. *Te Linde's Operative Gynecology*, 5th edn. (pp. 411–413). Ed. R. F. Mattingly. J. B. Lippincott Company, Philadelphia.
4. Griffen, W. O. (1974). Surgery of the gastro-intestinal tract in pregnancy. *Surgical Disease in Pregnancy.* (pp. 85–92). Eds. H. R. K. Barber and E. A. Graber. W. B. Saunders Co., Philadelphia.

7: Ovarian cysts and uterine fibroids complicating pregnancy incarcerated retroverted gravid uterus

1. Graber, E. A. (1974). Ovarian tumours in pregnancy. *Surgical Disease in Pregnancy* (pp. 428–437). Eds. H. R. K. Barber and E. A. Graber. W. B. Saunders Co., Philadelphia.
2. Taylor, E. S. (1972). Ovarian tumours in pregnancy. *Obstet. Gynecol. Survey* **27**, 43.

8: The control of haemorrhage in operative obstetrics

1. Miller, F. J., Mortel, R., Mann, W. J. and Jashan, A. E. (1976). Selective arterial embolisation for control of haemorrhage in pelvic malignancy: femoral and brachial catheter approaches. *The American Journal of Roentgenology, Radium Therapy and Nuclear Medicine* **126**, 5, 1028–1032.
2. Ring, E. G., Athanasouhs, C., Waltman, A. C., Margowes, M. N. and Baum, S. (1973). Arteriographic management of hemorrhage following pelvic fracture. *Radiology* **109**, 65–70.
3. Paster, S., Van Houten, F. X. and Adams, D. F. (1974). Percutaneous balloon catheterisation: a technique for the control of arterial hemorrhage caused by pelvic trauma. *Journal of the American Medical Associates* **230**, 573–575.
4. Dunn, D. C. (1981). Vascular Surgery – Annual Review. *Hospital Update* (p. 568). **7**, 6.
5. Allanson, D. J. (1980). Therapeutic embolisation. *Recent Advances in Surgery* (Vol. 10). Ed. S. Taylor. Churchill Livingstone, Edinburgh.
6. McNeese, S., Finck, E. and Yellin, A. E. (1980). Therapeutic embolisation. *American Journal of Surgery* **140**, 252.
7. Cotteel, P. (1981). Syndrome de defibrination aigue – données pratiques. De la Clinique du Docteur Cotteel, 1 Rue Hégel, Lille, France.

9: Caesarean section

1. Harley, J. M. G. (1980). Caesarean section. *Clinics in Obstetrics and Gynaecology* 7. No. 3. (pp. 529–557). Ed. I. MacGillivray. W. B. Saunders Co., Ltd., London.
2. Report on Confidential Enquiries into Maternal Deaths in England and Wales, 1973–1975. (1979). H.M.S.O., London.
3. Caesarean Childbirth, summary of an N.I.H. Consensus Statement. (1981). *British Medical Journal* **282**, 1600–1604.
4. Copies of the full report of the task force, containing a description and analysis of the literature and data on which this statement is based, may be obtained from the Office of Research Reporting, NICHD, Building 31, Room 2A34, NIH, 9000 Rockville Pike, Bethesda, Maryland 20205.
5. Easterday, C. L. (1974). Caesarean section. *Surgical Disease in Pregnancy*. Eds. H. R. K. Barber and E. A. Graber. W. B. Saunders Co., Philadelphia.
6. Philpott, R. H. (1980). Obstructed labour. *Clinics in Obstetrics and Gynaecology*. 7. No. 3. (p. 612). Ed. I. MacGillivray. W. B. Saunders Co., Ltd., London.

10: Hysterectomy for uterine rupture and post partum haemorrhage

1. Report on Confidential Enquiries into Maternal Deaths in England and Wales, 1973–1975 (1979). (pp. 88–92). H.M.S.O., London.
2. Groen, G. P. (1974). Uterine rupture in Nigeria. *Obstet. Gynecol.* **44**, 682–687.
3. Lawson, J. B. (1967). Rupture of the uterus. *Obstetrics and Gynaecology in the Tropics and Developing Countries* (p. 189). Eds. J. B. Lawson and D. B. Stewart. E. Arnold, London.
4. Mokgokong, E. T. and Marivate, M. (1976). Treatment of the ruptured uterus. *South African Medical Journal* **50**, 1621–1624.
5. Skelly, H. R., Duthie, A. M. and Philpott, R. H. (1976). Rupture of the uterus. *South African Medical Journal* **50**, 505–509.
6. Mickal, A., Begneaud, W. P. and Hawes, T. P. (1969). Pitfalls and complications of caesarean section hysterectomy. *Clinical Obstetrics and Gynecology* **12**, 660.
7. Barclay, D. L. (1970). Caesarean hysterectomy, a thirty years' experience. *Obstet. Gynecol.* **35**, 120.

11: Uterine trauma from automobile accidents, assault, and other external sources

1. Barno, A., Freeman, D. W. and Baker, M. P. (1962). Minnesota mortality study. *Minnesota Medicine* **45**, 847, 947.
2. Jimerson, S. and Crosby, W. M. (1977). Unpublished data reported in: Automobile injuries and blunt abdominal trauma (Crosby, W. M. 1979). *Trauma in Pregnancy* (pp. 101–106). Ed. H. J. Buchsbaum. W. B. Saunders Co., Philadelphia.
3. Buchsbaum, H. J. (1979). *Trauma in Pregnancy*. W. B. Saunders Co., Philadelphia.
4. Crosby, W. M. (1979). Automobile injuries and blunt abdominal trauma. *Trauma in Pregnancy* (pp. 126–129). Ed. H. J. Buchsbaum. W. B. Saunders Co., Philadelphia.
5. Golan, A. *et al.* (1980). Late pregnancy injuries – a report of 15 cases. *South African Medical Journal* **57**, 161.
6. Pepperell, R. J., Rubenstein, E. and MacIsaac, I. A. (1977). Motor car accidents during pregnancy. *Medical Journal of Australia* **1**, 203.
7. Huelke, D. F. and Gikas, P. W. (1968). Causes of death in automobile accidents. *Journal of the American Medical Association* **203**, 1100.

8. Crosby, W. M., Synder, R. G., Snow, C. C. *et al.* (1968). Impact injuries in pregnancy. 1. Experimental Studies. *Am. J. Obstet. Gynecol.* **101**, 108.
9. Crosby, W. M. and Costiloe, J. P. (1971). Safety of lap belt restraint for pregnant victims of automobile collisions. *N. Engl. J. Med.* **284**, 632.
10. Buchsbaum, H. J. (1979). Penetrating injury of the abdomen. *Trauma in Pregnancy*. W. B. Saunders Co., Philadelphia.
11. Shaftan, G. W. (1960). Indications for operation in abdominal trauma. *Annals of Surgery* **99**, 657.
12. Cornell, W. P., Ebert, P. A. and Zuidema, G. D. (1965). X-ray diagnosis of penetrating wounds of the abdomen. *Journal of Surgical Research* **5**, 142.

12: Management of cervical neoplasia in pregnancy

1. Abitol, M., Benjamin, F. and Gastillo, N. (1973). Management of abnormal cervical smear and carcinoma *in situ* of the cervix during pregnancy. *Am. J. Obstet. Gynecol.* **117**, 904.
2. Wanless, J. F. (1971). Carcinoma of cervix in pregnancy. *Am. J. Obstet. Gynecol.* **110**, 173.
3. Ortiz, R. and Newton, M. (1971). Management of abnormal cervical smears in pregnancy. *Am. J. Obstet. Gynecol.* **109**, 46.
4. McDonnell, J. M., Mylotte, M. and Gustafson, R. C. (1981). Colposcopy in pregnancy a 12-year experience. *Brit. J. Obstet. Gynecol.* **88**, 414.
5. Creasman, W. T., Rutledge, F. N. and Fletcher, G. A. (1970). Carcinoma of the cervix associated with pregnancy. *Obstet. Gynecol.* **36**, 495.
6. Thompson, J. D., Caputo, T. A. and Franklin, E. (1975). The surgical management of invasive cancer of the cervix in pregnancy. *Am. J. Obstet. Gynecol.* **121**, 853.
7. Di Saia, P. J. and Creasman, W. T. (1981). *Clinical Gynaecologic Oncology* (p. 79). Mosby & Co., St. Louis.
8. Morrow, C. P. and Townsend, D. E. (1981). *Synopsis of Gynaecologic Oncology* (2nd Edn.) (p. 93). John Wiley & Sons, New York.
9. Stafl, A. and Mattingley, R. F. (1973). Colposcopic diagnosis of cervical neoplasia. *Obstet. Gynecol.* **41**, 168.
10. De Petrillo, A. D., Townsend, D. E. and Morrow, C. P. *et al.* (1975). Colposcopic evaluation of the abnormal pap. test in pregnancy. *Am. J. Obstet. Gynecol.* **121**, 441.
11. Talebian, F., Krumholz, B. A. and Shayau, A. (1976). Colposcopic evaluation of the patients with abnormal smears during pregnancy. *Obstet. Gynecol.* **47**, 693.
12. Benedet, J. L., Boyes, D. A. and Nichols, T. (1977). Colposcopic evaluation of pregnant patients with abnormal cervical smears. *Brit. J. Obstet. Gynecol.* **84**, 517.
13. Ostergard, D. R. and Nieberg, R. K. (1979). Evaluation of abnormal cervical cytology during pregnancy with colposcopy. *Am. J. Obstet. Gynecol.* **134**, 756.
14. Lurain, J. R. and Gallup, D. G. (1979). management of abnormal smears in pregnancy. *Obstet. Gynecol.* **53**, 484.
15. Singer, A. and Kirkup, W. (1980). Colposcopy in the management of the pregnant patient with abnormal cervical cytology. *Brit. J. Obstet. Gynecol.* **87**, 322.

13: Gestational trophoblastic disease

1. Elston, C. W. and Bagshawe, K. D. (1972). The value of histological grading in the management of hydatidiform mole. *The Journal of Obstetrics and Gynecology of the British Commonwealth* **79**, 717–724.
2. Report on Confidential Enquiries into Maternal Deaths in England and Wales, 1973–1975. H.M.S.O., London.
3. Chun, D. and Ma, H. K. (1974). Choriocarcinoma in Hong Kong. *Journal of the Royal College of Surgeons of Edinburgh* **19**, 69.

4. Goldstein, D. P. (1974). Surgery of moles and chorio-carcinoma. *Surgical Diseases in Pregnancy* (pp. 494–508). Eds. H. R. K. Barber and E. A. Graber. W. B. Saunders Co., Philadelphia.

5. Editorial Comment, 31st August, 1974. (p. 54). *Brit. Med. J.* (1974).

6. Li, M. C., Hertz, R. and Spencer, D. B. (1956). Effects of methotrexate therapy upon choriocarcinoma and chorioadenoma. *Proc. Soc. Exp. Biol. Med.* **92**, 361–366.

7. Bagshawe, K. D. (1969). *Choriocarcinoma – The Clinical Biology of the Trophoblast and its Tumours*. Edward Arnold, London.

8. Brewer, J. I., Eckman, T. R., Dolkart, R. W., Torok, E. E. and Webster, A. (1971). Gestational trophoblastic disease. A comparative study of the results of therapy in patients with invasive mole and choriocarcinoma. *Am. J. Obstet. Gynecol.* **109**, 355–360.

9. Goldstein, D. P., Goldstein, P. R., Bottomley, P., Osathanondh, R. and Marean, A. R. (1976). Methotrexate with citrovorum factor rescue for non-metastatic gestational trophoblastic neoplasma. *Obstet. Gynecol.* **48** (3), 321–323.

10. Hammond, C. B., Hertz, R., Ross, G. T. *et al.* (1967). Primary chemotherapy for non-metastatic gestational trophoblastic neoplasms. *Am. J. Obstet. Gynecol.* **98**, 1–78.

11. Hammond, C. B., Borchert, L. G., Tyrey, L., Creasman, W. T. and Parker, R. T. (1973). Treatment of metastatic trophoblastic disease – good and poor prognosis. *Am. J. Obstet. Gynecol.* **115**, 451–457.

12. Bagshawe, K. D. (1976). Risk and prognostic factors in trophoblastic neoplasia. *Cancer* **38**, 1373–1385.

13. Goldstein, D. P., Pastorfide, G. B., Osanthanondh, R. *et al.* (1975). A rapid solid phase radioimmunoassay specific for human chorionic gonadotrophin in gestational trophoblastic disease. *Obstet. Gynecol.* **45**, 527–530.

14. Pastorfide, G. B., Goldstein, D. P. and Kosasa, T. S. (1974). The use of radioimmunoassay specific for human chorionic gonadotrophin in patients with molar pregnancy and gestational trophoblastic disease. *Am. J. Obstet. Gynecol.* **120**, 1025–1028.

15. Vaitukaitus, J., Braustein, G. D. and Ross, G. T. (1972). A radioimmunoassay which specifically measures human chorionic gonadotrophin in the presence of human LH. *Am. J. Obstet. Gynecol.* **113**, 751–758.

16. Pastorfide, G. B. and Goldstein, D. P. (1973). Pregnancy after hydatidiform mole. *Obstet. Gynecol.* **42**, 67–70.

17. Ross, G. T. (1976). Congenital anomalies among children born of mothers receiving chemotherapy for gestational trophoblastic neoplasms. *Cancer* **37**, Suppl. 2: 1043–1047.

18. Van Thiel, D. H., Ross, G. T. and Lipsett, M. B. (1970). Pregnancies after chemotherapy of trophoblastic neoplasms. *Science* **169** (952), 1326–1327.

19. Walden, P. A. M. and Bagshawe, K. D. (1976). Reproductive performance of women successfully treated for gestational trophoblastic tumors. *Am. J. Obstet. Gynecol.* **125** (8), 1108–1114.

20. Brewer, J. I., Eckman, R. R., Dolkart, R. W., Torok, E. E. and Webster, A. (1971). Gestational trophoblastic disease. A comparative study of the results of therapy in patients with invasive mole and choriocarcinoma. *Am. J. Obstet. Gynecol.* **109**, 355–360.

21. Goldstein, D. P. and Berkowitz (1979). Methotrexate with citrovorum factor rescue for gestational trophoblastic neoplasms. *Abstracts of International Symposium on Gestational Trophoblastic Tumours* (May 1979. p. 30). Postgraduate Medical Centre, Charing Cross Hospital, London.

22. Ma, H. K. and Wong, L. C. (1979). Treatment of gestational trophoblastic disease in Hong Kong. *Abstracts of International Symposium on Gestational Trophoblastic Tumours* (May 1979. p. 33). Postgraduate Medical Centre, Charing Cross Hospital, London.

23. Lewis, J., Ketchum, A. S. and Hertz, R. (1966). Surgical intervention during chemotherapy of gestational trophoblastic neoplasma. *Cancer* **19**, 517.

24. Goldstein, D. P. (1974). Surgery of moles and choriocarcinoma. *Surgical Diseases in Pregnancy* (pp. 494–508). Eds. H. R. K. Barber and E. A. Graber. W. B. Saunders Co., Philadelphia.

25. Ratnam, S. S. and Chew, S. C. (1979). Surgery for metastatic trophoblastic tumours. *Abstracts of International Symposium on Gestational Trophoblastic Tumours* (May 1979. p. 28). Postgraduate Medical Centre, Charing Cross Hospital, London.

26. Hammond, C. B., Weed, J. C. and Currie, J. L. (1980). The role of operation in the current therapy of gestational trophoblastic disease. *Am. J. Obstet. Gynecol.* **136**, 844.

15: Anaesthetic and resuscitative aspects of obstetric surgery

1. Baker, A. S., Ojemann, R. G. and Schwartz, M. N. *et al.* (1975). Spinal epidural abscess. *N. Engl. J. Med.* **293**, 463.

2. Archer, G. W. and Marx, G. F. (1974). *Brit. J. Anaesth.* **46**, 358.

3. Moir, D. D. (1970). *Brit. J. Anaesth.* **42**, 136.

4. Tunstall, M. E. and Hawksworth, G. M. (1981). Halothane uptake and nitrous oxide concentration. *Anaesthesia* **36**, 177.

5. Rothe, M. J., Davey, D. A. and Du Toit, H. J. (1968). *Anaesthesia* **23**, 585.

6. Hey, V. M. F. and Ostich, D. G. (1978). *Anaesthesia* **33**, 462.

7. Sellick, R. A. (1961). *Lancet* **11**, 404.

8. Bieniarz, J., Crottogini, J. J. and Curachet, E. *et al.* (1968). Aorta-caval compression in late human pregnancy. *Am. J. Obstet. Gynecol.* **100**, 203.

9. Crawford, J. S. Burton, M. and Davies P. (1973). *Brit. J. Anaesth.* **44**, 477.

10. Report on Confidential Enquiries into Maternal Deaths in England and Wales, 1973–1975. (1979) (pp. 38–47). H.M.S.O., London.

11. Browse, N. L. (1978). Diagnosis of deep vein thrombosis. In Thrombosis. Ed. D. Thomas. *British medical Bulletin* **34**, 2, 163.

12. Johnson, W. C., Patten, D. A. and Widrich, W. C. *et al.* (1974). *Am. J. Surg.* **127**, 424.

13. Bonnar, J. (1979). Venous thrombo-embolism and pregnancy. *Recent Advances in Obstetrics and Gynaecology* No. 13 (pp. 174). Eds. Sir John Stallworthy and Gordon Bourne. Churchill-Livingstone, Edinburgh.

14. Kakkar, V. V., Djazaeri, B. and Fok, J. (1982). Low molecular-weight heparin and prevention of post operative deep vein thrombosis. *Brit. Med. Journal* **284**, 375.

Combined index

This is a combined index for volumes 1–6. Individual volumes are referred to by Roman numerals (I–VI). All references are to page numbers.